The Mobile Lipid Clinic:
A Companion Guide

The Mobile Lipid Clinic: A Companion Guide

Second Edition

MICHAEL H. DAVIDSON, M.D., F.A.C.C., F.A.C.P.

Executive Medical Director
Radiant Research
Director of Preventive Cardiology and Professor
Rush University Medical Center
Chicago, Illinois

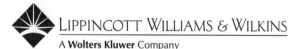

LIPPINCOTT WILLIAMS & WILKINS
A **Wolters Kluwer** Company
Philadelphia · Baltimore · New York · London
Buenos Aires · Hong Kong · Sydney · Tokyo

Project Manager: Melissa Jones, Silverchair Science + Communications, Inc.
Managing Editor: Jennifer Jett
Compositor: Silverchair Science + Communications, Inc.
Printer: Transcontinental Printing, Inc.

Printed in Canada

Library of Congress Cataloging-in-Publication Data

Davidson, Michael, 1956-
    The mobile lipid clinic : a companion guide / Michael H. Davidson.--2nd ed.
      p. ; cm.
    Includes bibliographical references and index.
    ISBN 0-7817-6088-7 (alk. paper)
      1. Lipids--Metabolism--Disorders. 2. Lipids--Metabolism--Disorders--Prevention.
3. Lipids--Metabolism--Disorders--Risk factors. I. Title.
    [DNLM: 1. Hyperlipidemia--therapy. 2. Lipoproteins--metabolism. 3. Risk Factors. WD
    200.5.H8 D253m 2005]
    RC632.L5D384 2005
    616.3'997--dc22
                                                                    2005009099

Care has been taken to confirm the accuracy of the information presented and to describe generally accepted practices. However, the authors, editors, and publisher are not responsible for errors or omissions or for any consequences from application of the information in this book and make no warranty, expressed or implied, with respect to the currency, completeness, or accuracy of the contents of the publication. Application of this information in a particular situation remains the professional responsibility of the practitioner.

The authors, editors, and publisher have exerted every effort to ensure that drug selection and dosage set forth in this text are in accordance with current recommendations and practice at the time of publication. However, in view of ongoing research, changes in government regulations, and the constant flow of information relating to drug therapy and drug reactions, the reader is urged to check the package insert for each drug for any change in indications and dosage and for added warnings and precautions. This is particularly important when the recommended agent is a new or infrequently employed drug.

Some drugs and medical devices presented in this publication have Food and Drug Administration (FDA) clearance for limited use in restricted research settings. It is the responsibility of health care providers to ascertain the FDA status of each drug or device planned for use in their clinical practice.

10 9 8 7 6 5 4 3 2 1

To Martha, and to Arin, David, Jeffrey, Jonathan,
and my parents

Contents

Acknowledgments

I want to thank Mary Lou Briglio for her excellent administrative and editorial support and Karen Ruzicka, M.S., R.D., for developing the dietary plans. I also want to thank Joe Scheese, Roy Furman, M.D., and Elise Furman of Scientific Software Tools for assistance in developing the Mobile Lipid Clinic™ software.

Introduction

My father died at the age of 47 of a myocardial infarction (MI). His death was not only a tremendous personal tragedy for his wife and six children, but his company also lost a valuable vice president, and his community in Dayton, Ohio, grieved for the loss of his tireless dedication to charitable organizations. My father was only one of millions of men and women to die from coronary heart disease (CHD) in 1973. In retrospect, 1973 was the peak year of CHD deaths in the United States. My father was a chemist, was not overweight, and was a non-smoker with a "normal" cholesterol of 250 mg per dL. His only known risk factor was that his father also died of an MI at age 63. Two days before his heart attack, he noticed severe chest discomfort running up a flight of stairs. He went immediately to the hospital and was admitted as a "rule out MI." After 2 days of serial electrocardiograms and negative cardiac enzymes, he was discharged home to spend the weekend with his family. Early the next morning, however, the severe chest pain resumed and did not abate when he lied down. Within an hour, a friend rushed him to the hospital where an electrocardiogram revealed a massive anterior wall MI. He went into cardiogenic shock and received the hospital's first intraaortic balloon pump, but despite other heroic measures, including emergency coronary bypass surgery, he died in less than 12 hours.

Since 1973, there has been a gradual decline in the death rate from CHD. This decline has been attributed, in part, to improved medical care. Today, a patient with an MI similar to my father's with thrombolytic therapy and/or acute angioplasty is likely to survive. However, the greatest contribution to the decline has been lifestyle changes. Reductions in dietary saturated fat and cigarette smoking are believed responsible for more than half of the decline in CHD deaths since 1973. The decline in CHD, however, has slowed and currently remains virtually flat for women. Obviously, considerable improvement is still necessary because CHD remains the leading killer for both men and women. As a cardiologist, I have marveled at the advancements in technology and therapeutics for the management of acute coronary events since the 1980s. However, an ancient Chinese proverb says it best: "Inferior doctors treat the full-blown disease; good doctors treat the disease before evident; and superior doctors prevent the disease." All physicians want to be "superior doctors." An MI should not represent the beginning of care, but rather the failure of care.

Despite tremendous advances in our understanding of the pathogenesis and treatment of atherosclerosis, the actual implementation of proven cardiovascular risk-management strategies has been difficult. CHD is a preventable disease, yet very effective treatments for the modification of risk factors remain underused. The goal of this book is to provide an easy-to-read resource on how to implement risk-reduction strategies, in conjunction with valuable tools such as personal digital assistant (PDA) software. There are many worthwhile and well-written resource books about the management and treatment of atherosclerotic disease. This book was written more as a "how-to" manual rather than focusing on detailed information. My hope is that combining a "how-to" strategy with the tools to implement the strategy will ultimately lead to more successful, "superior" doctors. I also know personally the ravages of CHD. The Talmud, written almost 2,000 years ago, says "one who saves a life saves an entire world." Saving at least one "entire world" is the objective of this book.

Introduction to the Second Edition

After publication of the first edition of *The Mobile Lipid Clinic: A Companion Guide* in 2002, I received comments about the Introduction, which described my father's premature death from a myocardial infarction at age 47. In the brief 2 years since the publication of the first edition, considerable new data and therapies have become available that are changing our treatment approaches to dyslipidemia. In addition, on a personal level, I have been deeply affected by my experiences with two new cases of premature heart disease. My younger brother, a family physician in Ohio, at age 44, developed unstable angina and underwent emergency coronary bypass surgery to four vessels. He was a vegetarian and nonsmoker with a total cholesterol of 150 mg per dL and a low-density lipoprotein cholesterol of 95 mg per dL but a very low high-density lipoprotein cholesterol of 25 mg per dL. He has subsequently recovered well from his surgery and has returned to his practice and is raising his four children with his wife.

The second case involves a man in his late 40s. He came to see me 5 years ago at the urging of his wife because both his father and brother died prematurely of coronary heart disease (CHD). He was found to have significant hyperlipidemia, and I initiated statin therapy with recommendations that he follow up with his primary care physician. I saw him several months later walking on the street to work, and I reiterated to him the importance of treatment and follow-up. Unfortunately, I found out recently that he died while bicycling along the lake shore in Chicago. Apparently, he did not continue on the statin prescription that I gave him 5 years ago and did not follow up with a primary care physician.

These two cases represent our challenge as clinicians to reduce the prevalence of CHD. My brother represents the patients who presently fall outside the guidelines for initiating lipid-lowering therapy yet developed premature CHD. New approaches to risk assessment and more aggressive therapeutic targets are emerging to help clinicians close the gap between those who need to receive lipid-altering therapy and the patients for whom the guidelines presently recommend to initiate treatment. The second case described above is perhaps a much more difficult challenge for physicians. For some reason, I failed to convince him of the importance of initiating and maintaining treatment to reduce his risk of heart disease. The problem with preventive medicine is that we can never know with certainty with an individual person whether our risk-modifying strategies actually reduced the development of CHD. This may explain why many patients are noncompliant with lipid-lowering therapies, because they either do not appreciate the need for treatment or believe that they will be spared from disease by good fortune or by engaging in other risk-modifying strategies. Somehow, as health professionals, we need to do a better job of educating and motivating our patients to initiate well-demonstrated life-saving measures. Therefore, our challenge is twofold: to effectively implement known risk-modifying therapies in our patients and to develop new strategies to decrease the residual risk in patients who we presently believe are receiving the appropriate treatment.

The second edition of *The Mobile Lipid Clinic: A Companion Guide* will hopefully help health professionals effectively deliver quality preventive cardiac care by providing a programmatic approach to the implementation of the various guidelines. This can be accomplished by integrating the Mobile Lipid Clinic™ software program, which will provide assistance in the identification, tracking, education, and motivation of patients at risk for CHD.

I turned 47 years old this year, the same age as my father when he died of a myocardial infarction. I envy those people who, due to the benefits of the longevity of their parents or grandparents, look forward to a long and productive life. I live with trepidation, but also with optimism for the benefits of lipid-altering therapy to hope for the wedding blessing of the Falashas of Ethiopia, "May you live to see your children's children and the children of their children."

Chapter 1

Implementation of the National Cholesterol Education Program Adult Treatment Panel III Guidelines

IDENTIFYING HIGH-RISK PATIENTS

The National Cholesterol Education Program Adult Treatment Panel III (NCEP ATP III) guidelines outline a nine-step approach to identifying high-risk patients and implementing the guidelines (Table 1.1). High-risk patients are identified by a fasting lipid profile (step 1). NCEP ATP III classifies an optimal low-density lipoprotein cholesterol (LDL-C) as less than 100 mg per dL and a desirable total cholesterol as less than 200 mg per dL. Along with assessing lipoprotein levels to determine high-risk status, the presence of clinical atherosclerosis, including peripheral arterial disease, abdominal aortic aneurysm, and symptomatic carotid artery disease, is then assessed (step 2). [In NCEP ATP III, clinical forms of atherosclerotic disease now represent a coronary heart disease (CHD) risk equivalent.] The presence of major risk factors is then determined (step 3). According to ATP III, major risk factors (exclusive of LDL-C) that modify LDL goals include cigarette smoking, hypertension (blood pressure greater than or equal to 140 per 90 mm Hg or on antihypertensive medication), low high-density lipoprotein cholesterol (HDL-C) (less than 40 mg per dL), family history of premature CHD, and age (men, 45 years or older; women, 55 years or older). If two risk factors are present, the global risk score is calculated (step 4).

Table 1.1. Nine-Step Approach to Implementation of the National Cholesterol Education Program Adult Treatment Panel III Guidelines

1. Determine fasting lipoprotein levels.
2. Identify presence of clinical atherosclerosis.
3. Determine presence of major risk factors.
4. If 2+ risk factors present, calculate global risk score.
5. Determine risk category and establish LDL-C goal.
6. Initiate TLC diet if LDL-C is above goal.
7. Add drug therapy if LDL-C continues to exceed initiation levels.
8. Identify metabolic syndrome and treat if present after 3 mo of TLC.
9. Treat elevated triglycerides to non-high-density lipoprotein goals.

LDL-C, low-density lipoprotein cholesterol; TLC, therapeutic lifestyle change.
From the Executive Summary of the Third Report of the National Cholesterol Education Program (NCEP) Expert Panel on Detection, Evaluation, and Treatment of High Blood Cholesterol in Adults (Adult Treatment Panel III). JAMA 2001;285:2486–2497, with permission.

CALCULATING THE GLOBAL RISK SCORE

The global risk score, which is calculated with the Framingham scoring, allows better targeting of intensive treatment to individuals who have multiple (2+) risk factors. The Framingham risk scoring system is used to estimate the 10-year CHD risk based on age, total cholesterol, smoking status, and systolic blood pressure. The total risk score sums the points for each risk factor, and the 10-year CHD risk is estimated from the total points. Individuals with multiple risk factors are divided into those with 10-year risk for CHD of greater than 20%, 10% to 20%, and less than 10%.

Figure 1.1. ➤ Calculating abbreviated risk score. Coronary heart disease (CHD) score sheet for men using total cholesterol (TC) or low-density lipoprotein cholesterol (LDL-C) categories. Uses age, TC (or LDL-C), high-density lipoprotein cholesterol (HDL-C), blood pressure, diabetes, and smoking. Estimates risk for CHD over a period of 10 years based on Framingham experience in men 30 to 74 years old at baseline. Average risk estimates are based on typical Framingham subjects, and estimates of idealized risk are based on optimal blood pressure; TC of 160 to 199 mg per dL (or LDL of 100 to 129 mg per dL), HDL-C of 45 mg per dL in men, no diabetes, and no smoking. Use of the LDL-C categories is appropriate when fasting LDL-C measurements are available. Note: When systolic and diastolic pressures provide different estimates for point scores, use the higher number. [a]Hard CHD events exclude angina pectoris. [b]Low risk was calculated for a person the same age, optimal blood pressure, LDL-C of 100 to 129 mg per dL or cholesterol of 160 to 199 mg per dL, HDL-C 45 mg per dL for men or 55 mg per dL for women, nonsmoker, and no diabetes. Risk estimates were derived from the experience of the Framingham Heart Study, a predominantly white population in Massachusetts. pts, points. (From Wilson PWF, D'Agostino RB, Levy D, et al. Prediction of coronary heart disease using risk factor categories. *Circulation* 1998;97:1837–1847, with permission.)

Step 1

Age		
Yr	LDL pts	Cholesterol pts
30–34	−1	[−1]
35–39	0	[0]
40–44	1	[1]
45–49	2	[2]
50–54	3	[3]
55–59	4	[4]
60–64	5	[5]
65–69	6	[6]
70–74	7	[7]

Step 2

LDL-C		
(mg/dL)	(mmol/L)	LDL ts
<100	<2.59	−3
100–129	2.60–3.36	0
130–159	3.37–4.14	0
160–190	4.15–4.92	1
≥190	≥4.92	2

Cholesterol		
(mg/dL)	(mmol/L)	Cholesterol pts
<160	<4.14	[−3]
160–199	4.15–5.17	[0]
200–239	5.18–6.21	[1]
240–279	6.22–7.24	[2]
≥280	≥7.25	[3]

Step 3

HDL-C			
(mg/dL)	(mmol/L)	LDL pts	Cholesterol pts
<35	<0.90	2	[2]
35–44	0.91–1.16	1	[1]
45–49	1.17–1.29	0	[0]
50–59	1.30–1.55	0	[0]
60	1.56	−1	[−2]

Step 4

Blood Pressure					
Systolic (mm Hg)	Diastolic (mm Hg)				
	<80	80–84	85–89	90–99	≥100
<120	0 [0] pts				
120–129		0 [0] pts			
130–139			1 [1] pts		
140–159				2 [2] pts	
≥160					3 [3] pts

Step 5

Diabetes		
	LDL pts	Cholesterol pts
No	0	[0]
Yes	2	[2]

Step 6

Smoker		
	LDL pts	Cholesterol pts
No	0	[0]
Yes	2	[2]

Step 7 (sum from steps 1–6)

Adding up the points	
Age	_____
LDL-C or cholesterol	_____
HDL-C	_____
Blood pressure	_____
Diabetes	_____
Smoker	_____
Point total	_____

Step 8 (determine CHD risk from point total)

CHD risk			
LDL pts total	10-yr CHD risk (%)	Cholesterol pts total	10-yr CHD risk (%)
>−3	1	—	—
−2	2	—	—
−1	2	[<−1]	[2]
0	3	[0]	[3]
1	4	[1]	[3]
2	4	[2]	[4]
3	6	[3]	[5]
4	7	[4]	[7]
5	9	[5]	[8]
6	11	[6]	[10]
7	14	[7]	[13]
8	18	[8]	[16]
9	22	[9]	[20]
10	27	[10]	[25]
11	33	[11]	[31]
12	40	[12]	[37]
13	47	[13]	[45]
≥14	≥56	[≥14]	[≥53]

Step 9 (compare to average person your age)

Comparative Risk			
Age (yr)	Average 10-yr CHD risk (%)	Average 10-yr hard[a] CHD risk (%)	Low[b] 10 yr CHD risk (%)
30–34	3	1	2
35–39	5	4	3
40–44	7	4	4
45–49	11	8	4
50–54	14	10	6
55–59	16	13	7
60–64	21	20	9
65–69	25	22	11
70–74	30	25	14

Key	
Relative Risk	
	Very low
	Low
	Moderate
	High
	Very high

Step 1

Age		
Yr	LDL pts	Cholesterol pts
30–34	−9	[−9]
35–39	−4	[−4]
40–44	0	[0]
45–49	3	[3]
50–54	6	[6]
55–59	7	[7]
60–64	8	[8]
65–69	8	[8]
70–74	8	[8]

Step 2

LDL-C		
(mg/dL)	(mmol/L)	LDL ts
<100	<2.59	<2
100–129	2.60–3.36	0
130–159	3.37–4.14	0
160–190	4.15–4.92	2
≥190	≥4.92	2

Cholesterol		
(mg/dL)	(mmol/L)	Cholesterol pts
<160	<4.14	[−2]
160–199	4.15–5.17	[0]
200–239	5.18–6.21	[1]
240–279	6.22–7.24	[1]
≥280	≥7.25	[3]

Step 3

HDL-C			
(mg/dL)	(mmol/L)	LDL pts	Cholesterol pts
<35	<0.90	5	[5]
35–44	0.91–1.16	2	[2]
45–49	1.17–1.29	1	[1]
50–59	1.30–1.55	0	[0]
≥60	1.58	−2	[−3]

Step 5

Diabetes		
	LDL pts	Cholesterol pts
No	0	[0]
Yes	4	[4]

Step 6

Smoker		
	LDL pts	Cholesterol pts
No	0	[0]
Yes	2	[2]

Step 7 (sum from steps 1–6)

Adding up the points	
Age	____
LDL-C or cholesterol	____
HDL-C	____
Blood pressure	____
Diabetes	____
Smoker	____
Point total	____

Step 8 (determine CHD risk from point total)

CHD risk			
LDL pts total	10-yr CHD risk (%)	Cholesterol pts total	10-yr CHD risk (%)
≤−2	1	[<−2]	[1]
−1	2	[−1]	[2]
0	2	[0]	[2]
1	2	[1]	[2]
2	3	[2]	[3]
3	3	[3]	[3]
4	4	[4]	[4]
5	5	[5]	[4]
6	6	[6]	[5]
7	7	[7]	[6]
8	8	[8]	[7]
9	9	[9]	[8]
10	11	[10]	[10]
11	13	[11]	[11]
12	15	[12]	[13]
13	17	[13]	[15]
14	20	[14]	[18]
15	24	[15]	[20]
16	27	[16]	[24]
≥17	≥32	[≥17]	[≥27]

Step 9 (compare to average person your age)

Comparative Risk			
Age (yr)	Average 10-yr CHD risk (%)	Average 10-yr hard[a] CHD risk (%)	Low[b] 10-yr CHD risk (%)
30–34	<1	<1	<1
35–39	<1	<1	1
40–44	2	1	2
45–49	5	2	3
50–54	8	3	5
55–59	12	7	7
60–64	12	8	8
65–69	13	8	8
70–74	14	11	8

Key	
Relative Risk	
	Very low
	Low
	Moderate
	High
	Very high

Step 4

Blood Pressure					
Systolic (mm Hg)	Diastolic (mm Hg)				
	<80	80–84	85–89	90–99	≥100
<120	3 [−3] pts				
120–129		0 [0] pts			
130–139			0 [0] pts		
140–159				2 [2] pts	
≥160					3 [3] pts

The original Framingham score (Figs. 1.1 and 1.2) holds value in the total CHD risk, as opposed to the modified global risk adopted by the NCEP ATP III, which allocates points to account for age-associated increases in serum cholesterol and the higher lifetime risk associated with high serum cholesterol and cigarette smoking. Therefore, the modified global risk score for young patients who smoke cigarettes or have high serum cholesterol will be much higher than the original Framingham score. Figure 1.3 compares the revised ATP III global risk score to the original Framingham equations. This revised ATP III global risk score will result in more young individuals achieving a high global risk score. The net impact is to include more young high-risk individuals into a more aggressive goal category. Additionally, due to the residual risk associated with treated hypertension, patients with the same blood pressure on treatment receive a higher point score.

Using the global risk scoring system, a 57-year-old male (8 points) nonsmoker (0 points) with no CHD, no diabetes, normal weight, a systolic blood pressure of 152/94 mm Hg (1 point), a total cholesterol level of 264 mg per dL (4 points), and an HDL-C level of 32 mg per dL (2 points) would have a CHD risk of 15 points, with a resultant 10-year CHD risk of 20% (Fig. 1.4). The new global risk score places emphasis on younger age and CHD risk, as well as lifetime risk. Calculation of the global risk score is essential in ATP III and adds a step to risk assessment beyond risk factor counting.

Once the risk category is determined, the LDL-C goal is established (step 5). For CHD and CHD risk equivalents, the LDL-C goal is less

◄ **Figure 1.2.** Calculating abbreviated risk score. Coronary heart disease (CHD) score sheet for women using total cholesterol (TC) or low-density lipoprotein cholesterol (LDL-C) categories. Uses age, TC (or LDL-C), high-density lipoprotein cholesterol (HDL-C), blood pressure, diabetes, and smoking. Estimates risk for CHD over a period of 10 years based on Framingham experience in women 30 to 74 years old at baseline. Average risk estimates are based on typical Framingham subjects, and estimates of idealized risk are based on optimal blood pressure, TC of 160 to 199 mg per dL (or LDL of 100 to 129 mg per dL), HDL-C of 55 mg per dL in men, no diabetes, and no smoking. Use of the LDL-C categories is appropriate when fasting LDL-C measurements are available. Note: When systolic and diastolic pressures provide different estimates for point scores, use the higher number. [a]Hard CHD events exclude angina pectoris. [b]Low risk was calculated for a person the same age, optimal blood pressure, LDL-C of 100 to 129 mg per dL or cholesterol of 160–199 mg per dL, HDL-C of 45 mg per dL for men or 55 mg per dL for women, nonsmoker, and no diabetes. Risk estimates were derived from the Framingham Heart Study, a predominantly white population in Massachusetts. pts, points. (From Wilson PWF, D'Agostino RB, Levy D, et al. Prediction of coronary heart disease using risk factor categories. *Circulation* 1998;97:1837–1847, with permission.)

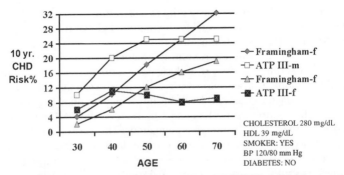

Figure 1.3. Graph comparing Adult Treatment Panel III (ATP III) global risk scores to the old Framingham scores. BP, blood pressure; CHD, coronary heart disease; f, female; HDL, high-density lipoprotein; m, male.

Age (Yrs)	Pts
20-34	-9
35-39	-4
40-44	0
45-49	3
50-54	6
55-59	8
60-64	10
65-69	11
70-74	12
75-79	13

Systolic Blood Pressure	Treated	Untreated
<120	0	0
120-129	0	1
130-139	1	2
140-159	1	2
≥ 160	2	3

Total Cholesterol (mg/dL)	20-39	40-49	50-59	60-69	70-79
<160	0	0	0	0	0
160-199	4	3	2	1	0
200-239	7	5	3	1	0
240-279	9	6	4	2	1
280	11	8	5	3	1

Cigarette Smoking	20-39	40-49	50-59	60-69	70-79
Nonsmoker	0	0	0	0	0
Smoker	8	5	3	1	1

HDL-C (mg/dL)	Pts
> 60	-1
50-59	0
40-49	1
< 40	2

57 yo male
Nl weight
BP 152/94
FBS 118
Tchol 264
TG 350
HDL-C 32
LDL-C 162
Nonsmoker
No DM
No CHD

CHD Risk	
Pts	10-Yr CHD Risk
< 0	< 1%
0	1%
1	1%
2	1%
3	1%
4	1%
5	2%
6	2%
7	3%
8	4%
9	5%
10	6%
11	8%
12	10%
13	12%
14	16%
15	20%
16	25%
≥ 17	≥ 30%

Figure 1.4. Assessing coronary heart disease (CHD) risk in men. The shaded areas indicate point (Pt) values for a 57-year-old male nonsmoker with no CHD, no diabetes mellitus (DM), normal (Nl) weight, a systolic blood pressure (BP) of 152/94 mm Hg, a total cholesterol (Tchol) level of 264 mg per dL, and a high-density lipoprotein cholesterol (HDL-C) level of 32 mg per dL. FBS, fasting blood sugar; LDL-C, low-density lipoprotein; TG, triglycerides.

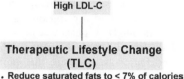

Figure 1.5. The essential features of the TLC diet in the treatment of hypercholesterol-emia. LDL-C, low-density lipoprotein cholesterol.

than 100 mg per dL; for individuals with multiple (2+) risk factors, the LDL-C goal is less than 130 mg per dL; and for individuals with 0 to 1 risk factors, the LDL-C goal is less than 160 mg per dL. The therapeutic lifestyle change (TLC) diet is then initiated (step 6) based on risk category and LDL-C goal. The essential features of TLC are outlined in Figure 1.5. For individuals with CHD or CHD risk equivalents (10-year risk greater than 20%), TLC is initiated for an LDL-C level greater than or equal to 100 mg per dL.

Drug therapy is added when the LDL-C continues to exceed initiation levels (step 7). For individuals with CHD or CHD risk equivalents, drug therapy is initiated for LDL levels greater than or equal to 100 mg per dL, with the goal of attaining an LDL-C level of less than 100 mg per dL and an optional goal of less than 70 mg per dL for very-high-risk patients. When drugs are prescribed, attention to TLC should continue to be maintained and reinforced.

Individuals with metabolic syndrome should be identified and treated with drug therapy after 3 months of TLC (step 8). Factors characteristic of the metabolic syndrome include abdominal obesity, atherogenic dyslipidemia (elevated triglyceride, small LDL particles, low HDL-C), raised blood pressure, insulin resistance (with or without glucose intolerance), and prothrombotic and proinflammatory states. ATP III recognizes the metabolic syndrome as a secondary target of risk-reduction therapy.

As elevated triglycerides are also an independent risk factor for CHD, individuals with elevated triglycerides should be treated to achieve the target goal for LDL-C (step 9). In addition to weight reduction and increased physical activity, drug therapy can be considered in high-risk individuals with elevated triglycerides (greater than 200 mg per dL) to achieve the non–HDL-C goals.

Achieving ATP III goals is a relatively complex, step-by-step process that requires some challenging tools to ensure that physicians and other health professionals adhere closely to the guidelines. Simply speaking, guidelines that are not implemented do not work. Thus, it will be a challenge to come up with tools to ensure compliance with ATP III standards.

MOTIVATING THE PATIENT: CARDIOVASCULAR RISK–ASSOCIATED AGE

One useful means to explain the significance of the 10-year Framingham score to patients is by using the cardiovascular (CV) risk–associated age. The CV risk–associated age is calculated based on gender-related age points, HDL-C level, total cholesterol level, systolic blood pressure, smoking status, presence of diabetes mellitus, and electrocardiographic left ventricular hypertrophy (Table 1.2). The points for each risk factor are added, and the CV risk–associated age equivalent is determined based on the summed points. The calculations can be shared with the patient to demonstrate that by lowering total cholesterol, raising HDL-C, and lowering triglycerides, the CV risk–associated age and risk of CHD can decrease. Instilling motivation is probably more likely if a patient is counseled that a decrease in CV risk–associated age from 68 years to 53 years can be achieved with lipid modification than if informed that his or her risk can be reduced from 14% to 8%. The effect of modifying other risk factors, such as smoking and hypertension, can also be demonstrated. The CV risk–associated age can be used to determine a patient's NCEP ATP III goals and to motivate the patient to adhere to the recommended treatment program.

ADHERENCE: ACHIEVING GOALS AND PROMOTING COMPLIANCE

There are essentially six key elements to promoting adherence to the ATP III guidelines (Table 1.3). The first essential element is identifying high-risk patients. This can be done in a number of ways, including the traditional office-based physician visit, which is where patients are most likely to access the physician. However, many medical offices are not set up to do screening of high-risk patients in a formal way. Establishing algorithms in the office to obtain a standard lipid profile, blood pressure, fasting glucose, and waist circumference (which is key for the

Table 1.2. Cardiovascular Age Equivalency

Step 1: Find points for each risk factor

Women

Age (yr)	Pts	Age (yr)	Pts
30	-12	47-48	5
31	-11	49-50	6
32	-9	51-52	7
33	-8	53-55	8
34	-6	56-60	9
35	-5	61-67	10
36	-4	68-74	11
37	-3		
38	-2		
39	-3		
40	0		
41	1		
42-43	2		
44	3		
45-46	4		

Men

Age (yr)	Pts	Age (yr)	Pts
30	-2	57-59	13
31	-1	60-61	14
32-33	0	62-64	15
34	1	65-67	16
35-36	2	68-70	17
37-38	3	71-73	18
39	4	74	19
40-41	5		
42-43	6		
44-45	7		
46-47	8		
48-49	9		
50-51	10		
52-54	11		
55-56	12		

HDL-C (mg/dL)	Pts
25-26	7
27-29	6
30-32	5
33-35	4
36-38	3
39-42	2
43-46	1
47-50	0
51-55	-1
56-60	-2
61-66	-3
67-73	-4
74-80	-5
81-87	-6
88-96	-7

Total-C (mg/dL)	Pts
139-151	-3
152-166	-2
167-182	-1
183-199	0
200-219	1
220-239	2
240-262	3
263-288	4
289-315	5
316-330	6

SBP (mm Hg)	Pts
98-104	-2
105-112	-1
113-120	0
121-129	1
130-139	2
140-149	3
150-160	4
161-172	5
173-185	6

Other	Pts[a]
Cigarettes	4
Diabetic (male)	3
Diabetic (female)	6
ECG-LVH	9

Step 2: Sum points for all risk factors (subtract minus points from total)

$$\overline{Age} + \overline{HDL\text{-}C} + \overline{Total\text{-}C} + \overline{SBP} + \overline{Smoker} + \overline{Diabetes} + \overline{ECG\text{-}LVH} = \overline{Point\ total}$$

continued

Table 1.2. Continued

Step 3: Calculated cardiovascular age risk equivalent

Points	Age (yr) Women	Age (yr) Men	Points	Age (yr) Women	Age (yr) Men	Points	Age (yr) Women	Age (yr) Men
-12	30	<30	4	47–48	39	18	>74	71–73
-11	31	<30	5	49–50	40–41	>19	>74	74
-9	32	<30	6	51–52	42–43			
-8	34	<30	7	53–55	44–45			
-6	35	<30	8	56–60	46–47			
-5	36	<30	9	61–67	48–49			
-4	37	<30	10	68–74	50–51			
-3	37	<30	11	>74	52–54			
-2	38	30	12	>74	55–56			
-1	39	31	13	>74	57–59			
0	40	32–33	14	>74	60–61			
1	41–43	34	15	>74	62–64			
2	44	35–36	16	>74	65–67			
3	45–46	37–38	17	>74	68–70			

ECG-LVH, electrocardiographic left ventricular hypertrophy; HDL-C, high-density lipoprotein cholesterol; Pts, points; SBP, systolic blood pressure.
aZero points for each "no."

Table 1.3. Implementation of the National Cholesterol Education Program Adult Treatment Panel III Guidelines: Six Essential Elements to Promoting Adherence

1. Identify high-risk patients
2. Calculate global risk
3. Determine goals
4. Initiate therapy
5. Motivate and educate the patient to maintain compliance
6. Patient follow-up and tracking of progress

metabolic syndrome diagnosis) and then screening for secondary causes of dyslipidemia can be instrumental in identifying high-risk patients in the office setting. Training other health care professionals, such as nurse case managers or advanced practice nurses, to screen for important risk factors, such as hypertension, cigarette smoking, diabetes, clinical atherosclerosis, and family history of CV disease, can also facilitate prompt recognition of patients at increased risk for CHD, as well as trigger the appropriate screening tests for those patients.

Treatment on an inpatient basis during hospitalization is an additional way to manage patients who are identified as high risk for CHD. The hospital is a proven entry point for many high-risk individuals; however, this approach is mostly secondary prevention in nature. Yet, the hospitalized patient can be provided with intensive efforts aimed at increasing adherence. The Cardiac Hospitalization Atherosclerosis Management Program illustrated that use of a formal algorithm in hospitalized patients can make a difference when it comes to making sure that patients are, for instance, discharged on statins, aspirin, beta blockers, and angiotensin-converting enzyme inhibitors, if appropriate, and in ensuring long-term compliance. Initiation of atherosclerosis therapy in the hospital setting has been shown to result in higher utilization rates both at the time of discharge and during long-term follow-up (Fig. 1.6). Hospital-based treatment protocols such as the Cardiac Hospitalization Atherosclerosis Management Program have the potential to significantly increase use of indicated therapies to manage coronary artery disease. Additional research has shown that prescription of therapy at the time of initial angiographic diagnosis of CHD improves long-term medication compliance, with nearly twice as many patients taking prescribed medications at follow-up (Fig. 1.7).

The use of chart stickers or inserts has also proven to be beneficial in identifying high-risk patients. In ATP II, a simple chart sticker was put on top of patient charts that can potentially have the new global risk score listed and can serve as another way to identify high-risk individuals. Patients at high risk for CV disease can also be

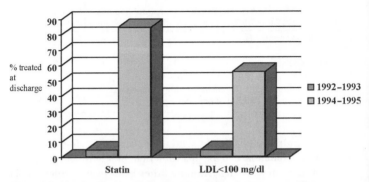

Figure 1.6. The Cardiac Hospitalization Atherosclerosis Management Program. Compliance at 12 months. LDL, low-density lipoprotein.

identified through the diagnostic billing code system and hospital databases.

Other strategies aimed at improving identification of high-risk patients include teaching physicians to implement lipid treatment guidelines, using reminders to prompt physicians to attend to lipid management, and identifying a patient advocate in the medical office, such as a nurse case manager or advanced practice nurse, to help deliver or prompt care.

Public screenings, targeted screenings in locations such as shopping malls and pharmacies, and corporate screening programs can all serve

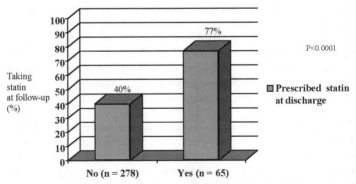

Figure 1.7. Graph illustrating that in-hospital initiation of lipid therapy improves long-term compliance.

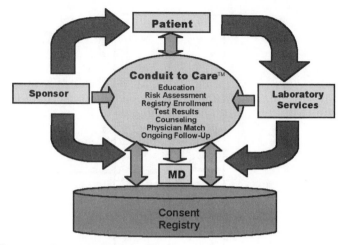

Figure 1.8. The patient management system.

to identify individuals at risk for CHD. In ATP III, primary prevention is highlighted as offering the greatest opportunity for reducing the burden of CHD. One aim of primary prevention is to reduce long-term risk (longer than 10 years) as well as short-term risk (10 years or less).

In addition to identifying individuals at risk for CHD, the ATP III guidelines place an increased emphasis on screening noncoronary atherosclerosis patients—for instance, those patients with peripheral arterial disease, carotid artery disease, or abdominal aortic aneurysm. Essentially, none of these patients should leave the hospital without aggressive risk factor identification and modification. After hospitalization, coordinated patient management can facilitate continued follow-up and an integrated approach to care (Fig. 1.8).

A global risk assessment is necessary to target patients most likely to benefit from risk modification and improve cost effectiveness. The number needed to treat (NNT) to prevent one event over a 5- or 10-year period is often used to evaluate the benefits of risk modification. The basic principle of risk modification is that the higher the risk, the greater the potential for benefit. Assuming a generous 50% reduction in CHD clinical events with risk modification, if the baseline risk is decreased from 20% to 10% for every 100 patients treated, ten fewer patients will have events, or the NNT to prevent one event is ten. If the risk is 2% over 10 years and the risk is reduced to 1% with intervention,

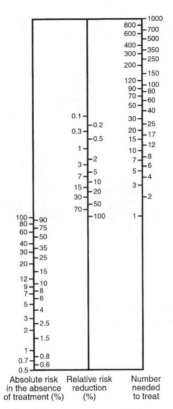

Figure 1.9. Nomogram for calculating the number needed to treat. (Published with permission.)

then, for every 100 patients treated, only one event would be prevented; therefore, the NNT is 100. Cost for each year of life saved is based on the NNT analysis. Figure 1.9 provides a nomogram for converting the global risk score into NNT.

The Framingham global risk score has limitations, and, because the study was conducted in a mostly white population, the applicability to other ethnic groups is not certain. Family history of CHD is not part of the equation because this variable did not add significantly to the predictive value of the equation. The lack of additive predictive value of family history may be due to the difficulty in assessing a true family his-

Table 1.4. Effects of a Single Risk Factor or Age on Global Risk

	50-yr-old man	50-yr-old man	60-yr-old man
Cholesterol	310	210	210
Triglycerides	150	150	150
High-density lipoprotein	45	45	45
Cigarette smoker	No	No	No
Glucose	Normal	Normal	Normal
Blood pressure (mm Hg)	120/80	152/92	120/80
Global risk: 10-yr probability of coronary heart disease	12%	12%	12%

tory of premature CHD. A parent who died of premature CHD but was also a heavy cigarette smoker may not have passed on a genetic predisposition for CHD to his or her children. Genetic causes of hyperlipidemia or low HDL-C, which result in familial premature CHD, would already be incorporated into the Framingham score. The Framingham score is approximately 80% predictive of future CHD events and other lipid parameters [e.g., lipoprotein(a)], inflammatory markers [e.g., C-reactive protein (CRP)], and noninvasive imaging of atherosclerosis [e.g., electron beam computed tomography (EBCT) and carotid ultrasound] may provide additional predictive value.

Patients, as well as physicians, do not appreciate the magnitude of risk associated with multiple risk factors. Table 1.4 presents three cases of men with the same Framingham risk score. The purpose of this comparison is to demonstrate the effects of a single risk factor or age on global risk.

Basically, a single risk factor is equivalent to adding 100 mg per dL points to the total cholesterol or 10 years of age-equivalent risk. A 50-year-old man with a total cholesterol of 210 mg per dL and an elevated blood pressure of 142/92 mm Hg has a 10-year CHD risk equivalent to that of a 60-year-old man with the same lipid profile but a normal blood pressure. A 50-year-old man with a total cholesterol of 210 mg per dL and hypertension also has a risk equivalent to that of a normotensive 50-year-old man with a total cholesterol of 310 mg per dL. Therefore, the Framingham risk score provides the data to convert the 10-year absolute risk into a more meaningful educational tool for the patient. A 50-year-old hypertensive man with a total cholesterol of 210 mg per dL may not fully comprehend the significance of a 10% 10-year risk of CHD, but may better understand his risk if informed that he has a risk equivalent to that of a 60-year-old man or a normotensive man his age with a total cholesterol of 310 mg per dL.

The CV risk–associated age equivalency is provided in Table 1.2. The 10-year CHD absolute risk is converted into an age for a person with an equivalent risk without the presence of significant risk factors. Due to widespread public education, most patients understand the risk associated with serum cholesterol for heart disease. A patient may think that a total cholesterol of 210 mg per dL is not seriously elevated, but a cholesterol of 310 mg per dL is reason for alarm. Therefore, converting a patient's global risk into a CV age or cholesterol equivalent is more likely to ascertain that the patient understands the clinical significance of his or her risk factor profile.

The ATP III guidelines, although continuing to focus on LDL as the primary target of treatment, have modified the therapeutic approach to include more patients who are at high risk for CHD but do not yet have clinical evidence of CHD for the more aggressive goal of LDL less than 100 mg per dL. The CHD risk equivalent category includes diabetic patients, patients with a 10-year absolute risk of 20% or higher, and patients with noncoronary clinical atherosclerosis (peripheral vascular disease, transient ischemic attacks, or cerebral vascular events) (Fig. 1.10). Diabetes is considered a CHD risk equivalent because it confers a high risk of new CHD at least equivalent to that of a nondiabetic with a prior myocardial infarction (Fig. 1.11). Although these data are known for type 2 diabetic patients, the high risk most likely applies to type 1 diabetic patients as well. The guidelines also identify individuals with the metabolic syndrome that is defined as having at least three of the five criteria listed in Table 1.5 as candidates for intensified TLC. The patient with the metabolic syndrome should be treated

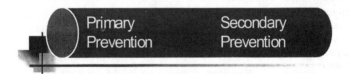

Primary   Secondary
Prevention   Prevention

Ways to sharpen identification of high-risk patients
(Identify the "CHD risk-equivalent" patients)

- Non-coronary atherosclerosis (e.g. TIA, CVA, PAD)
- Diagnosis of type 2 diabetes
- Global risk assessment (>20% 10-yr risk)

Figure 1.10. The coronary heart disease (CHD) risk continuum. Primary and secondary prevention. CVA, cerebrovascular accident; PAD, peripheral arterial disease; TIA, transient ischemic attack.

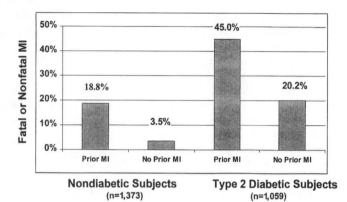

Figure 1.11. Incidence of myocardial infarction (MI) during a 7-year follow-up in a Finnish population. (From Haffner SM, Lehto S, Ronnemaa T, et al. Mortality from coronary heart disease subjects with type 2 diabetes in non-diabetic subjects with and without previous myocardial infarction implications for treatment of hyperlipidemia in diabetic subjects without prior myocardial infarction. *N Engl J Med* 1998;339:229–234, with permission.)

Table 1.5. Clinical Identification of the Metabolic Syndrome

Risk factor	Defining level
Abdominal obesity[a]	
Waist circumference[b]	
Men	>102 cm (>40 in.)
Women	>88 cm (>35 in.)
Triglycerides	≥150 mg/dL
High-density lipoprotein cholesterol	
Men	<40 mg/dL
Women	<50 mg/dL
Blood pressure	≥130/≥85 mm Hg
Fasting glucose	≥110 mg/dL

[a]An overweight state and obesity are associated with insulin resistance and the metabolic syndrome. However, the presence of abdominal obesity is more highly correlated with the metabolic risk factors than is an elevated body mass index. The simple measure of waist circumference is recommended, however, to identify the body weight component of the metabolic syndrome.

[b]Some men can develop multiple metabolic risk factors when the waist circumference is only marginally increased [e.g., 94 to 102 cm (37 to 40 in.)]. Such patients may have strong genetic contribution to insulin resistance, and they should benefit from changes in life habits, similar to men with categorical increases in waist circumference.

to an LDL or non-HDL goal as specified by his or her risk factor status, but added consideration should be given to body weight reduction and physical exercise.

The other significant change involves the use of non-HDL as a secondary target for patients with serum triglycerides greater than or equal to 200 mg per dL. Non-HDL is simply the total cholesterol minus the HDL or the LDL plus very-low-density lipoprotein (VLDL). VLDL is calculated by dividing the fasting triglyceride level by five. The calculated LDL by the Friedewald formula is

$$LDL = total\ cholesterol - \left[\left(\frac{HDL + triglycerides}{5}\right)\right]$$

This formula is accurate if chylomicrons are absent. Chylomicrons are formed when fat is absorbed postprandially but cleared within 12 hours in most people. If triglycerides are greater than 500 mg per dL, the patient is often not fully fasted for 12 hours or has prolonged clearance of chylomicrons, and, therefore, the calculation of VLDL equal to triglycerides divided by 5 is inaccurate. Chylomicrons have a ratio of triglycerides to cholesterol of 10:1 or more, which explains the inaccuracy of the Friedewald formula when triglycerides exceed 500 mg per dL (see Chapter 2). Non-HDL, however, combines the LDL with the other cholesterol-containing particles (VLDL, intermediate-density lipoproteins, and chylomicrons, if present). Non-HDL correlates closely with apolipoprotein B (Apo B) (0.95 correlation) and, therefore, potentially represents all the atherogenic lipoproteins. Apo B or non-HDL has been shown to be more predictive than LDL in many of the outcome trials and is significantly better at identifying risk in patients with hypertriglyceridemia. Figure 1.12 compares the CV event rates of non-HDL versus LDL in the Scandinavian Simvastatin Survival Study (4S). Both parameters are fairly linear, with non-HDL as linear, if not more linear, than LDL. Apo B is perhaps the most linear, as demonstrated in Figure 1.13.

Table 1.6 presents two lipid profiles demonstrating the benefits of non-HDL over LDL in patients with hypertriglyceridemia. Both patients have the same total cholesterol, HDL, and LDL/HDL ratio. However, based on the Prospective Cardiovascular Münster (PRO-CAM) study, Patient A has approximately twice the risk of Patient B (Fig. 1.14). According to the PROCAM trial, the hypertriglyceridemic subgroup (triglycerides greater than or equal to 200 mg per dL) with an elevated LDL/HDL cholesterol ratio had the highest risk of atherosclerotic CHD. Although only 4.3% of participants in the PROCAM

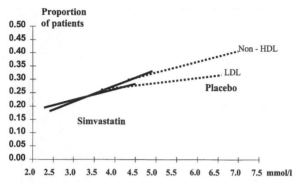

Figure 1.12. Major coronary events on treatment. Non–high-density lipoprotein (HDL) versus low-density lipoprotein (LDL). (Adapted from 4S Trial; Davidson MH. Introduction: utilization of surrogate markers of atherosclerosis for the clinical development of pharmaceutical agents. *Am J Cardiol* 2001;87:1A–7A.)

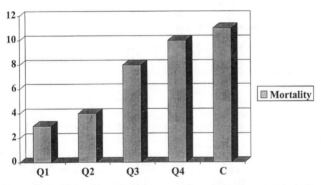

Figure 1.13. The relation of mortality in Scandinavian Simvastatin Survival Study to the decrease in apolipoprotein B.

Table 1.6. Benefits of Non–High-Density Lipoprotein (HDL) over Low-Density Lipoprotein (LDL) in Patients with Hypertriglyceridemia

	Patient A	Patient B
Total cholesterol	250 mg/dL	250 mg/dL
Triglycerides	350 mg/dL	100 mg/dL
HDL	30 mg/dL	30 mg/dL
LDL	150 mg/dL	200 mg/dL
LDL/HDL	5.0 mg/dL	6.7 mg/dL
Non-HDL	220 mg/dL	220 mg/dL

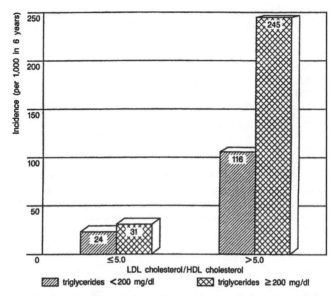

Figure 1.14. Results and conclusions of the Prospective Cardiovascular Münster Study. Coronary heart disease risk according to triglycerides and low-density lipoprotein (LDL) or high-density lipoprotein (HDL) cholesterol.

study were in this subgroup, it accounted for one-fourth of the CHD events observed.

The ATP III sets the goal for non–HDL-C in persons with high serum triglycerides at 30 mg per dL higher than that for LDL-C on the premise that a VLDL cholesterol level of less than or equal to 30 mg per dL (triglycerides of 150 mg per dL divided by 5) is normal. Table 1.7 summarizes the ATP III guidelines.

The European guidelines also use the Framingham risk score to determine the eligibility of patients for therapeutic intervention. Patients with CHD, clinical noncoronary atherosclerosis, or a 2% or greater 10-year risk should be treated with lipid-lowering drugs (if dietary therapy fails) to an LDL goal of less than 3.0 mmol per L (115 mg per dL). The 2% 10-year risk calculation is determined by evaluating the risk factor or a color-coded chart (Figs. 1.15 through 1.18). Color charts allow for the easy determination of high-risk patients without the use of adding up point scales or the need for a risk calculator. However, the European guidelines only account for relatively short-

Table 1.7. Summary of Adult Treatment Panel III Guidelines

	LDL goal (mg/dL)	If triglycerides >200 mg/dL, non–high-density lipoprotein goal (mg/dL)
Low risk		
<2 Risk factors	<160	<190
Moderate risk		
≥2 Risk factors	<130	160
Moderate high risk		
≥2 Risk factors; 10–20% 10-yr risk	<100	<130
High risk	<100	<130
CHD, peripheral arterial disease, abdominal aortic aneurysm		
>50% carotid stenosis		
Diabetes[a]		
>20% 10-yr risk		
Creatinine >1.5 mg/dL[b]		
10–20% 10-yr risk plus high-sensitivity C-reactive protein >2.0[c]		
Very high risk		
CHD plus:	<70[d]	<100[d]
Diabetes		
Metabolic syndrome		
Cigarette smoking		
Acute coronary syndrome		

CHD, coronary heart disease; LDL, low-density lipoprotein.
[a]American Diabetes Association recommends that all type 2 diabetic patients age >80 years should lower LDL by at least 30%, even if baseline LDL is less than 100 mg/dL.
[b]High risk by National Kidney Foundation guidelines.
[c]High risk by American Heart Association/Centers for Disease Control and Prevention guidelines.
[d]Adult Treatment Panel III optional goal.

term risk (10 years) and do not factor in as much as the NCEP ATP III concept of lifetime risk. To account somewhat for lifetime risk, the European guidelines recommend that for evaluating risk, the patient's age should be adjusted to 60 years. For patients with less than 2% annual risk of CHD (after correction to age 60 years), the European guidelines recommend lifestyle changes only, and drug therapy is not indicated unless the patient has a very high serum cholesterol or familial hypercholesterolemia.

The Framingham Heart Study has also developed a stroke risk prediction chart (Table 1.8). Patients are often more concerned about the risk for stroke than CHD. The stroke risk equation does not include cholesterol due to a lack of association between this risk factor and

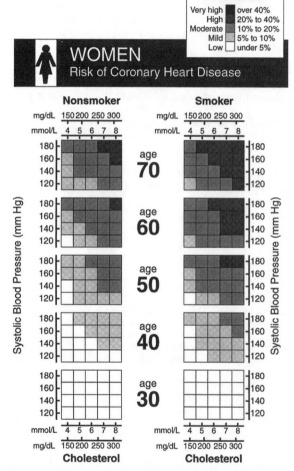

Figure 1.15. Risk of coronary heart disease in women smokers and nonsmokers.

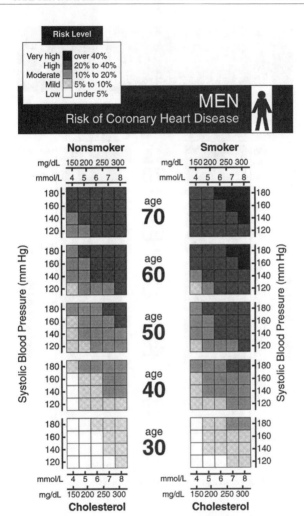

Figure 1.16. Risk of coronary heart disease in men smokers and nonsmokers.

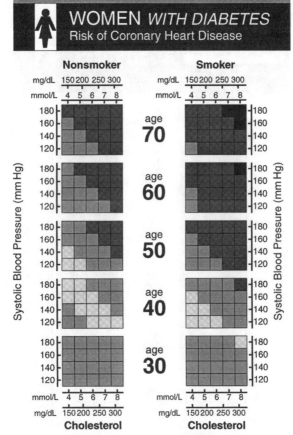

Figure 1.17. Risk of coronary heart disease in women with diabetes; smokers and nonsmokers.

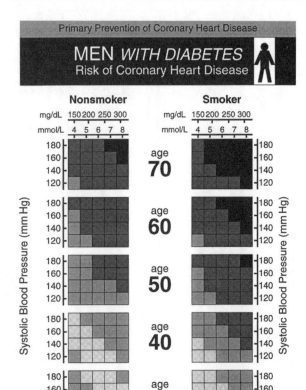

Figure 1.18. Risk of coronary heart disease in men with diabetes; smokers and non-smokers.

Table 1.8. Stroke Risk Factor Prediction Chart

Step 1: Find points for each risk factor

Men

Age (yr)	SBP	HYP RX	Diabetes	Cigs	CVD	AF	LVH
		No = 0 / Yes = 2	No = 0 / Yes = 2	No = 0 / Yes = 3	No = 0 / Yes = 3	No = 0 / Yes = 4	No = 0 / Yes = 6
54–56 = 0	95–105 = 0						
57–59 = 1	106–116 = 1						
60–62 = 2	117–126 = 2						
63–65 = 3	127–137 = 3						
66–68 = 4	138–148 = 4						
69–71 = 5	149–159 = 5						
72–74 = 6	160–170 = 6						
75–77 = 7	171–181 = 7						
78–80 = 8	182–191 = 8						
81–83 = 9	192–202 = 9						
84–85 = 10	203–213 = 10						

Women

Age (yr)	SBP	HYP RX	Diabetes	Cigs	CVD	AF	LVH
		No = 0 / If yes see below	No = 0 / Yes = 3	No = 0 / Yes = 3	No = 0 / Yes = 2	No = 0 / Yes = 6	No = 0 / Yes = 4
54–56 = 0	95–104 = 0						
57–59 = 1	105–114 = 1						
60–62 = 2	115–124 = 2						
63–65 = 3	125–134 = 3						
66–68 = 4	135–144 = 4						
69–71 = 5	145–154 = 5						
72–74 = 6	155–164 = 6						
75–77 = 7	165–174 = 7						
78–80 = 8	175–184 = 8						
81–83 = 9	185–194 = 9						
84–86 = 10	196–204 = 10						

If currently under antihypertensive therapy, add the following points, depending on SBP level

SBP	95–104	105–114	115–124	125–134	135–144	145–154
Points	6	5	5	4	3	3

SBP	155–164	165–174	175–184	185–194	195–204
Points	2	1	1	0	0

Step 2: Sum points for all risk factors

$$\overline{\text{Age}} + \overline{\text{SBP}} + \overline{\text{HYP RX}} + \overline{\text{Diabetes}} + \overline{\text{Cigs}} + \overline{\text{CVD}} + \overline{\text{AF}} + \overline{\text{LVH}} = \overline{\text{Point total}}$$

Step 3: Look up risk corresponding to point total

Men 10-yr

Pts	Probability (%)	Pts	Probability (%)	Pts	Probability (%)
1	2.6	11	11.2	21	41.7
2	3.0	12	12.9	22	46.6
3	3.5	13	14.8	23	51.8
4	4.0	14	17.0	24	57.3
5	4.7	15	19.5	25	62.8
6	5.4	16	22.4	26	68.4
7	6.3	17	25.5	27	73.8
8	7.3	18	29.0	28	79.0
9	8.4	19	32.9	29	83.7
10	9.7	20	37.1	30	87.9

Women 10-yr

Pts	Probability (%)	Pts	Probability (%)	Pts	Probability (%)
1	1.1	11	7.6	21	43.4
2	1.3	12	9.2	22	50.0
3	1.6	13	11.1	23	57.0
4	2.0	14	13.3	24	64.2
5	2.4	15	16.0	25	71.4
6	2.9	16	19.1	26	78.2
7	3.5	17	22.8	27	84.4
8	4.3	18	27.0		
9	5.2	19	31.9		
10	6.3	20	37.3		

Step 4: Compare to average 10-yr risk

Average 10-yr probability by age

Men		Women	
55–59	5.9%	55–59	3.0%
60–64	7.8%	60–64	4.7%
65–69	11.0%	65–69	7.2%
70–74	13.7%	70–74	10.9%
75–79	18.0%	75–79	15.5%
80–84	22.3%	80–84	23.9%

AF, history of atrial fibrillation; Cigs, smokes cigarettes; CVD, history of myocardial infarction, angina pectoris, coronary insufficiency, intermittent claudication, or congestive heart failure; Diabetes, history of diabetes; HYP RX, under antihypertensive therapy; LVH, left ventricular hypertrophy; Pts, points; SBP, systolic blood pressure.

From Framingham Heart Study and the American Heart Association, with permission.

stroke in the Framingham study. However, the statin trials have demonstrated a significant reduction in stroke rates in patients with CHD.
The stroke risk prediction chart may also help motivate patients to
modify other important risk factors, such as hypertension or cigarette
smoking.

Noninvasive imaging techniques to assess preclinical atherosclerosis
have become popular tools to enhance CHD risk predictability. The
EBCT to assess coronary calcium is a relatively widely available, moderate-
cost technology for evaluating the atherosclerotic plaque burden. Calcium scores do predict future coronary events; however, the superiority
of calcium scores predicting CHD events over the Framingham risk
score is uncertain. Most evidence suggests that the calcium score percentile for an individual's age is the best predictor of future events;
therefore, a combination of the Framingham risk score with the coronary calcium score percentile by age may provide an enhancement of
risk prediction. Table 1.9 lists the coronary calcium score by sex and
age and provides percentile rankings. Grundy has advocated adding
points to the Framingham score to adjust for a high percentile of coronary calcium for an individual's age. A person in the 90th percentile of
coronary calcium would receive three more points, whereas a person

Table 1.9. Calcium Score Nomogram for 9,728 Consecutive Subjects

Patient age group yr (n)	Calcium score			
	25th percentile	50th percentile	75th percentile	90th percentile
Men (5,433)				
35–39 (479)	0	0	2	21
40–44 (859)	0	0	11	64
45–49 (1,066)	0	3	44	176
50–54 (1,085)	0	16	101	320
55–59 (853)	3	41	187	502
60–64 (613)	14	118	434	804
65–70 (478)	28	151	569	1,178
Women (4,295)				
35–39 (288)	0	0	0	4
40–44 (589)	0	0	0	9
45–49 (822)	0	0	0	23
50–54 (903)	0	0	0	66
55–59 (693)	0	0	33	140
60–64 (515)	0	4	87	310
65–70 (485)	0	24	123	362

*From Davidson MH. Introduction: utilization of surrogate markers of atherosclerosis for the clini-
cal development of pharmaceutical agents. Am J Cardiol 2001; 87(4A):1A–7A, with permission.*

Table 1.10. Adjusting Framingham Age Points for Coronary Calcium Score

Percentile of calcium score	Point adjustment[a]
0–24th	–2
25–49th	–1
50–74th	+1
75–89th	+2
≥90th	+3

[a]The adjustment shown should be substituted for the age score of a given patient, whether man or woman.

with a low calcium score would have points deducted from the score (Table 1.10). Rather than using a biologic age, the EBCT may provide a more accurate means of aging the coronary arteries. This concept of combining the Framingham score to the EBCT coronary calcium percentile as a means of enhancing risk predictability needs further testing in a clinical trial.

Obesity is a growing problem in the United States and throughout the developing world. Although obesity is not part of the Framingham score, patients who are obese usually have metabolic syndrome or diabetes with high triglycerides, low HDL, and hypertension, which contribute to a higher score and are associated with marked increase in progression of atherosclerosis. Obesity is best defined by body mass index (BMI) rather than weight because of significant height variability. BMI is highly predictive of the future development of diabetes. Table 1.11 shows the marked increase in risk of developing diabetes as BMI increases. Color-coded charts, as shown in Figure 1.19, are available to quickly evaluate BMI to define patients who are clinically obese.

Table 1.11. Body Mass Index at Age 18 and Age-Adjusted Risk of Diabetes Among a Cohort of U.S. Women Aged 30–55 Yr in 1976 and Followed for 8 Yr

Body mass index at age 18 yr (kg/m^2)	Age-adjusted relative risk
<19	1.0
19.0–19.9	0.7
20.0–20.9	0.9
21.0–21.9	1.2
22.0–22.9	1.6
23.0–23.9	1.8
24.0–24.9	2.1
25.0–26.9	3.3
27.0–28.9	4.2
≥29.0	6.1

BMI TABLE

HEIGHT (ft/in)	WEIGHT (lb) 120	130	140	150	160	170	180	190	200	210	220	230	240	250	260	270	280	290	300	310	320	330
4'5"	30	33	35	38	40	43	45	48	50	53	55	58	60	63	65	68	70	73	75	78	80	83
4'6"	29	31	34	36	39	41	43	46	48	51	53	55	58	60	63	65	68	70	72	75	77	80
4'7"	28	30	33	35	37	40	42	44	46	49	51	53	56	58	60	63	65	67	70	72	75	77
4'8"	27	29	31	34	36	38	40	43	45	47	49	52	54	56	58	61	63	65	67	69	72	74
4'9"	26	28	30	32	35	37	39	41	43	45	48	50	52	54	56	58	61	63	65	67	69	71
4'10"	25	27	29	31	33	36	38	40	42	44	46	48	50	52	54	56	59	61	63	65	67	69
4'11"	24	26	28	30	32	34	36	38	40	42	44	46	48	50	53	55	57	59	61	63	65	67
5'0"	23	25	27	29	31	33	35	37	39	41	43	45	47	49	51	53	55	57	59	61	62	64
5'1"	23	25	26	28	30	32	34	36	38	40	42	43	45	47	49	51	53	55	57	59	60	62
5'2"	22	24	26	27	29	31	33	35	37	38	40	42	44	46	48	49	51	53	55	57	59	60
5'3"	21	23	25	27	28	30	32	34	35	37	39	41	43	44	46	48	50	51	53	55	57	58
5'4"	21	22	24	26	27	29	31	33	34	36	38	39	41	43	45	46	48	50	51	53	55	57
5'5"	20	22	23	25	27	28	30	32	33	35	37	38	40	42	43	45	47	48	50	52	53	55
5'6"	19	21	23	24	26	27	29	31	32	34	36	37	39	40	42	44	45	47	48	50	52	53
5'7"	19	20	22	23	25	27	28	30	31	33	34	36	38	39	41	42	44	45	47	49	50	52
5'8"	18	20	21	23	24	26	27	29	30	32	33	35	36	38	40	41	43	44	46	47	49	50
5'9"	18	19	21	22	24	25	27	28	30	31	32	34	35	37	38	40	41	43	44	46	47	49
5'10"	17	19	20	22	23	24	26	27	29	30	32	33	34	36	37	39	40	42	43	44	46	47
5'11"	17	18	20	21	22	24	25	27	28	29	31	32	33	35	36	38	39	40	42	43	45	46
6'0"	16	18	19	20	22	23	24	26	27	28	30	31	33	34	35	37	38	39	41	42	43	45
6'1"	16	17	18	20	21	22	24	25	26	28	29	30	32	33	34	36	37	38	40	41	42	44
6'2"	15	17	18	19	21	22	23	24	26	27	28	30	31	32	33	35	36	37	39	40	41	42
6'3"	15	16	18	19	20	21	23	24	25	26	27	29	30	31	32	34	35	36	37	39	40	41
6'4"	15	16	17	18	19	21	22	23	24	26	27	28	29	30	32	33	34	35	37	38	39	40
6'5"	14	15	17	18	19	20	21	23	24	25	26	27	28	30	31	32	33	34	36	37	38	39
6'6"	14	15	16	17	18	20	21	22	23	24	25	27	28	29	30	31	32	34	35	36	37	38
6'7"	14	15	16	17	18	19	20	21	23	24	25	26	27	28	29	30	32	33	34	35	36	37
6'8"	13	14	15	16	18	19	20	21	22	23	24	25	26	27	29	30	31	32	33	34	35	36
6'9"	13	14	15	16	17	18	19	20	21	23	24	25	26	27	28	29	30	31	32	33	34	35
6'10"	13	14	15	16	17	18	19	20	21	22	23	24	25	26	27	28	29	30	31	32	33	35

Less risk → More risk

Figure 1.19. Body mass index (BMI) table.

EMERGING THERAPEUTIC STRATEGIES

Although lipid-lowering therapy has demonstrated significant CV event reduction across a wide spectrum of at-risk populations, there remains a relatively high residual risk of morbidity or mortality in patients with diabetes or the metabolic syndrome. There is a well-recognized linear relationship between LDL-C levels and the event rates in all of the major statin secondary prevention trials; however, in the diabetic subgroups, the event rates in the statin-treated patients exceed those of the nondiabetic placebo patients (Fig. 1.20). A similar relationship exists for the subgroup of patients with low HDL and elevated triglycerides, two major features of the metabolic syndrome. In the Heart Protection Study (HPS) subgroup of patients with low HDL (less than 35 mg per dL), simvastatin had an event rate of 22.5% compared to an event rate of 20.9% for patients taking placebo with a higher HDL (greater than or equal to 43 mg per dL). Patients with hypertriglyceridemia (triglycerides greater than or equal to 354 mg per dL on simvastatin) had an event rate of 23.2% compared to 23.7% for placebo patients with triglycerides less than 177 mg per dL. Therefore, patients with low HDL or high triglycerides on statin therapy have a residual risk of CV events comparable to placebo patients with normal levels of HDL and triglycerides.

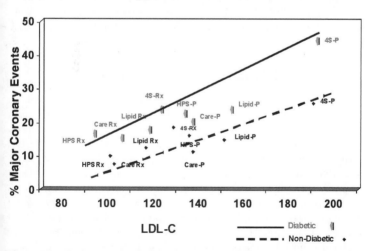

Figure 1.20. Statin risk reduction in diabetic and nondiabetic patients. LDL-C, low-density lipoprotein cholesterol; HPS, heart protection study; Rx, therapy; 4S, Scandinavian Simvastatin Survival Study.

The clinical significance of the high residual risk in patients with metabolic syndrome or diabetes is of growing importance due to the increasing prevalence of obesity and the associated comorbidities in the world. Therefore, new strategies are emerging to better define the therapeutic targets and the implementation of therapies to achieve these more aggressive goals.

EMERGING TARGETS OF THERAPY

The NCEP ATP III established an LDL goal of less than 100 mg per dL and a non-HDL goal (for patients with triglycerides greater than 200 mg per dL) of 130 mg per dL for patients at high risk for CV events. The American Diabetic Association (ADA) recommends three lipid goals (LDL less than 100 mg per dL, triglycerides less than 150 mg per dL, and HDL greater than 40 mg per dL) for patients with diabetes. Due to the results of the HPS study, which demonstrated the benefits of statin therapy, even in patients with LDL less than 100 mg per dL at baseline, simvastatin received a label change approved by the U.S. Food and Drug Administration to recommend the initiation of the 40-mg dose for all high-risk patients, regardless of the baseline LDL level. Therefore, evidence-based medicine would support the implementation of statin therapy for all high-risk patients regardless of the LDL level. A more difficult clinical question to answer based on the available trial data is the appropriate target level for LDL in high-risk patients.

ADULT TREATMENT PANEL III UPDATE

Since the publication of ATP III in 2001, five major clinical trials of statin therapy with clinical endpoints have been published. These five trials extended the benefits of statin therapy across a wide spectrum of at-risk populations and emphasized the importance of adhering to an LDL-C goal of less than 100 mg per dL in high-risk individuals. Two of these trials, HPS and the Pravastatin or Atorvastatin Evaluation and Infection Therapy (PROVE-IT) trial, supported an even more aggressive LDL-C goal for patients at very high risk for CHD events. The ATP III revised the guidelines to recommend a therapeutic optional goal of LDL less than 70 mg per dL and non-HDL less than 100 mg per dL for patients at very high risk. The definition of *very high risk* was left deliberately up to clinical judgment. However, factors that favor the definition of *very high risk* include established CVD plus (a) multiple risk factors (especially diabetes); (b) several poorly controlled risk factors (especially continued ciga-rette smoking); (c) multiple risk factors of the metabolic syndrome [especially high triglycerides greater than or equal to 200 mg per dL plus non-HDL-C greater than or equal to 130 mg per dL with low HDL (less than 40 mg per dL)]; and (d), on the basis of PROVE-IT, patients with acute coronary syndromes. Although not specifically stated, the intent of the revised ATP III report suggests that CVD with recurrent events with an LDL less than 100 mg per dL should also be considered for the optional therapeutic goal of LDL less than 70 mg per dL.

The revised ATP III also encouraged continued focus on non-HDL for patients with elevated triglycerides and low HDL, thereby recom-mending niacin or fibrates in addition to statins for patients at their LDL goal but not yet at their non-HDL goals. When initiating LDL-lowering therapy in a person of high risk or modestly high risk, a reduction in LDL-C of at least 30% to 40% beyond dietary therapy should be achieved, if feasible.

In addition, for patients with a Framingham 10-year risk of 10% to 20%, therapeutic goals of LDL less than 100 mg per dL and non-HDL less than 130 mg per dL should be considered an option based on the results of the Anglo-Scandinavian Cardiac Outcomes Trial. Therefore, the revised ATP III report basically divides patients into five categories across the risk continuum: very high to high, modestly high, and mod-erate to low risk (Table 1.7).

There were some noticeable differences between the revised ATP III recommendations from some of the professional organizations. In a divergence from the ADA guidelines, ATP III did not recommend a target goal of HDL greater than 40 mg per dL and triglycerides less than 150 mg per dL for diabetics. Also, for patients with diabetes with-out CVD, ATP III did not yet endorse the ADA concept of starting on LDL-lowering drugs when LDL-C is less than 100 mg per dL at baseline to lower LDL by at least 30% but, rather, left the decision to treat up to clinical judgment. ATP III also did not mention the National Kidney Foundation recommendation that patients with renal impairment (creatinine greater than 1.5 mg per dL) be classified as high risk.

The revised ATP III guidelines have formally endorsed the concept of "the lower the better," especially for very-high-risk patients. The panel also recognized the potential challenges of achieving the optional thera-peutic target LDL-C of less than 70 mg per dL and non-HDL less than 100 mg per dL. The benefits of aggressive lipid control are well docu-mented in clinical trials, but achieving improved outcomes in the at-risk population remains an elusive goal in many patients.

Table 1.12. Ongoing Statin Treatment Trials

Trial	N	Population	Treatment	Duration (yr)	Primary outcome
TNT	10,000	CHD	Atorvastatin, 10 mg, vs. atorvastatin, 80 mg, to target low-density lipoprotein of 100 mg/dL vs. 75 mg/dL	5	Coronary death, nonfatal myocardial infarction, death
SEARCH	10,000	CHD	Simvastatin, 20 mg, vs. simvastatin, 80 mg	5	Cardiac events
IDEAL	7,600	CHD	Simvastatin, 20–40 mg, vs. atorvastatin, 80 mg	5.5	Cardiac events
JUPITER	15,000	C-reactive protein	Rosuvastatin, 20 mg, vs. placebo	5	Cardiac events

CHD, coronary heart disease; IDEAL, Incremental Decrease in Events through Aggressive Lipid Lowering; JUPITER, Justification for the Use of Statins in Primary Prevention: An Intervention Trial Evaluating Rosuvastatin; SEARCH, Study of Effectiveness of Additional Reductions in Cholesterol and Homocysteine; TNT, Treating to New Targets.

There are three large-scale clinical trials under way to evaluate the clinical benefits of an LDL of approximately 70 mg per dL compared to an LDL of 100 mg per dL (Table 1.12). These trials, which are due to be completed over the next 2 years, are likely to officially lower the therapeutic LDL targets (rather than optional) if significant clinical benefits are demonstrated.

RATIO GOALS

A total cholesterol/HDL goal has been advocated by the Canadian guidelines (Table 1.13) (Appendix E). These guidelines are similar to the NCEP ATP III recommendation in that goals for LDL-C are more aggressive according to the risk classification. However, rather than non-HDL targets, the Canadian guidelines have a total cholesterol/HDL ratio less than 4.0. The advantage of this approach is that for patients with low HDL, more aggressive LDL-lowering or HDL-raising may be necessary to achieve both targets. As greater reduction in LDL-C is usually easier to achieve with the present therapies than significantly raising HDL, a ratio target of more than 4.0 may frequently require reducing LDL-C levels to less than 75 mg per dL in patients with low HDL. For example, a patient with an HDL of 30 mg per dL and triglycerides of 150 mg per dL would require a target total cholesterol of 120 mg per dL and an LDL-C of 60 mg per dL. For patients with higher HDL levels, an LDL lower than 100 mg per dL would most likely result in a ratio goal of less than 4.0. Therefore, by including a ratio target, the Canadian guidelines appropriately require more aggressive LDL-lowering in patients with low HDL based on clinical trials that have demonstrated that this subpopulation has a significantly higher residual risk of events on statin therapy. The ratio has been shown to be a better epidemiologic predictor of CV events than LDL and also appears to significantly improve event prediction on statin

Table 1.13. Canadian Guidelines: Cholesterol Goals

Risk level	Low-density lipoprotein goal (mg/dL)	Total cholesterol/high-density lipoprotein ratio
Low	160	<6.0
Moderate	130	<5.0
High[a]	100	<4.0

[a]High risk includes coronary heart disease, peripheral vascular disease, and diabetes ≥20% 10-year risk.
Adapted from Genest, et al. Can Med Assoc J 2003;169:921–924.

therapy. Thus, rather than having a more aggressive LDL goal for all patients, a ratio goal of less than 4.0 in conjunction with an LDL-C goal of less than 100 mg per dL may sufficiently identify the higher-risk patients who deserve more aggressive lipid-altering interventions.

The argument against a ratio target is based on a lack of evidence supporting HDL-raising as a therapeutic target, and, thus, there is a concern that a ratio target would inappropriately emphasize the benefits of increasing HDL. However, because raising HDL by more than 25% with existing therapies is difficult, the most likely means to achieve a ratio goal of less than 4.0 would still require more aggressive LDL-C lowering.

Another ratio target that has been evaluated is the Apo B/AI ratio. The Apo B/AI ratio is a better predictor of events in large population observational trials, such as the high Apo B, low Apo AI, and improvement in the prediction of fatal myocardial infarction (AMORIS) study (Fig. 1.21), and the best predictor of events on statin therapy, according to the Air Force/Texas Coronary Atherosclerosis Prevention Study trial. The Canadian guidelines also included an Apo B/AI ratio of less than 0.7 as an appropriate target. Apo B measurements are most useful in patients with hypertriglyceridemia because it incorporates all the atherogenic lipoproteins. Non-HDL correlates better with Apo B than LDL, especially in patients with hypertriglyceridemia. The main reason the Apo B/AI ratio predicts better than the total cholesterol/HDL is that, in the hypertriglyceridemic population and in those with small dense LDL (Apo B/LDL greater than 1.0), the Apo B level is signifi-

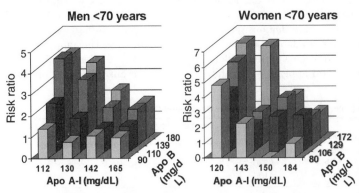

Figure 1.21. Relative risk ratios of fatal myocardial infarction by quartiles of apolipoprotein (Apo) B and Apo A-I. (From Walldius G, et al. *Lancet* 2001;358:2026–2033, with permission.)

cantly more predictive of CV events than the total cholesterol level. Apo measurements are not universally available and are more expensive than a standard lipid profile to determine than the total cholesterol/HDL ratio and, therefore, the utilization of the Apo B/AI ratio on a therapeutic target will require additional justification based on a cost-benefit analysis. However, to define a therapeutic benefit of a lipid-altering treatment, putative changes in the Apo B/AI ratio may be useful for demonstrating an enhanced benefit of a therapy and may provide a helpful lipid surrogate endpoint for regulatory approval for novel therapies.

C-REACTIVE PROTEIN

High-sensitivity CRP (hs-CRP) has evolved as an important predictor of CV events and is highly correlated with the metabolic syndrome. The more the five criteria of the metabolic syndrome are present, the more likely the hs-CRP will be elevated (Fig. 1.22). According to the American Heart Association/Centers for Disease Control and Prevention's Scientific Statement on Markers of Intervention and Cardiovascular Disease, the patient with an intermediate Framingham ATP III 10-year risk score of 10% to 20% with an LDL level below the cutpoint for initiation of drug therapy is the most appropriate patient in whom to measure CRP level. The basis for this recommendation is that in this

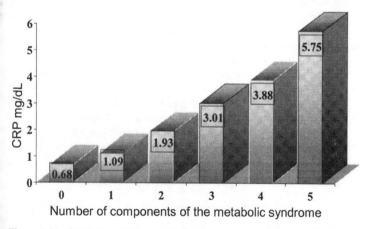

Figure 1.22. Graph illustrating the correlation between C-reactive protein (CRP) and the metabolic syndrome. (From Ridker, et al. *Circulation* 2003;107:391, with permission.)

intermediate risk group, an elevated CRP level would provide a rationale to initiate lipid-lowering therapy. In patients already known to be at high risk, such as those with diabetes, CHD, or a greater than 20% Framingham 10-year risk score, measuring CRP level would not be necessary because the initiation of lipid-lowering therapy is clearly indicated. The AHA/Centers for Disease Control and Prevention panel considered recommending more widespread testing of CRP level, such as in those patients with a family history of CHD or the metabolic syndrome, but considered the evidence inadequate at this time. For patients with CHD, more aggressive treatment of LDL in those with an elevated CRP has not yet been demonstrated to be beneficial in clinical trials. As more evidence accumulates regarding the benefits of CRP testing, the recommendation as to which patients will benefit from testing is likely to broaden.

Although the value of hs-CRP to identify high-risk patients for treatment is well documented, the use of this inflammatory marker as a therapeutic target is uncertain. Reduction in hs-CRP is only weakly correlated with lowering of LDL-C. Although all statins appear to lower hs-CRP, approximately one-third of patients taking statin therapy have a negligible reduction, and ezetimibe monotherapy does not lower hs-CRP but, in combination with a statin, appears to double the hs-CRP reduction. The Reversing Atherosclerosis with Aggressive Lipid Lowering trial found that atorvastatin, 80 mg, lowered hs-CRP by 35% compared to 8% for pravastatin, 40 mg. These data suggest the possibility that despite reductions in lipid levels, hs-CRP may remain elevated if other risk factors are stimulating the inflammatory process, and perhaps more aggressive lipid control or further modification of other risk factors is necessary. Therefore, lowering hs-CRP to a therapeutic target of less than 1.0 mg per dL may indicate adequate management of the various risk factors. Proving this hypothesis will require more intensive investigation. The ongoing Justification for the Use of Statins in Primary Prevention: An Intervention Trial Evaluating Rosuvastatin (JUPITER) (Table 1.12), which is evaluating the effects of rosuvastatin, 20 mg, or placebo in 15,000 patients with LDL less than 130 mg per dL and hs-CRP greater than 2.0, will hopefully shed light on this important issue.

GLOBAL RISK GOAL

A modified form of the Framingham risk score is used by multiple international guidelines to stratify patients into risk groups for determining thresholds for the initiation of therapy and goals of treatment. Using the Framingham score as a therapeutic target is problematic for two reasons. First, this global risk formula was based on observational data, and, although some intervention trials have shown good correlation with the Framingham equation, there is a concern that the score may not adequately assess risk for patients on treatment. Second, age and sex are powerful contributors to the overall Framingham score, and these nonmodifiable risk factors make the Framingham score difficult to use clinically. An alternative is a global risk score that attempts to incorporate the divergent guidelines that have been established in the United States for the various risk factors. A hypothetical global risk score that includes the recommendations of NCEP ATP III; the Seventh Report of the Joint National Committee on Prevention, Detection, Evaluation, and Treatment of High Blood Pressure (JNC 7); and the ADA is shown in the following formula:

Goal <4.0 = total cholesterol /HDL + (glycosylated hemoglobin – 7.0) + (systolic blood pressure – 130/10 mm Hg) + number of cigarette packs/day

This hypothetical global risk goal has the advantage of targeting all the major modifiable risk factors simultaneously, as opposed to an isolated approach for each risk factor. In the past, due to the influence of separate risk factor treatment guidelines and the marketing of drugs for individual risk factors, the therapeutic approach of risk factor modification has become a silo phenomenon. A global risk goal would encourage clinicians to evaluate and treat the major risk factors in more of a united fashion to achieve an overall therapeutic target. The proposed hypothetical global risk score would also encourage more aggressive lipid control of the total cholesterol/HDL ratio if a patient continues to smoke despite all efforts for cessation or has a glycosylated hemoglobin that remains elevated above 7.0 mg per dL after maximal therapy. A global risk score may be impossible to achieve in a significant percentage of the high-risk populations, but this concept is an attempt to better coordinate the management of all of the major modifiable risk factors.

EXPANDING THE DEFINITION OF HIGH-RISK PATIENTS

According to NCEP ATP III, the definition of high risk includes patients with clinical atherosclerosis, diabetes, and those without these conditions but with an adapted Framingham 10-year risk of absolute CHD greater than 20%. There are already two accepted modifications of the guidelines based on the HPS. NCEP ATP III allows for clinical judgment in the initiation of lipid-lowering therapy for patients at high risk with an LDL between 100 mg per dL and 130 mg per dL. Based on the HPS results demonstrating a benefit regardless of the baseline LDL, the clinical judgment zone at 100 to 130 mg per dL should no longer exist, and, for patients with baseline LDL less than 100 mg per dL, consideration should be given for the initiation of treatment. Although this high-risk group is already estimated to include 20 million people in the United States and is likely to grow as the population ages and becomes more obese, there is increasing interest in identifying a higher-risk primary prevention population to target for more aggressive lipid-lowering goals. The AHA/Centers for Disease Control and Prevention recommendation to use hs-CRP screening in patients with a Framingham 10-year risk of 10% to 20% may identify another significant portion of the population that requires the more aggressive LDL goal of less than 100 mg per dL, as opposed to the present goal of less than 130 mg per dL (Fig. 1.23). Based on the hs-CRP observational data, a Framingham 10-year risk of 5% or greater in conjunction with an hs-CRP level in the borderline risk range (1.0 to 3.0 mg per L) confers a substantially higher relative risk. These data would support a high-risk classification for patients with a Framingham 10-year risk of 5% or greater in conjunction with an hs-CRP level of 2.0 mg per L or greater. Because an hs-CRP of 2.0 mg per L is approximately the

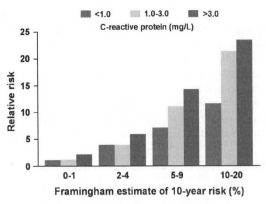

Figure 1.23. High-sensitivity C-reactive protein adds prognostic information at all levels of the Framingham risk score. (From Ridker, et al. *N Engl J Med* 2002;347: 1557, with permission.)

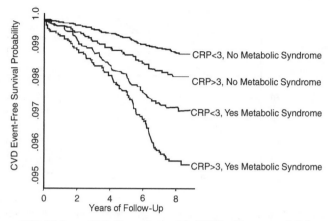

Figure 1.24. High-sensitivity C-reactive protein (CRP) adds prognostic information to the Adult Treatment Panel III definition of metabolic syndrome. n = 14,719. CVD, cardiovascular disease. (From Ridker, et al. *Circulation* 2003;107:391–397, with permission.)

median level for adult Americans, this strategy could potentially result in a significant increase in the U.S. population that would be classified as high risk for more aggressive treatment.

An alternative strategy is the screening of patients with any of the five criteria for the metabolic syndrome (i.e., visceral obesity, low HDL, hypertriglyceridemia, hypertension, or impaired fasting glucose) for elevated hs-CRP. This strategy would approximate the screening of patients with a Framingham score of 5% or greater; however, because the score is so influenced by age and sex, this approach would probably incorporate younger Americans. In patients with the metabolic syndrome, hs-CRP remains an important predictor of CV events (Fig. 1.24). Thus, rather than a blanket recommendation to treat all patients with the metabolic syndrome to an LDL goal of less than 100 mg per dL regardless of the risk classification, perhaps a more cost-effective approach would be to only consider patients with the metabolic syndrome as high risk if they have an hs-CRP of 2.0 or greater or a Framingham score of 20% or greater. The JUPITER trial should provide important insights into the utility of hs-CRP as a screening measure to identify patients who require more aggressive risk modification. The issue regarding the risk classification of metabolic syndrome

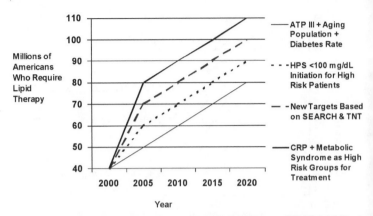

Figure 1.25. Graph illustrating the growing need for lipid therapy. ATP III, Adult Treatment Panel III; CRP, C-reactive protein; HPS, Heart Protection Study; SEARCH, Study of Effectiveness of Additional Reductions in Cholesterol and Homocysteine; TNT, Treating to New Targets.

patients remains a difficult challenge, as more than 40% of the older adult population already has the metabolic syndrome, and this figure is likely to grow significantly over the next decade. Evidence-based trials, which include cost-effectiveness evaluations, will likely be necessary to establish the appropriate treatment recommendations for this growing at-risk population.

As the clinical trial data accumulate regarding the benefits of lipid-lowering treatment for an expanding definition of high-risk individuals targeted for aggressive goals of therapy, the size of this population is likely to challenge the available resources. Figure 1.25 illustrates the potential magnitude of the problem facing the medical community over the next decades as an aging, increasingly more obese population is combined with evidence-based information that supports more widespread use of aggressive interventions.

MOBILE LIPID CLINIC™

The Mobile Lipid Clinic™ is a personal digital assistant (PDA) software program for the Palm™ or for the personal computer with Microsoft software that allows the health professional the ability to calculate, and, if desired, store a patient's CV risk information. The program was designed to help the health professional not only track patient data, but also educate the patient on the importance of global risk assessment. The program will calculate the 10-year Framingham score for the patient; convert the score to an adjusted CV risk age equivalent; provide a goal probability of risk for the patient; determine the ATP III goal, the percent LDL reduction to achieve the ATP III goal, and adjustment of risk for the calcium score; and calculate the BMI with the relative risk of developing diabetes (see Appendix C for instructions).

SELECTED READING

Abbott RD, Wilson PWF, Kannel WB, et al. High density lipoprotein cholesterol, total cholesterol screening, and myocardial infarction. *Arteriosclerosis* 1988;8:207–211.

Anderson KM, Castelli WP, Levy DL. Cholesterol and mortality: 30 years of follow-up from the Framingham study. *JAMA* 1987;257: 2176–2180.

Assmann G, Schulte H, Funke H, et al. The emergence of triglycerides as a significant independent risk factor in coronary artery disease. *Eur Heart J* 1998;19[Suppl M]:M8–M14.

Austin MA, Hokanson JE, Edwards KL. Hypertriglyceridemia as a cardiovascular risk factor. *Am J Cardiol* 1998;81(4A):7B–12B.

Executive Summary of the Third Report of the National Cholesterol Education Program (NCEP) Expert Panel on Detection, Evaluation, and Treatment of High Blood Cholesterol in Adults (Adult Treatment Panel III). *JAMA* 2001;285:2486–2497.

Frost PH, Havel RJ. Rationale for use of non-high-density lipoprotein cholesterol rather than low-density lipoprotein cholesterol as a tool for lipoprotein cholesterol screening and assessment of risk and therapy. *Am J Cardiol* 1998;81(4A):26B–31B.

Grundy SM. Cholesterol-lowering trials: a historical perspective. In: Grundy SM, ed. *Cholesterol-lowering therapy: evaluation of clinical trial evidence.* New York: Marcel Dekker Inc, 2000:1–44.

Grundy SM. Cholesterol management in the era of management care. *Am J Cardiol* 2000;85[Suppl]:3A–9A.

Grundy SM, Cleeman JI, Merz CN, et al. Implications of recent clinical trials for the National Cholesterol Education Program Adult Treatment Panel III guidelines. *Circulation* 2004;110:227–239.

Grundy SM, Pasternak R, Greenland P, et al. Assessment of cardiovascular risk by use of multiple risk-factor assessment equations: a statement for healthcare professionals from the American Heart Association and the American College of Cardiology. *Circulation* 1999;100:1481–1492.

Haffner SM, Lehto S, Ronnemaa T, et al. Mortality from coronary heart disease in subjects with type 2 diabetes in nondiabetic subjects with and without previous myocardial infarction implications for treatment of hyperlipidemia in diabetic subjects without prior myocardial infarction. *N Engl J Med* 1998;339:229–234.

Lloyd-Jones DM, Larson MG, Beiser A, et al. Lifetime risk of developing coronary heart disease. *Lancet* 1999;353:89–92.

Pekkanen J, Linn S, Heiss G, et al. Ten-year mortality from cardiovascular disease in relation to cholesterol level among men with and without preexisting cardiovascular disease. *N Engl J Med* 1990;322:1700–1707.

Rossouw JE, Lewis B, Rifkind BM. The value of lowering cholesterol after myocardial infarction. *N Engl J Med* 1990;323:1112–1119.

Wilson PWF, D'Agostino RB, Levy D, et al. Prediction of coronary heart disease using risk factor categories. *Circulation* 1998;97:1837–1847.

Chapter 2

Lipoprotein Metabolism and the Pathogenesis of Atherosclerosis

Atherosclerosis is the result of an inflammatory response to oxidized apolipoprotein (Apo) B–containing lipoprotein, especially low-density lipoprotein cholesterol (LDL-C). Figures 2.1 through 2.7 provide a step-by-step guide to the formation of advanced atherosclerotic plaque.

LIPOPROTEIN METABOLISM

The understanding of lipoprotein metabolism is critical for the characterization of the various genetic abnormalities that result in dyslipidemia and also provides a better knowledge base for the proper use of therapeutic interventions. The following is a step-by-step guide to understanding lipoprotein metabolism and genetic causes of dyslipidemia.

LIPOPROTEIN STRUCTURE

Cholesterol ester and triglycerides are *hydrophobic* (water-fearing) neutral lipids and, therefore, must be transported through the plasma inside the core of a *hydrophilic* (water-loving) sphere. The basic lipoprotein structure consists of a sphere with a core of cholesterol ester, triglyceride, and a surface of phospholipid-free cholesterol proteins called *apolipoproteins*. Apolipoproteins are analogous to a zip code that directs the lipoprotein to the various receptors.

There are five basic lipoproteins: chylomicrons, very-low-density lipoproteins (VLDLs), intermediate-density lipoproteins (IDLs), LDLs, and high-density lipoproteins (HDLs). Each of these lipoproteins differs in their content of triglycerides, cholesterol, and apolipoproteins (Fig. 2.8).

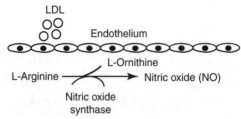

Figure 2.1. A healthy endothelium—the lining of the arterial wall. A healthy endothelium contains the enzyme nitric oxide synthase that converts the amino acid L-arginine into nitric oxide. Nitric oxide is a powerful vasodilator and protects the endothelium from cell adhesion and the penetration of low-density lipoprotein cholesterol (LDL-C) particles. If the endothelium is damaged due to risk factors such as cigarette smoking, hypertension, or diabetes, this results in the destruction or impairment of the nitric oxide synthase. Therefore, the protection of nitric oxide to prevent cell adhesion or LDL-C penetration is lost, and a greater concentration of LDL-C is now below the endothelium in the subendothelial space.

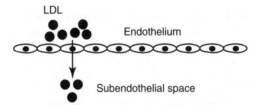

Figure 2.2. Low-density lipoprotein cholesterol (LDL-C) penetration of the endothelium. Atherosclerosis develops from the amount of LDL in the subendothelial space that becomes oxidized rather than the amount of LDL in the blood. This phenomenon explains why a single risk factor, such as hypertension, is approximately equivalent in coronary heart disease risk to a 100 mg per dL increase in serum cholesterol. The presence of a risk factor, by causing endothelial cell damage, allows greater LDL-C penetration into the subendothelial space, and after the LDL-C becomes oxidized, stimulates the inflammatory response, leading to atherosclerosis.

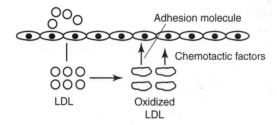

Figure 2.3. Oxidation of low-density lipoprotein cholesterol (LDL-C) and the release of chemotactic and cell adhesion molecules. Oxidation of the apoprotein B–containing lipoproteins is a critical step in the formation of foam cells, the inflammatory cells that lead to the development of atherosclerotic plaque. Butter becoming rancid or iron rusting are both oxidative processes. Once LDL-C has penetrated into the subendothelial space, oxidation is enhanced, and the particles are modified structurally. These oxidized particles with modified membranes become antigenic oxidized particles similar to a foreign body reaction. Consequently, these antigenic oxidized particles stimulate the release of chemotactic factors and adhesion molecules.

Chylomicron Metabolism—The Exogenous Pathway

Chylomicrons are formed from dietary fat and cholesterol. Chylomicrons are assembled in the intestines after the absorption of fat. They are secreted initially into the lacteals of the intestinal villi and join the lymphatic circulation to enter the blood via the thoracic duct. The chylomicrons are composed mostly of triglycerides along with dietary cholesterol, and on the surface are the apolipoproteins Apo B48, Apo E, and Apo CII. Apo B48 is an abbreviated version of B100 made in the intestines. Once in the blood, the chylomicrons account for the postprandial rise in triglycerides. Usually, fat absorption is generally complete within a few hours of food ingestion; therefore, after a fat load, the triglyceride rise in the blood lasts postprandially for approximately 4 to 10 hours. The rate of postprandial chylomicron clearance is perhaps an indicator of coronary artery disease risk. Once in the blood, the chylomicrons are acted on by the enzyme lipoprotein lipase on the capillary wall that is activated by Apo CII. Lipoprotein lipase liberates the triglyceride from the chylomicrons, forming free fatty acids that are used for energy or deposit in fat stores. Once most or all of the triglyceride is removed from the chylomicron, a much smaller remnant is formed that is cleared from the liver by B/E receptor. The chylomicrons are too large to pass through the endothelium and induce foam cell formation, but there is evidence that chylomicron remnants may be atherogenic.

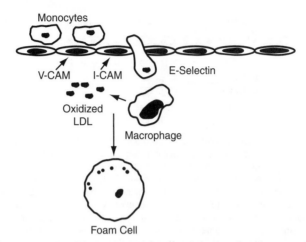

Figure 2.4. These chemotactic factors (monocyte chemotactic protein-1, macrophage colony-stimulating factor) recruit monocytes to the endothelial cell surface, and the adhesion molecules [intracellular adhesion molecule (I-CAM), vascular cell adhesion molecule (V-CAM), E-selectin] cause the adhesion of the monocyte to the endothelium and also promote the penetration of the monocyte through the endothelial cell layer into the subendothelial space. In the subendothelial space, the monocytes transform into macrophages and engulf the oxidized low-density lipoprotein (LDL) particles. The oxidized LDL particles are recognized by the receptor CD36 on the macrophage. As more oxidized LDL particles are incorporated into the macrophage, they appear more "foaming," hence the name *foam cells*. As more foam cells form, they coalesce, forming a fatty streak visible on the arterial wall. These fatty streaks, over time, progress to advanced lesions with a fibrous cap made from collagen and a lipid core.

The clearance rate of chylomicrons for individuals is variable. Obesity, high triglyceride levels in the fasting state, low HDL-C, diabetes, and, perhaps, other as-yet undetermined factors are associated with slow clearance of postprandial chylomicrons. The impairment of lipoprotein to lipase appears to explain the variability in postprandial chylomicron clearance. High triglycerides in the fasting state may competitively inhibit lipoprotein lipase, and, therefore, after a postprandial fat load, the enzyme is not as freely available to break down the chylomicrons. From an evolutionary perspective, slow clearance of dietary fat may be protective against starvation. Certain populations, such as the Asian Indians and Pima Indians that are predisposed to hypertriglyceridemia and diabetes,

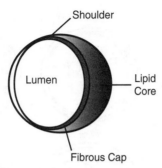

Figure 2.5. As the lipid core expands, the lumen of the artery does not narrow initially but, rather, there is a compensatory remodeling of the artery.

have developed a higher prevalence for the genes that slow postprandial fat clearance.

Endogenous Lipoprotein Metabolism

The majority of the blood cholesterol comes from the endogenous production of lipoprotein from the liver rather than from dietary

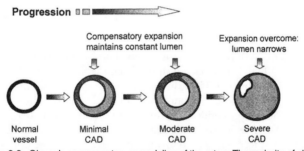

Figure 2.6. Glagov's compensatory remodeling of the artery. The majority of clinical events (myocardial infarctions, unstable angina, sudden death) occur when a nonstenotic lesion (less than 70% stenosis) abruptly ruptures. The atherosclerotic plaques usually rupture at the shoulder regions where the shear stress is at the highest and plaque contains the most inflammatory foam cells. These foam cells secrete cytokines that either break down collagen (matrix metalloproteinase-1) or inhibit the synthesis of collagen. The net result is a thinning of the fibrous cap. Over time, with rough shear stress, the fibrous cap may break, exposing the underlying lipid core to the lumen. The lipid core, by releasing tissue factors, stimulates thrombosis, leading to the development of an acute coronary event. CAD, coronary artery disease. (Adapted from Glagov et al. *N Engl J Med*.)

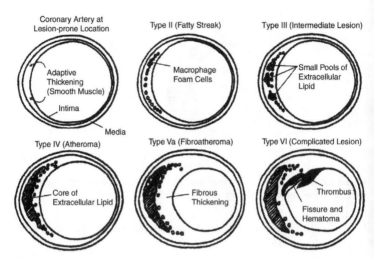

Figure 2.7. Plaque rupture and coronary thrombosis—sequence of events. The foam cells also secrete other cytokines, such as interleukin-6 (IL-6), that stimulate the liver to produce C-reactive protein (CRP). These inflammatory markers, such as intracellular adhesion molecule, vascular cell adhesion molecule, E-selectin, IL-6, and CRP, are potentially useful as surrogate blood tests for foam cell formation. (Adapted from Ambrose and Weinrauch 1996. Copyright 1996, AMA. Figure was adapted from Stary et al. 1995.)

sources. The liver is the main organ for lipoprotein production and clearance. VLDL is synthesized in the liver, mediated by the microsomal transfer protein (MTP) that assembles triglycerides and cholesterol with Apo B and E with phospholipid. Lipogenesis is the synthesis of fatty acids (triglycerides are three fatty acids attached together) from glucose. This process is regulated by insulin, and the hypertriglyceridemia that frequently accompanies diabetes is, in part, due to the oversynthesis of fatty acids in the liver. Cholesterol is synthesized from acetyl-coenzyme A (CoA), with the enzyme hepatic 3-methylglutaryl (HMG)-CoA reductase as the rate-limiting step in converting HMG-CoA into mevalonate. The liver uses cholesterol to produce bile salts, with the enzyme 7-hydroxylase as the catalyst. Acylcholesterol acyltransferase (ACAT) converts free cholesterol into cholesterol ester for incorporation with triglycerides and Apo in the formation of VLDL. The liver also removes cholesterol from the blood as LDL via the LDL receptor (Fig. 2.9).

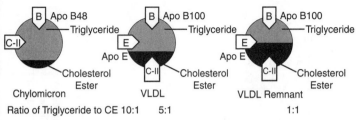

Ratio of Triglyceride to CE 10:1   5:1   1:1

Lipoproteins without significant triglyceride content

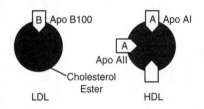

Figure 2.8. Lipoprotein content—triglyceride-containing lipoproteins. Knowing the lipoproteins that contain triglycerides and the ratio of triglyceride-to-cholesterol ester (CE) is very helpful in interpreting the lipid profile of a patient. If triglycerides are elevated, that indicates that chylomicrons, very-low-density lipoproteins (VLDLs), or intermediate-density lipoproteins are increased in the plasma. The triglyceride to cholesterol ratio in the lipoproteins provides a helpful clinical hint to which triglyceride-containing lipoproteins may be elevated. Even without lipoprotein electrophoresis, the culprit lipoprotein causing the dyslipidemia can be differentiated by understanding the basic composition of these various lipoproteins. Apo, apoprotein; HDL, high-density lipoprotein; LDL, low-density lipoprotein.

The liver, therefore, represents the primary target to modify lipoprotein metabolism. By blocking bile-acid reabsorption from the intestine, bile-acid sequestrants induce the liver to produce more bile acids that require cholesterol, thereby upregulating LDL receptors to increase LDL-C removal from the blood. Statins or HMG-CoA reductase inhibitors block the rate-limiting step in cholesterol synthesis, thus also upregulating LDL receptors. MTP inhibitors block the assembly of VLDL, and ACAT inhibitors also may inhibit the production of VLDL by blocking the conversion of free cholesterol to cholesterol ester needed to be incorporated into VLDL before secretion. Hepatic MTP or ACAT inhibitors are in clinical development, and their safety or efficacy has not yet been determined.

Once VLDL is secreted from the liver into the plasma enriched in triglycerides, the particle is acted on by lipoprotein lipase that liberates

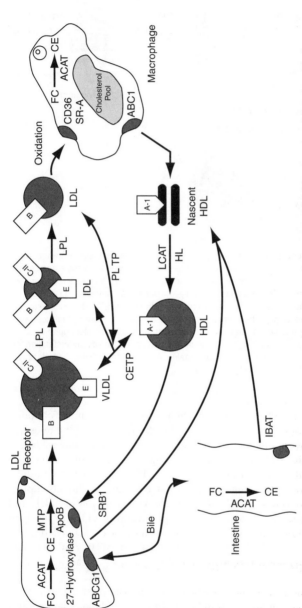

Figure 2.9. Lipoprotein metabolism. ABC1, adenosine triphosphate-binding cassette G1 transport; ACAT, acylcoenzyme A: cholesterol acyltransferase; Apo, apolipoprotein; CE, cholesterol ester; CETP, cholesterol ester transfer protein; FC, free cholesterol; HDL, high-density lipoprotein; LPL, lipoprotein lipase; MTP, microsomal triglyceride transfer protein; PLTP, phospholipid transfer protein; SR, scavenger receptor.

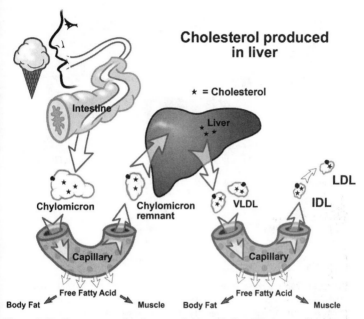

Figure 2.10. Exogenous and endogenous lipid metabolism. IDL, intermediate-density lipoprotein; LDL, low-density lipoprotein; VLDL, very-low-density lipoprotein. (Images © 2001 medmovie.com™. All rights reserved. Used with permission.)

the fatty acids for energy or fat storage. A VLDL remnant particle or IDL is further catabolized by hepatic lipases to produce a triglyceride-depleted lipoprotein called LDL (Fig. 2.10). If triglycerides are high, the LDL particle may receive triglycerides from other lipoproteins via cholesterol ester transfer protein (CETP), and this more triglyceride-enriched LDL is further degraded to a small, dense LDL particle.

LDL has three basic fates: it can return to the liver via the LDL receptor, it can move to other cells for hormone production or as part of the cell membranes, or it may infiltrate an impaired endothelium and become oxidized, stimulating the production of foam cells (Fig. 2.11).

HIGH-DENSITY LIPOPROTEIN METABOLISM

HDL is thought to protect against atherosclerosis by promoting the efflux of excess cholesterol from cells and returning that cholesterol to

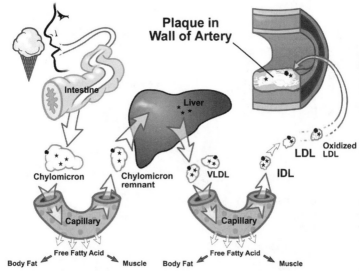

Figure 2.11. Pathogenesis of atherosclerosis. IDL, intermediate-density lipoprotein; LDL, low-density lipoprotein; VLDL, very-low-density lipoprotein. (Images © 2001 medmovie.com™. All rights reserved. Used with permission.)

the liver for excretion into the bile. This process is known as *reverse cholesterol transport*. HDL may also decrease atherosclerosis by inhibiting LDL oxidation and stimulating prostacyclin. The structure and metabolism of HDL is complex. HDL, similar to other lipoproteins, is composed of phospholipids, cholesterol, a small amount of triglycerides, and apoproteins. The major apolipoprotein is AI, which is synthesized and secreted by both the intestines and the liver. A discoid nascent Apo AI–containing HDL particle, which is cholesterol depleted, interacts with peripheral cells and acquires cholesterol and phospholipid through a transport process facilitated by the cellular protein adenosine triphosphate–binding cassette protein 1 (ABC1). Unesterified cholesterol is esterified to cholesterol ester within the HDL particle by the enzyme lecithin-cholesterol acyl transferase, which is activated by Apo AI. The cholesterol ester within the HDL can be taken up selectively by the liver through the action of the scavenger receptor B1 (SR-B1) (Fig. 2.12), or the cholesterol ester can be exchanged for triglycerides from the Apo B–containing particles via CETP (Fig. 2.13).

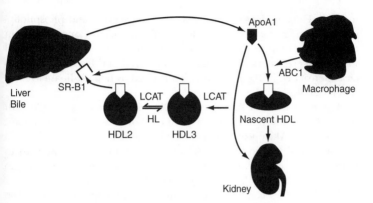

Figure 2.12. High-density lipoprotein (HDL) metabolism. ABC1, adenosine triphosphate–binding cassette protein 1; Apo, apolipoprotein; LCAT, lecithin cholesterol acyltransferase; SR-B1, scavenger receptor B1.

Conversely, the phospholipid transfer protein mediates the transfer of phospholipids from Apo B–containing particles to HDL. HDL metabolism is also affected by several members of the lipoprotein lipase gene family. The hydrolysis of triglycerides in chylomicrons and VLDL by lipoprotein lipase results in the transfer of lipids and apolipoproteins

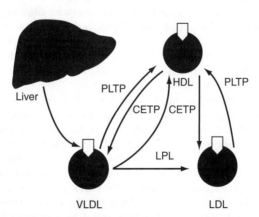

Figure 2.13. Transfer proteins. CETP, cholesterol ester transfer protein; HDL, high-density lipoprotein; LDL, low-density lipoprotein; LPL, lipoprotein lipase; PLTP, phospholipid transfer protein; VLDL, very-low-density lipoprotein.

to HDL. Hepatic lipase hydrolyzes HDL triglyceride and phospholipids, generating smaller lipid-depleted HDL particles. Consequently, in the presence of hypertriglyceridemia, cholesterol in HDL is exchanged with triglyceride-enriched lipoproteins for triglycerides, and the triglyceride-enriched HDLs are further hydrolyzed by hepatic lipase to form smaller HDLs.

A mutant form of Apo AI called *Apo AI-milano* is associated with reduced HDL levels but not increased cardiovascular risk. The mutant form of Apo AI appears to be more efficient in reverse cholesterol transport, and infusion of Apo AI-milano in animal models appears to markedly decrease atherosclerosis. Infusions of Apo AI-milano into humans are presently being evaluated in clinical trials.

Apo AII is the second most abundant apolipoprotein after Apo AI. Apo AII appears to inhibit the activity of Apo AI and, therefore, is considered to be a proatherogenic protein, but the mechanism is not well understood. Apo AIV, similar to Apo AI, appears to activate lecithin-cholesterol acyltransferase and promote cellular cholesterol efflux. HDL also contains Apo E, which also appears to be antiatherogenic by promoting the uptake of HDL by the liver. Therefore, the upregulation of the expression of Apo AI, Apo AIV, or Apo E and the downregulation of Apo AII are potential targets to improve reverse cholesterol transport.

SR-B1 mediates the selective uptake of HDL cholesterol ester by hepatocytes and steroidogenic cells without removal of Apo AI. SR-B1, therefore, appears to allow the HDL particle to unload its cholesterol into the liver, depleting its cholesterol content and allowing the particle to return to the peripheral cells to pick up more cholesterol. Upregulating SR-B1, therefore, appears to lower HDL cholesterol but may improve reverse cholesterol transport. In animal models, overexpression of SR-B1 decreases the development of atherosclerosis while lowering HDL levels.

CETP mediates the transfer of cholesterol ester from HDL to VLDL. This shunt pathway, from an evolutionary perspective, allows cholesterol ester to return to VLDL more quickly than to the liver via SR-B1 and is then synthesized into VLDL. The monkey and the rabbit also have CETP and, similar to the human, have low HDL and high LDL. The mouse and the dog lack CETP and have high HDL and lower LDL. Transgenic mice given the CETP gene develop a more human lipid profile with a lower HDL and higher LDL. There are Japanese families that are CETP deficient and have very high levels of HDL, but it is unclear if they have reduced cardiovascular risk. Alcohol also appears to raise HDL by inhibiting CETP. Therefore, CETP inhibition increases HDL, but the potential benefit on atherosclerosis in humans remains uncertain. In cholesterol-fed rabbits given oral CETP inhibitors or a vaccine to create anti-CETP antibodies, atherosclerosis is markedly decreased. Oral CETP inhibition and a CETP vaccine are presently in human trials to raise HDL and determine the effects on atherosclerosis.

Perhaps the most attractive means to raise HDL and promote reverse cholesterol transport is to upregulate ABC1. By upregulating ABC1, more cholesterol would be removed from the macrophages and into nascent HDL. Thus, a combination of upregulating ABC1, inhibiting CETP, and upregulating SR-B1 may theoretically induce profound regression of atherosclerosis.

INHERITED LIPID DISORDERS: A SIMPLIFIED APPROACH

Genetic disorders may account for up to 80% of patients with premature coronary heart disease (CHD). Understanding lipid disorders and their clinical implication is helpful in identifying the patients at greatest risk for CHD. In addition, screening for genetic lipid disorders provides an opportunity to include family members in a CHD prevention program who may have otherwise not been aware of their increased risk. A strong family history of premature CHD is often a source of much anxiety for a patient, and, if the genetic disorder can be correctly diagnosed and effectively treated, the patient is frequently relieved of the anxiety.

Lipoproteins are classified by their content. Lipoproteins also vary in size and Apo content as the particle is metabolized. As previously noted, there are five basic families of lipoproteins: chylomicrons, VLDL, IDL, LDL, and HDL. Almost all triglycerides are found in chylomicrons, VLDL, and IDL. Genetic disorders that increase the plasma levels of these three lipoproteins thus result in hypertriglyceridemia (Table 2.1). Often, the ratio of the triglyceride to the cholesterol level in the serum can provide a clue to which triglyceride-rich particles are elevated. Chylomicrons, VLDL, and IDL have a ratio of triglycerides to cholesterol in each particle of 10:1, 5:1, and 1:1, respectively (Fig.

Table 2.1. Increased Triglycerides

Increased chylomicrons: Lipoprotein lipase or apoprotein CII deficiency
  Increased very-low-density lipoproteins: Familial combined hyperlipidemia or familial hypertriglyceridemia
Increased intermediate-density lipoproteins: Familial dysbeta lipoprotein

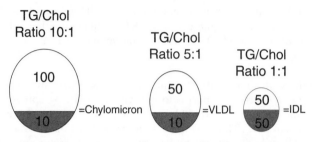

Figure 2.14. Triglyceride (TG) and cholesterol (Chol) composition of the various classes of lipoproteins. IDL, intermediate-density lipoprotein; VLDL, very-low-density lipoprotein.

2.14). Thus, when chylomicrons are elevated, the serum triglycerides are usually ten times higher than the serum total cholesterol. However, if the triglycerides are only twice as high as the total cholesterol, then VLDL is usually the culprit elevated lipoprotein, and if both triglycerides and total cholesterol are equally elevated, the patient has an increase in IDL or a combination of high VLDL and LDL (Table 2.2). Another way to screen for elevated chylomicrons is to place a tube of the patient's serum or plasma in the refrigerator overnight and look for the creamy layer of chylomicrons on the surface (Fig. 2.15).

To simplify lipoprotein metabolism, an easy way to understand the structure of lipoproteins is to use the analogy of a boat. A lipoprotein is analogous to a boat filled with fat people (triglycerides) and thin people (cholesterol) directed to its location (receptor) by a captain (Apo) (Fig. 2.16). Chylomicrons, VLDL, and LDL have different compositions of fat people (triglycerides), thin people (cholesterol), and captains (Apo) (Fig. 2.17). Chylomicrons are large boats filled

Table 2.2. Examples of Triglyceride Disorders

	Example A: Elevated chylomicrons	Example B: Elevated very-low-density lipoprotein	Example C: Elevated intermediate-density lipoprotein
Cholesterol	350 mg/dL	350 mg/dL	500 mg/dL
Triglycerides	3,000 mg/dL	700 mg/dL	450 mg/dL
High-density lipoprotein	30 mg/dL	30 mg/dL	30 mg/dL
Triglyceride/cholesterol ratio	10:1	5:1	1:1

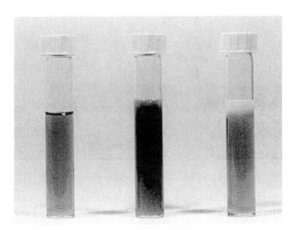

Figure 2.15. Chylomicron layer on the surface of plasma.

with a large number of fat people (triglycerides) that are formed postprandially after fat ingestion. Apo CII on the surface of the chylomicrons activates lipoprotein lipase on the capillary surface to break down the triglycerides into free fatty acids for energy use or, if not used, deposited in fat stores (Fig. 2.18). The remaining particle is called the *chylomicron remnant*, which is relatively devoid of triglyceride but potentially rich in cholesterol that is removed from the circulation by the liver, but also may be a substrate for atherosclerosis. Apo

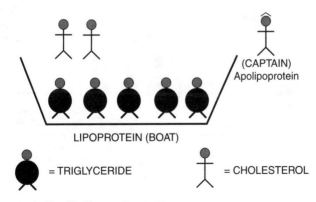

Figure 2.16. Simplified lipoprotein structure.

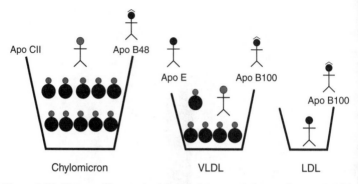

Figure 2.17. Classes of lipoproteins (simplified structures). Apo, apolipoprotein; LDL, low-density lipoprotein; VLDL, very-low-density lipoprotein.

CII is the plank of the boat, and lipoprotein lipase is like alligators in the water that break down the triglycerides into free fatty acids. Therefore, if Apo CII or lipoprotein lipase is deficient or impaired, this can lead to marked inhibition of chylomicron clearance, causing hyperchylomicronemia syndrome. This syndrome is characterized by distinctive eruptive xanthomas, markedly lipemic serum, and lipemic retinalis (Fig. 2.19). Hypothyroidism and diabetes can aggravate lipoprotein lipase impairment.

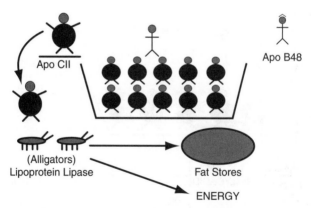

Figure 2.18. Chylomicron metabolism. Apo, apolipoprotein.

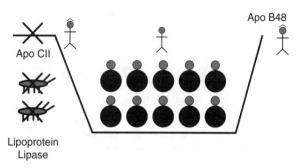

Figure 2.19. Hyperchylomicronemia syndrome. Apo, apolipoprotein.

VLDL is synthesized in the liver and represents the endogenous rather than exogenous source of triglycerides and cholesterol in the blood. VLDL is assembled in the hepatocytes by MTP by combining Apo B-100 with triglycerides, cholesterol, and phospholipid. The VLDL boat is similar to the chylomicron, but much smaller in size and with less fat (triglycerides) and thin (cholesterol) people, with Apo B-100 as the captain (Fig. 2.20). Familial hypertriglyceridemia, a dominant genetic disorder in which all the family members have only isolated hypertriglyceridemia (Fig. 2.21), occurs due to the secretion of enlarged VLDL particles. Because the VLDL particles are enlarged rather than more plentiful, the

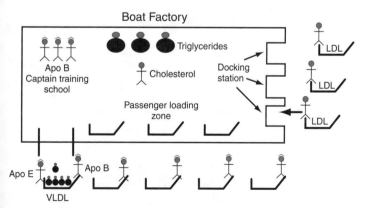

Figure 2.20. Very-low-density lipoprotein (VLDL) boat factory. Apo, apolipoprotein; LDL, low-density lipoprotein.

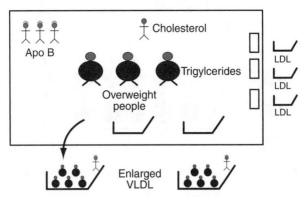

Figure 2.21. Familial hypertriglyceridemia. Apo, apolipoprotein; LDL, low-density lipoprotein; VLDL, very-low-density lipoprotein.

Apo B level is often normal, and the ratio of Apo B to LDL is less than 1.0. HDL is often normal, and the risk of CHD is only slightly above average.

The more common and potentially much higher risk for CHD VLDL disorder is familial combined hyperlipidemia (FCH). In this disorder, Apo B is overproduced, resulting in the secretion of more VLDL particles rather than enlarged VLDL particles (Fig. 2.22). These abun-

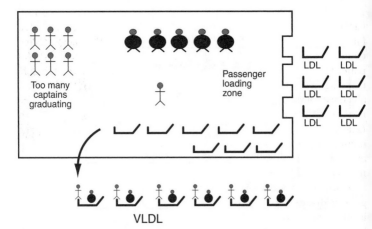

Figure 2.22. Familial combined hypertriglyceridemia. LDL, low-density lipoprotein; VLDL, very-low-density lipoprotein.

Table 2.3. Importance of Non–High-Density Lipoprotein (HDL) Cholesterol

Total cholesterol mg/dL	210	210
Triglycerides mg/dL	300	100
HDL mg/dL	25	25
LDL mg/dL	125	165
Total cholesterol/HDL	8.4	8.4
Non-HDL mg/dL	185	185
LDL/HDL	5	6.6
Coronary heart disease risk/1,000 patients/ 8 yr	246	118

LDL, low-density lipoprotein.

dant VLDL particles oversaturate the ability of lipoprotein lipase to break down all the triglycerides, resulting in triglyceride-enriched LDL, which are further metabolized by hepatic lipase to form dense LDL particles. The more prevalent VLDL particles also exchange their triglycerides for cholesterol in HDL mediated by CETP, resulting in lower HDL-C levels. The net result of this autosomal dominant disorder is a combined elevation of both triglycerides and LDL, with low HDL and significantly increased risk of premature CHD. Because the serum triglyceride is usually greater than 200 mg per dL, non-HDL is a better target for treatment because this value includes all the triglyceride-rich particles, as well as LDL (Table 2.3). In addition, because the LDL is small and dense, the total LDL level may not be significantly elevated, and the Apo B/LDL ratio is frequently greater than or equal to 1.0. This genetic disorder is important to diagnosis because the risk of CHD is very high. Asian Indians have a high incidence of FCH. Among family members, the lipid profile can vary from pure hypercholesterolemia to combined hyperlipidemia to isolated hypertriglyceridemia. In patients with hypertriglyceridemia, measuring Apo B can help confirm the diagnosis because patients with familial hypertriglyceridemia usually have a normal Apo B level. Patients with FCH also may have a corneal arcus and xanthelasma but almost never have tendon xanthomas (Fig. 2.23). The disorder may not be as evident in childhood or in premenopausal women. Weight gain, especially visceral fat increase, usually worsens the condition, and patients are at much higher risk for the metabolic syndrome and type 2 diabetes.

Familial dysbetalipoproteinemia (type 3) is a rare but important genetic disorder to diagnose properly. Familial dysbetalipoproteinemia is due to an accumulation of VLDL remnant or IDL. These patients are homozygous for the Apo E2:E2 genotype, which is present in 1% of the population. Normally, Apo E2:E2 is associated with a low incidence of

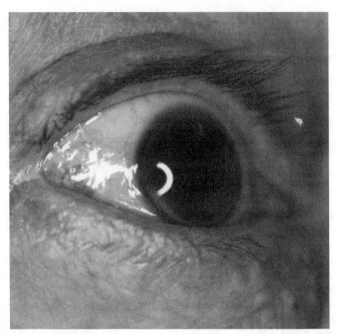

Figure 2.23. Eye of a patient with familial combined hyperlipidemia. Note the corneal arcus and xanthelasma.

dyslipidemia, which suggests, under normal conditions, having their genotype result in more effective lipoprotein clearance. However, when FCH is present, this appears to overwhelm the more effective but slower clearance of the Apo E2:E2 genotype. The result of the combination of FCH plus Apo E2:E2 is the rare disorder (1 in 10,000) characterized by VLDL remnant accumulation with tuberoeruptive xanthomas on the elbows and palms. Another hallmark physical finding is the presence of an orange discoloration in the creases of the palms. Often, the total cholesterol is very high (greater than 300 mg per dL) and the triglycerides are elevated to an equally high level.

Familial hypercholesterolemia (FH) causes severe elevations of LDL levels due to the impairment or absence of the LDL receptor. The LDL boats have no docking stations and, thus, accumulate in the blood (Fig. 2.24). The LDL receptor, discovered by Drs. Brown and Goldstein, is a complex protein that contains a binding domain to Apo B that is tightly

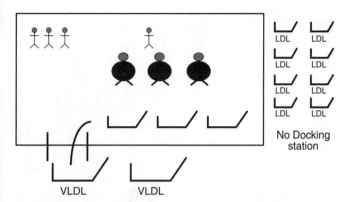

Figure 2.24. Familial hypercholesterolemia. LDL, low-density lipoprotein; VLDL, very-low-density lipoprotein.

coiled (Fig. 2.25). Therefore, a mutation of even one amino acid in the binding domain can unravel the coil and impair the ability of the receptor to bind Apo B. Most of the mutations are in the binding domain, but many other mutations have been identified. Patients with FH have severe elevation of LDL, and the disorder is present at birth. Homozygous FH (1 in 1,000,000) patients have no normal LDL receptors, the LDL levels often exceed 1,000 mg per dL at birth, and these children develop severe atherosclerosis at an early age. The much more common heterozygous FH (1 in 500) patients have one-half the number of nor-

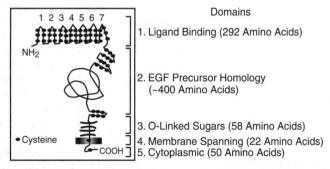

Figure 2.25. The human low-density lipoprotein receptor. EGF, epidermal growth factor.

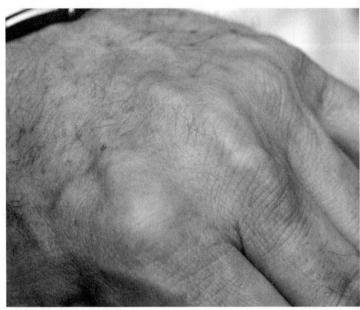

Figure 2.26. Hand of a patient with familial hyperlipidemia. Note the xanthoma present on the knuckles.

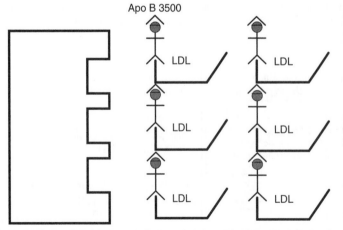

Figure 2.27. Familial defective apolipoprotein B (Apo B) 3500. LDL, low-density lipoprotein.

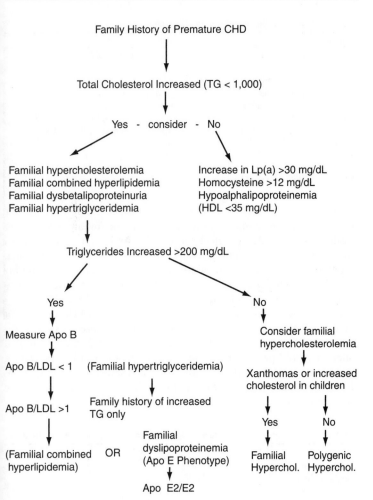

Figure 2.28. Algorithm for diagnosis of genetic lipid disorders. Apo, apolipoprotein; HDL, high-density lipoprotein; hyperchol., hypercholesterolemia; LDL, low-density lipoprotein.

Table 2.4. Types and Causes of Genetic Disorders

Genetic disorders	Defect
Hyperchylomicronemia	Lipoprotein lipase, Apo CII
Familial	
Dysbetalipoproteinemia	Apo E
Hypertriglyceridemia	Enlarged very-low-density lipoprotein
Combined hyperlipidemia	Apo B overproduction
Hypercholesterolemia	Low-density lipoprotein receptors
Hypoalphalipoproteinemia	Apo AI, high-density lipoprotein
Defective Apo B	Apo B
Lp(a)	Lp(a)

Apo, apolipoprotein; Lp(a), lipoprotein(a).

mal LDL receptors and develop LDL levels between 200 and 400 mg per dL. On physical examination, the pathognomonic findings are tendon xanthomas on the Achilles heel and knuckles of the hands (Fig. 2.26). These patients also commonly develop a corneal arcus and xanthelasma, which are also present in patients with FCH. FH is more commonly found in French Canadians, Lebanese Christians, South African Afrikaners, and Jews of Lithuanian descent.

Familial defective Apo B is due to accumulation of LDL because of a defective Apo B rather than impaired LDL receptors. The captain (Apo B) is blinded and cannot dock the boats (Fig. 2.27). Familial defective Apo B patients have the Apo B mutation Apo B 3500. There is some evidence the LDL elevations are not as severe as FH, but, often, the clinical manifestations are identical (e.g., xanthomas with severe LDL elevations).

Table 2.5. Increased Coronary Artery Disease Risk and Lipoprotein Abnormalities

Abnormality	Risk	Prevalence
Familial heterozygous	3×	<1
Familial combined	4×	15
Lp(a)	3–5×	33
Hyperapolipoprotein B	3×	30–80
ATHS gene (low-density lipoprotein pattern B)	3×	15 (Premenopausal women) 50 (Postmenopausal women) 40 (General population)
ATHS gene + Lp(a)	9×	~20
Familial defective Apo B[a]	?	<1
Hypoalphalipoproteinemia	3×	5–10

ATHS, atherosclerosis susceptibility; Lp(a), lipoprotein(a).
[a]Not apparent from routine lipid profile.

Familial hypoalphalipoproteinemia is due to an impairment in HDL synthesis. HDL levels are usually less than 35 mg per dL but may be lower than 25 mg per dL. This disorder is dominantly inherited and often does not respond well to HDL-raising therapies such as exercise, niacin, or alcohol. This relatively common genetic disorder may explain up to one-third of patients with premature CHD.

Lipoprotein(a) and homocystinemia are also relatively common genetic causes of premature CHD. These disorders are discussed in more detail in Chapter 5. Tables 2.4 and 2.5 provide a summary of the various inherited lipid disorders and their prevalence and risk of CHD. Figure 2.28 provides an algorithm to follow to properly diagnose the correct disorder.

SELECTED READING

Grundy SM. Hypertriglyceridemia, atherogenic dyslipidemia, and the metabolic syndrome. *Am J Cardiol* 1998;81(4A):18B–25B.

Mahley RW, Weisgraber KH, Innerarity TL, et al. Genetic defects in lipoprotein metabolism. Elevation of atherogenic lipoproteins caused by impaired catabolism. *JAMA* 1991;265(1):78–83.

Chapter 3

Therapeutic
Lifestyle Changes*

Therapeutic lifestyle changes is a term coined by the National Cholesterol Education Program Adult Treatment Panel III (NCEP ATP III) to incorporate a multifaceted nonpharmacologic approach to reducing the risk for coronary heart disease (CHD). The essential features of the therapeutic lifestyle changes are the following:

1. Reduction of saturated fat to less than 7% of total calories
2. Less than 200 mg per day of dietary cholesterol
3. Optional increases in plant sterols 2 g per day and viscous soluble fiber to enhance low-density lipoprotein (LDL) lowering
4. Weight reduction
5. Increased physical activity

A helpful pneumonic is SCOPE:

*S*aturated fat reduction to less than 7% of calories
*C*holesterol decrease to 200 mg per day
*O*besity treatment
*P*lant sterols and viscous soluble fiber
*E*xercise

Many physicians consider dietary therapy a waste of time. However, dietary therapy can be quite effective if the correct therapy is applied

---

*This chapter contains dietary advice that deviates somewhat from the National Cholesterol Education Program Adult Treatment Panel III recommendations, especially in regard to the use of low-carbohydrate diets to treat hypertriglyceridemia or the metabolic syndrome. The use of low-carbohydrate diets is controversial and deserves further clinical investigation. I decided to include my own recommendations regarding certain aspects of dietary therapy based on my experience as a lipid specialist while treating patients. When my views differed significantly from the various national expert panels, I have also provided their recommendations.

Table 3.1. Dietary Intervention for Abnormal Lipoproteins

Abnormal lipoprotein	Dietary intervention
Elevated chylomicrons	Reduce total fat intake
Increased low-density lipoprotein	Reduce saturated fat to <7% of calories
	Cholesterol intake <200 mg/d
	Soluble viscous fiber
	Plant sterol/stanols
	Soy protein
High triglycerides	Reduce simple carbohydrates
	Lower glycemic load
Low high-density lipoprotein	Decrease transfatty acid
	Increase alcohol intake (moderately)

to specific patient abnormalities, especially with the assistance of registered dietitians. As with the drug treatment of dyslipidemia, dietary therapy may also vary depending on the type of lipoprotein abnormality (Table 3.1). The following is a targeted dietary therapeutic approach based on the type of dyslipidemia present.

HIGH LOW-DENSITY LIPOPROTEIN

With the exception of familial hypercholesterolemia, most patients with elevated LDL have dietary saturated fat intolerance. Therefore, dietary treatment should be targeted to saturated fat reduction to less than 7% of calories. Dietary studies have determined that reducing saturated fat to less than 7% of calories is necessary to have a significant reduction in LDL. The Seven Countries Study (Fig. 3.1) is the best evidence that saturated fat is the main culprit for inducing hypercholesterolemia around the world. Three intervention studies, the Boeing Fat Intervention Trial (BEFIT), Diet Alternative, and DELTA, demonstrated the benefits of lowering LDL by approximately 10% by decreasing saturated fat to less than 7% of calories.

The MEDFICTS (*M*eats, *E*ggs, *D*airy, *F*ried foods, *In* baked goods, *C*onvenience foods, *T*able fats, *S*nacks) dietary assessment questionnaire is an easy to administer survey that can identify the source of overconsumption of saturated fat in most patients (Fig. 3.2). Once the sources of saturated fat are identified, the challenge is to have the patient adhere to recommended dietary changes. One successful approach is to have the patient tell, or, ideally, write down for the physician or health professional the past 1 to 2 days of dietary intake. After reviewing the dietary intake, the patient can be informed of the various changes that will reduce his or her saturated fat intake.

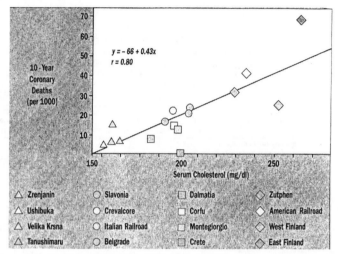

$$y = -66 + 0.43x$$
$$r = 0.80$$

Figure 3.1. Seven Countries Study. Epidemiologic evidence supporting high levels of serum cholesterol as a major reason for coronary heart disease.

Example:

Breakfast	Saturated fat (g)	Cholesterol (mg)	Calories
2 eggs cooked in butter	6.0	500	200
2 slices of bacon	2.7	11	86
1 slice of toast with butter	2.5	0	112
One 8 oz glass of whole milk	16.8	33	150
1 cup of coffee with Half & Half	1.1	6	20
Total	**14.1**	**550**	**568**

Substitute breakfast			
2 egg whites or egg substitute cooked	1.0	0	96
2 slices of lean turkey bacon	0.2	11	45
1 slice of toast with low-fat margarine	1.0	0	112
One 8 oz glass of skim milk	0.3	4	86
1 cup of coffee with skim milk	0	0	8
Total	**2.5**	**15**	**357**

For almost every high-saturated-fat food, there is an alternative low-fat food that will most likely be an acceptable alternative for patients. The Mobile Lipid Clinic™ program automatically prints out a list of

Name:_____

Date:_____

MEDFICTS: Dietary Assessment Questionnaire

(**M**eats, **E**ggs, **D**airy, **F**ried foods, **I**n baked goods, **C**onvenience foods, **T**able fats, **S**nacks)

Directions: For each food category for both group 1 and group 2 listings: Please check a box in the "Weekly Consumption" column and in the "Serving Size" column. If patient rarely or never eats the food listed, please check only the "Weekly Consumption" box.

FOOD CATEGORY	WEEKLY CONSUMPTION			SERVING SIZE			SCORE
	Rarely/ Never	3 or less	4 or more	Small	Average	Large	For office use
M Meats Average amounts per day: 6 oz (equal in size to 2 decks of playing cards) Base your estimate on the food you consume the most of							
Group 1 Beef Steak, chuck blade, ground beef, meatloaf, corned beef	☐	■ 3 pts	■ 7 pts	■ × 1 pt	■ 2 pts	■ 3 pts =	_____
Processed Meats Regular hamburger, fast food hamburger, bacon, lunch meat, sausage, hot dogs, knockwurst							
Pork & Others Pork shoulder, pork chops, roast, pork ribs, ground pork, regular ham, lamb steaks, ribs, chops, organ meats, poultry with skin							
Group 2 Lean cuts of beef Sirloin tip, flank steak, round steak, rump roast, chuck arm roast	☐	☐	☐	☐	☐	+ ■ 6 pts =	_____
Low-fat processed meats Low-fat lunch meat, low-fat hot dogs, Canadian bacon							
Poultry, fish, meat Poultry without skin, fish, seafood, lamb flank, leg-shank, sirloin, roast, lean ham cured and fresh, pork loin chops, tenderloin, veal chops, cutlets, roast, venison							
E Eggs Weekly consumption is expressed as times/week				How many eggs do you eat each time?			
Group 1 Whole eggs, yolks	☐	■ 3 pts	■ 7 pts	≤1 1 pt	2 2 pts	≥3 3 pts =	_____
Group 2 Egg whites, egg substitutes (1/2 cup = 2 eggs)	☐	☐	☐	≤1	2	≥3	

+ Score 6 points if this box is checked.

Comments: _____ Total _____

Figure 3.2. MEDFICTS questionnaire for evaluation of compliance to National Cholesterol Education Program Step 1 and 2 diets. pts, points. (From the National Cholesterol Education Program, with permission.)

	WEEKLY CONSUMPTION			SERVING SIZE			SCORE
FOOD CATEGORY	Rarely/ Never	3 or less	4 or more	Small	Average	Large	For office use
D **Dairy**							
Milk Average serving: 1 cup							
Group 1 Whole milk, 2% milk, 2% buttermilk, yogurt (whole milk)	☐	3 pts	7 pts	× 1 pt	2 pts	3 pts =	___
Group 2 Skim milk, 1% milk, skim milk-buttermilk, yogurt (nonfat & low-fat)	☐	☐	☐	☐	☐	☐	
Cheese Average serving: 1 oz							
Group 1 Cream cheese, cheddar, monterey jack, colby, swiss, american processed, blue cheese Regular cottage cheese and ricotta (½ cup)	☐	3 pts	7 pts	× 1 pt	2 pts	3 pts =	___
Group 2 Low-fat and fat-free cheeses, skim milk mozzarella, string cheese Low-fat and fat-free cottage cheese, and skim milk ricotta (½ cup)	☐	☐	☐	☐	☐	☐	
Frozen desserts Average serving: ½ cup							
Group 1 Ice cream, milk shakes	☐	3 pts	7 pts	× 1 pt	2 pts	3 pts =	___
Group 2 Ice milk, frozen yogurt	☐	☐	☐	☐	☐	☐	
F **Fried foods** Average serving: see below							
Group 1 French fries, fried vegetables: (½ cup) Fried chicken, fish, and meat: (3 oz) Check meat category also	☐	3 pts	7 pts	× 1 pt	2 pts	3 pts =	___
Group 2 Vegetables, not deep fried Meat, poultry, or fish prepared by baking, broiling, grilling, poaching, roasting, stewing	☐	☐	☐	☐	☐	☐	
I In baked goods Average serving: 1							
Group 1 Doughnuts, biscuits, butter rolls, muffins, croissants, sweet rolls, danish, cakes, pies, coffee cakes, cookies	☐	3 pts	7 pts	× 1 pt	2 pts	3 pts =	

Comments: _____   Total _____

Figure 3.2. *Continued*

FOOD CATEGORY	WEEKLY CONSUMPTION			SERVING SIZE			SCORE
	Rarely/ Never	3 or less	4 or more	Small	Average	Large	For office use
Group 2 Fruit bars, low-fat cookies/cakes/pastries, angel food cake, homemade baked goods with vegetable oils	☐	■ 3 pts	■ 7 pts	× 1 pt	■ 2 pts	■ 3 pts =	
C Convenience foods Average serving: see below							
Group 1 Canned, packaged, or frozen dinners: e.g., pizza (1 slice) Macaroni and cheese (approximately 1 cup), pot pie (1), cream soups (1 cup)	☐	■ 3 pts	■ 7 pts	× 1 pt	■ 2 pts	■ 3 pts =	___
Group 2 Diet/reduced calorie or reduced fat dinners (1 dinner)	☐	☐	☐	☐	☐	☐	
T Table fats Average serving: see below							
Group 1 Butter, stick margarine: 1 pat Regular salad dressing or mayonnaise, sour cream: 1–2 tbsp	☐	■ 3 pts	■ 7 pts	× 1 pt	■ 2 pts	■ 3 pts =	___
Group 2 Diet and tub margarine, low-fat and fat-free salad dressings Low-fat and fat-free mayonnaise	☐	☐	☐	☐	☐	☐	
S Snacks Average serving: see below							
Group 1 Chips (potato, corn, taco), cheese puffs, snack mix, nuts, regular crackers, regular popcorn, candy (milk chocolate, caramel, coconut)	☐	■ 3 pts	■ 7 pts	× 1 pt	■ 2 pts	■ 3 pts =	___
Group 2 Air-popped or low-fat popcorn, low-fat crackers, hard candy, licorice, fruit rolls, bread sticks, pretzels, fat-free chips Fruit	☐	☐	☐	☐	☐	☐	

Comments: _____ Total ____

[Note frequent use of foods high in fat or saturated fat (e.g., coffee creamer, whipped topping)]

Directions for scoring:	Key	Score from p 1 + ____
Multiply weekly consumption points (3 or 7) by serving size points (1, 2, 3) for Group 1 foods only except for a large serving of Group 2 meats	40–70 Step I diet less than 40 Step II diet	Score from p 2 + ____ Final score ____
Example: ■ 3 pts ✓ 7 pts 1 pt 2 pts ✓ 3 pts 3 × 7 = 21 points	■ Foods high in fat, saturated fat, and/or cholesterol.	
Add score on pages 1–3 to get final score		

Figure 3.2. *Continued*

high-saturated-fat foods along with alternative foods, plus a 7-day diet plan that adheres to less than 7% of calories from saturated fat and less than 200 mg per day of dietary cholesterol. The benefits of a low dietary cholesterol intake on reducing serum cholesterol are less well established. Clinical studies with eggs have failed to demonstrate a significant increase in serum cholesterol with consuming up to two egg yolks per day (approximately 500 mg per day of dietary cholesterol). Commercially available Omega-Tech Eggs are from chickens fed a special diet containing omega-3 fatty acids. Clinical trials show they do not increase serum cholesterol and provide approximately 200 to 500 mg per day of omega-3 fatty acids.

There are three additional options to add to the diet to enhance LDL reduction: plant sterols, viscous soluble fiber, and soy protein. The cumulative benefits of all three dietary factors may lower LDL by approximately 20%, and, in conjunction with a low-saturated-fat diet, the total LDL reduction may approach 30% (Table 3.2). A 20% to 30% reduction in LDL is sufficient for many patients to obviate the need for drug therapy. Plant sterols as either stanol esters (Benecol™), or as sterols (Take Control™), are probably the most effective additional dietary ingredients to lower cholesterol. Several studies have demonstrated the benefits of both plant sterols and stanols in lowering LDL by 7% to 14% (see Plant Sterols and Stanol Esters).

Soluble viscous fibers also lower LDL by approximately 5% to 10% depending on the daily amount consumed. There have been many studies to verify the LDL-lowering effects of both β-glucan in oat cereal and psyllium (Figs. 3.3 and 3.4). Initially, the water solubility of the fiber was thought to cause the LDL-lowering effect, but nonviscous, water-soluble fibers, such as gum arabic, were shown not to lower LDL. To significantly lower LDL, a person should consume between 10 and 25 g per day of oat fiber or psyllium.

The benefits of soy protein on lowering LDL cholesterol are less firmly established than those of viscous fiber and plant sterols, but,

Table 3.2. Therapeutic Lifestyle Diet Plus

	Low-density lipoprotein cholesterol reduction (%)
Saturated fat <7%	8–10
Dietary cholesterol <200 mg/d	3–5
Adjuncts	
Dietary fiber	3–5
Plant stanol/sterol	5–15
Soy protein	5
Cumulative	20–30

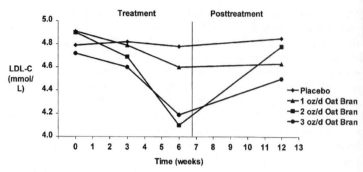

Figure 3.3. Short-term dose effects of oat bran on low-density lipoprotein cholesterol (LDL-C). (From Davidson, et al. *JAMA* 1991;265:1833, with permission.)

based on cumulative studies demonstrating a modest LDL reduction, the U.S. Food and Drug Administration (FDA) approved soy protein, at least 25 g per day (or four servings equal to 25 g per day noted on the food label), for the reduction of cardiovascular risk. In a metaanalysis of 38 soy protein studies, an overall mean of 9% LDL reduction was noted, with a range of 3.3% to 24%. For dietary studies, metaanalyses tend to overestimate the benefits of a food product because negative studies are less likely to be submitted or accepted for publication.

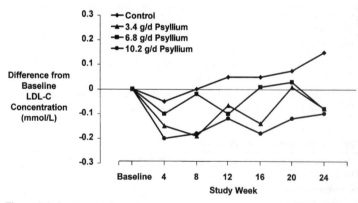

Figure 3.4. Long-term effects of psyllium food on low-density lipoprotein cholesterol (LDL-C) in hypercholesterolemic patients. (From Davidson MH, Makai KC, Kong JC, et al. Long-term effects of consuming foods containing psyllium seed husk on serum lipids in subjects with hypercholesterolemia. *Am J Clin Nutr* 1998;67:367, with permission.)

Table 3.3. Ways to Use or Add Soy in Foods

Soy food	Suggestions for use
8 oz plain soy milk (8 g[a])	In place of milk on cereal or cooking
8 oz flavored soy milk (6 g)	Drink with meals or as a snack
½ cup soy ground crumbles (9 g)	Use in recipes in place of ground meat
1 soy burger (10 g)	Instead of a hamburger
⅓ cup soy nuts (10 g)	As a snack
2 tbsp soy nut butter (8 g)	On a sandwich or on crackers
1 soy protein bar (14 g)	As a snack or a dessert
1 soy breakfast link (6.5 g)	In place of breakfast meat
¼ cup soy flour (8 g)	Replace part of flour in recipes with soy flour
½ cup tofu (10 g)	Add to stir fry or soups
¼ cup soy protein powder (12 g)	Add to a smoothie

[a]Grams of soy protein.

The FDA, for its review of health claim petition, usually selects only the studies that are well controlled with adequate sample sizes.

Soy protein contains isoflavones or phytoestrogens that may cause LDL reduction. However, other research suggests that the amino acid content of soy protein is responsible for hypocholesterolemia activity. Soy protein is mostly incorporated into low-fat foods, and there may be a substitution phenomenon in which hyperlipidemics who eat more soy protein will eat less fat-enriched foods. These theories regarding the hypocholesterolemic effects of soy protein are still being evaluated.

The most difficult challenge with increasing the amount of soy protein in the diet is the paucity of food products containing adequate soy amounts. A glass of soy milk contains approximately 7 to 8 g of soy protein. There are other products, such as tofu, soybean curd, and vegetable burgers, that contain approximately 7 to 8 g of soy protein per serving. These food items are becoming more widely available, but for most Americans, they remain difficult food products to develop a taste for. (Table 3.3 lists available food items containing soy protein.) The Mobile Lipid Clinic™ software program can print two versions of a low-saturated-fat diet. The first version is a standard diet with less than 7% of calories from saturated fat. The second version incorporates more than 20 g per day of viscous fiber and 2 g per day of plant sterols. If the first version does not adequately lower LDL to recommended goals, the second version may provide additive effects (see Appendix A).

An alternative to reducing total fat in the diet, and usually saturated fat as well, is to increase the amount of monounsaturated and polyunsaturated fats. In fat-restrictive diets, many patients compensate by eating more calories from simple carbohydrates, which results in an

Table 3.4. Seven Countries Study: Dietary Intake and Mortality Rates in Selected Cohorts

	Crete	Mediterranean[a]	Zutphen, Netherlands	U.S. railroad
Mortality[b]				
Total	514	1,090	1,091	1,153
Coronary heart disease	9	184	420	574
Serum cholesterol (mmol/L)	5.3	5.0	6.0	6.1
Food intake (g/d)[c]				
Bread	380	416	252	97
Legume	30	18	2	1
Fruit	464	130	82	233
Meat	35	140	138	273
Fish	18	34	12	3
Edible fat	95	60	79	33
Alcohol	15	43	3	6

[a]n = 9 cohorts.
[b]Ten years per 10,000 men aged 50 to 69 years.
[c]Evaluated in the 1960s.

increased glycemic load, leading to potential hypertriglyceridemia (HTG) and obesity. An attractive alternative to a low-fat diet is the Mediterranean diet. The Mediterranean diet is rich in complex carbohydrates and fiber, and the fat source is primarily monounsaturated fatty acids as found in olive oil. The Seven Countries Study, which was started in the early 1960s, demonstrated that Crete (an island off of Greece) showed the lowest mortality from CHD and all causes. The Crete diet was not a low-fat diet; in fact, the fat intake was almost three times as much as that of the U.S. population (Table 3.4). The major difference was the intake of olive oil. A more recent survey of CHD mortality also demonstrated a much lower CHD mortality among the Mediterranean populations compared to Northern Europe or the United States (Table 3.5). In the Lyon Diet Study, 605 postmyocardial infarction (MI) patients were randomly assigned to a Mediterranean-type diet versus an American Heart Association Step I diet. After a period of 4 years on the diet, although there were no differences in plasma lipids, the Mediterranean diet showed a 70% reduction in cardiac death and nonfatal MI (Fig. 3.5). There is also evidence that olive oil reduces the risk of diabetes and obesity, which may relate to the lower glycemic load of the Mediterranean diet. Olive oil also inhibits the oxidation of LDL both *in vitro* and *ex vivo*. Olive oil contains phenolic compounds that, in addition to small amounts of vitamin E, provide the antioxidant effect. The phenolic content is most highly concentrated in extra-virgin olives, but the content varies considerably

Table 3.5. Coronary Heart Disease Mortality Rates in Europe and the United States in the 1990s[a]

Sweden	291.3
Denmark	278.6
Great Britain and Northern Ireland	266.6
Finland	262.8
Germany	221.4
Ireland	220.5
Austria	208.9
United States	188.1
Netherlands	134.4
Luxembourg	129.2
Italy	126.4
Belgium	119.5
Greece	115.1
Portugal	92.1
France	85.0
Spain	89.5

[a]Non–age-adjusted mortality rates per year per 100,000 persons; data from 1992–1994.
From Statistisches Jahrbuch *1998*, with permission.

due to climate and production techniques. The Mediterranean diet is also rich in wine, legumes, cereals, fruit, and vegetables that also provide antioxidant effects. Red wine, compared to white wine, contains many more flavonoids that are potent antioxidants. The net result of the Mediterranean diet is a diet rich in antioxidants, low in saturated

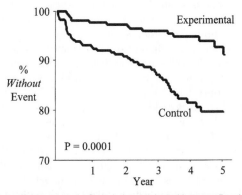

Figure 3.5. Lyon diet heart study. Cumulative survival without cardiac death and nonfatal myocardial infarction. (From de Lorgeril M, et al. *Circulation* 1999;99:779–785, with permission.)

fat, and with a low glycemic index (GI). Thereby, many Americans may prefer a Mediterranean diet over a low-fat diet to reduce CHD risk. A major challenge regarding the dietary counseling of patients interested in a Mediterranean diet is portion size control. The Italian and Greek restaurants in the United States provide portion sizes much larger than those consumed in Europe. The Mobile Lipid Clinic™ software program can print out a 7-day Mediterranean meal plan that provides the appropriate portion sizes (see Appendix A).

HIGH TRIGLYCERIDES OR METABOLIC SYNDROME

Patients with HTG usually have carbohydrate intolerance with one important exception. Patients with severe HTG due to hyperchylomicronemia have lipoprotein lipase impairment and cannot adequately clear postprandial fat intake. Because the dietary therapy is different for hyperchylomicronemia, it is important to recognize and treat this disorder appropriately. Patients with hyperchylomicronemia usually have triglycerides greater than 1,000 mg per dL; eruptive xanthomas on any part of the body but most commonly on the trunk, back, and buttocks; and, possibly, a history of pancreatitis. The serum or plasma of these patients, if left in the refrigerator overnight, has a creamy layer on top that is indicative of chylomicrons. Although hyperchylomicronemic syndromes are relatively rare, if a patient with this disorder is put on a low-carbohydrate diet, he or she will increase his or her total fat intake, and this may exacerbate the hyperchylomicronemia. The treatment for this disorder is total fat restriction to less than 10 g per day until the chylomicrons can clear properly and the diet may be slightly liberalized, but to no more than 10% of calories from fat. Often, these patients have another disorder, such as diabetes or hypothyroidism, which, if corrected, may help improve chylomicron clearance.

Most patients with HTG, however, have an overproduction of endogenous (rather than exogenous or dietary) triglycerides or very-low-density lipoprotein (VLDL). High carbohydrates stimulate the synthesis of VLDL triglycerides by the liver. The exact mechanism by which carbohydrates increase VLDL synthesis is not yet well understood, but, clearly, patients with high VLDL levels respond to carbohydrate restriction. The true culprit for the increased VLDL may not be carbohydrates per se but, rather, the glycemic load. The GI of foods is simply a ranking of foods based on their immediate effect on blood sugar levels. Simple carbohydrates that are rapidly digested and absorbed have the highest GI, but complex carbohydrates, protein, and fat are digested more slowly and, thus, release glucose more gradually into the blood. Therefore, to lower the glycemic load, the diet should be increased in the percent of calories from complex carbohydrates, protein, fat, or a combination of all three. GI may affect appetite and explain the rationale behind the increasing obesity rate despite a reduction in fat intake. One potential hypothesis is that a high glycemic load increases insulin secretion and insulin, or the drop in glucose that insulin induces increases neuropeptide Y production, increasing appetite. The net result of a high GI diet is an increase in hunger; therefore, an increase in caloric intake and subsequent weight gain. Many of the popular diets, such as Atkins, Protein Power, Carbohydrate Addict, Sugar Busters, and the South Beach Diet, rely on increasing the protein or fat in the diet while reducing the carbohydrates to reduce the glycemic load. In these popular press books, insulin is considered the culprit cause of weight gain, but the true cause of weight loss with these diets may be the better control of appetite with the consequent reduction in caloric intake. The Glucose Revolution and Dr. Dean Ornish's Eat More, Weigh Less diet plans rely on increasing the amounts of complex carbohydrates rather than protein and fat to lower the GI. All the popular diets can be placed into a continuum from a low GI diet to a moderate GI diet with the addition of more complex carbohydrates. Table 3.6 lists the food allowed and disallowed on each diet.

The Atkins diet represents the extreme of the low-carbohydrate diets. Atkins recommends 20 g or less of carbohydrates during the induction phase. Reducing caloric intake by 500 kcal per day should result in approximately 1 to 2 lb of weight loss per week (there are 3,500 kcal per lb). However, on the Atkins diet, the initial weight loss is approximately 4 to 6 lb in the first week. The difference is due to the diet-induced diuresis when carbohydrate intake is restricted to less than 20 g per day. Glycogen stores are mobilized in the liver and muscle. Each gram of glycogen is mobilized with approximately 2 g of water. Therefore, the 500 g of stored glycogen results in approximately 1 kg, or approximately 2 lb, of water loss when mobilized. Another effect is the generation of ketone bodies due to the catabolism of dietary and endogenous fat. Atkins advises readers to use urine dipsticks to check for the excretion of ketones to verify the diet is working. Ketone excretion also increases water loss, but ketones also suppress appetite, and this may explain, at least partially, the decreased hunger experienced by people on this diet. Long-term ketosis may lead to dehydration, constipation, and kidney stones. In addition, because Atkins allows unlimited consumption of high-fat foods and the exclusion of fruits, grains, and many vegetables, the long-term health effects of this diet are uncertain. However, a

Table 3.6. Food Allowances for Atkins, Sugar Busters, and Ornish/Pritikin Diets

	Carbo/g/ serving	Atkins	Sugar Busters	Ornish/ Pritikin
Proteins				
Cheeses	1	√	√	X
Cheese omelet	2	√	√	X
Eggs (2)	6	√	√	X
Fish and seafood	0	√	√	••
Poultry	0	√	√	••
Pork, lamb, veal	0	√	√	••
Fried chicken	13	√	X	X
Red meat, lean cuts	0	√	••	••
Bacon, cold cuts, marble beef, lamb	0	√	••	X
Cottage cheese	6	√	√	••
Whole milk	11	√	√	X
Skim milk	12	√	√	√
Soy milk	8	√	√	√
Nuts	5.4	√	√	X
Peanuts	5.4	√	√	X
Cashews	8.3	√	√	X
Almonds	5.5	√	√	X
Brazil nuts	5.5	√	√	X
Macadamia, raw	3.5	√	√	X
Walnuts	4.2	√	√	√
Yogurt (plain)	13	X	√	√
Yogurt (sugar-free)	13	X	√	√
Fats				
Butter	Trace	√	√	X
Cream cheese (1 oz)	1	√	√	X
Sour cream (1 tbsp)	1	√	√	X
Vegetable oil	0	√	√	X
Canola oil	0	√	√	X
Olive oil	0	√	√	X
Vegetables				
Artichokes	11.9	√	√	√
Asparagus	2.2	√	√	√
Bean sprouts	5.6	√	√	√
Beets	12.2	√	√	√
Bell peppers	7.2	√	√	√
Broccoli	7	√	√	√
Brussels sprouts	9.9	√	√	√
Carrots	7	X	••	√
Cabbage	4.9	√	√	√
Cauliflower	4	√	√	√
Celery	1.6	√	√	√
Corn	16.2	X	X	√

continued

Table 3.6. *Continued*

	Carbo/g/ serving	Atkins	Sugar Busters	Ornish/ Pritikin
Cucumber	3.6	√	√	√
Eggplant	8.2	√	√	√
Endive	2.1	√	√	√
Lettuce	1.6	√	√	√
Mushrooms	3.1	√	√	√
Mustard greens	5.6	√	√	√
Okra	9.6	√	√	√
Olives				
Green, large	0.5	√	√	√
Oil cured	2.3	√	√	√
Onion	14.8	X	√	√
Parsnip	23.1	X	√	√
Peas	19.4	X	√	√
Potatoes (baked)	32.8	X	√	√
Pumpkin (fresh)	7.0	X	√	√
Radishes	2.9	√	√	√
Sauerkraut	9.4	√	√	√
Spinach	2.4	√	√	√
Squash	5.5	√	√	√
Sweet potatoes (baked)	37.0	X	√	√
Sweet pickles	20	X	√	√
B & G (1 Tbsp)	4	√	√	√
Vlasic	3	√	√	√
Gherkins	10	√	√	√
Tofu (2-in. cube)	2.9	√	√	√
Tomatoes	5.8	√	√	√
Turnips	8.6	√	√	√
Fruits (fresh)				
Apples	10.0	X	••	√
Apricots	13.7	X	••	√
Avocados				
California	6.5	√	√	••
Florida	13.5	√	√	••
Bananas	26.4	X	X	√
Blackberries	18.6	X	••	√
Blueberries	22	••	••	√
Boysenberries	22.2	X	••	√
Cherries	14.7	••	••	√
Dates	58.3	X	••	√
Figs	10.2	X	••	√
Grapefruit	10.3	X	••	√
Grapes	9	X	••	√

continued

Table 3.6. *Continued*

	Carbo/g/ serving	Atkins	Sugar Busters	Ornish/ Pritikin
Kiwi	18	X	••	√
Lemon	6	X	••	√
Melons				
Honeydew (1 cup cubed)	13.1	X	••	√
Watermelon (1 cup diced)	10.2	X	X	√
Cantaloupe [5-in. dia. (½)]	20.4	X	••	√
Nectarines	23.6	X	••	√
Oranges	16	X	••	√
Peaches	9.7	X	••	√
Pears				
Bartlett	25.1	X	••	√
Bosc	22	X	••	√
D'Anjou	31	X	••	√
Pineapple	21.2	X	••	√
Plums	17.8	X	••	√
Raspberries	21	X	••	√
Strawberries	12.5	X	••	√
Raisins	7	X	••	√
Tangerines	11.7	X	••	√
Beans (general)	32.1	X	••	√
Cereals				
All Bran extra fiber	22	X	√	√
Bran buds	24	X	√	√
100% Bran	24	X	√	√
Oat bran	15	X	√	√
Shredded wheat	38	X	√	√
Multi-grain Cheerios	23	X	√	√
Oatmeal	27	X	√	√
Cream of Wheat	25	X	√	√
Instant hot cereals				
Cream of Wheat (1 pkg)	21	X	√	√
Instant grits (½ cup)	33	X	X	√
Maypo (½ cup)	36	X	√	√
Oatmeal (1 pkg)	19	X	√	√
Corn or rice-based cereals (1 cup)	26	X	X	√
Grits	32	X	X	X
Bread, white	14.1	X	X	√
Bread, whole wheat	11	X	••	√
Bread, rye	13	X	••	√
Corn bread	27.5	X	X	√
Pancake, buckwheat	17.4	X	••	√

continued

Table 3.6. *Continued*

	Carbo/g/ serving	Atkins	Sugar Busters	Ornish/ Pritikin
Pancake				
Dry mix (6-in. dia)	23.7	X	X	√
Frozen Aunt Jemima (3)	40	X	X	√
Peanut butter (natural, no sugar added)	3	••	√	X
Beverages (no sugar added)				
Diet drinks	0	√	√	√
Coffee	0	√	√	√
Tea	0	√	√	√
Apple juice	29.5	X	X	√
Grape juice	42	X	X	√
Grapefruit juice	23	X	••	√
Orange juice	27	X	••	√
Tomato juice	10.4	X	••	√
Soups (no sugar added)				
Noodle soups				
Chicken noodle (1 cup)	7.9	X	••	••
Rice-based soups	15	X	X	√
Chicken w/rice (1 cup)	5.8	X	••	√
Condiments				
Hot sauce	.1	√	√	√
Ketchup	3.8	••	••	√
Mayonnaise	0	√	√	√
Mustards	.3	√	√	√
Vinegar	.9	√	√	√
Pasta (white, 1 cup)	39.1	X	X	√
Pasta (whole wheat, 2 oz)	40	X	X	√
Rice (white)	49.6	X	X	√
Risotto	37	X	X	√
Flour products				
Crackers				
Ritz (5)	10	X	X	√
Townhouse (5)	9	X	X	√
Pastries				
Danish (5 oz)	64.8	X	X	X
Doughnuts				
Cake	29.8	X	X	X
Yeast-leavened glazed	22	X	X	X
Pies (apple, 1/8)	45	X	X	X
Muffins (Sara Lee blueberry)	30	X	X	X
Cookies				
Snackwells	21	X	X	X
Chips Ahoy (3)	23	X	X	X
Oreos (3)	23	X	X	X

continued

Table 3.6. *Continued*

	Carbo/g/ serving	Atkins	Sugar Busters	Ornish/ Pritikin
Ice cream (Ben & Jerry's vanilla, 1/2 cup)	21	X	X	X
Sugar-free Jello	0	X	X	X
Puddings	63.4	X	X	X
Frozen yogurt (Ben & Jerry's low-fat cherry, 1/2 cup)	31	X	X	X
Candy bars:				
Almond Joy	28	X	X	X
KitKat	26	X	X	X
Milk chocolate	25	X	X	X
Milky Way	43	X	X	X
Snickers	35	X	X	X
3 Musketeers	46	X	X	X
Reeses (1.6 oz)	25	X	X	X
York Peppermint Patty (1.5 oz)	34	X	X	X
Raisinets	31	X	X	X

√, allowed; X, not allowed; • •, allowed in moderation.

misconception among many health professionals is that Atkins does not advocate a ketotic diet for longer than 4 weeks. After the 4-week induction phase, more carbohydrates are added to the diet, and the maintenance phase continues with a lower-carbohydrate diet, but includes the intake of fruits, vegetables, and grains in moderation.

The Atkins diet may cause an increase in LDL-cholesterol (LDL-C), but if the weight loss is significant, LDL may actually decrease, and triglycerides often decrease dramatically. For patients with HTG (without hyperchylomicronemia), a modification of the Atkins diet can provide similar reductions in triglyceride levels without increasing saturated fat significantly and avoiding ketosis. The vast majority of nutrition experts do not believe the short-term weight loss induced by ketosis is worth the risk, especially in diabetics and patients with CHD.

The Sugar Busters diet by H. C. Steward and Drs. Bethea, Andrews, and Balart focuses almost entirely on the exclusion of simple carbohydrates from the diet. This diet allows, in moderation, intake of high-fat and -protein foods. This diet is also the most generous of the low-carbohydrate diets in allowing most fruit and high-fiber foods.

The Zone diet by Dr. Barry Sears is a lower-carbohydrate diet, but not really a low-carbohydrate diet. The Zone diet advocates a combination of carbohydrates, fat, and protein in every meal to lower the glycemic load and reduce insulin secretion. The Zone diet involves a fairly complex strategy of starting a meal with a low-fat source of protein, such as skinless poultry, fish, lean red meat, egg whites, low-fat dairy products, or soy sources of protein. The next step is to add "favorable" carbohydrates, such as vegetables (except for corn, carrots, rice, or potatoes), fruit (except bananas and raisins), and selected grains, such as oatmeal and barley. To complete the meal, the diet recommends the addition of nonsaturated fats, such as olive oil, almonds, avocados, and fish oils, and the avoidance of fatty red meat, egg yolks, organ meats, and processed foods (rich in trans fats). The Zone diet also advocates eating five times per day; three meals and two snacks.*

The South Beach Diet by Arthur Agatson, M.D., a cardiologist, advocates a low-carbohydrate and low-saturated-fat diet. This diet represents a healthier alternative to Atkins by restricting the unlimited consumption of high-saturated-fat foods. South Beach recommends severe carbohydrate restriction initially (for the first 2 weeks), but more complex carbohydrates are added to the diet in the long-term.

The Mobile Lipid Clinic™ has a 50 g carbohydrate, low-saturated-fat diet that provides a two-page summary for patients. Alternatively, a low glycemic diet sheet is available that incorporates more high-complex-carbohydrate diets (see Appendix A).

LOW HIGH-DENSITY LIPOPROTEIN

The nonpharmacologic management of low levels of HDL involves weight loss, exercise, smoking cessation, and, potentially, moderate increase in ethanol intake.

Weight Control

There is a clear association between body mass index (BMI) and HDL-cholesterol (HDL-C). Approximately 25% of men and 7% of women

---

*In my opinion, all of these diets, if used properly, significantly reduce triglyceride levels. In my experience, the best strategy to treat HTG is to start with a 50-g-per-day carbohydrate diet for approximately 2 weeks (see modified Atkins) before reevaluating the lipid profile. The triglyceride levels should be dramatically improved. After 2 weeks, the diet can be liberalized to allow more complex carbohydrates as advocated by the Protein Power or Zone diet books. The Real Age Diet (HarperCollins, 2001), written by Drs. Michael Roizen and John LaPuma (also a gourmet chef), provides a thorough and scientific discussion of each diet and how to improve the diet's overall health benefits. This book uses years of age ("real age") to motivate patients to evaluate all the health effects of the total diet.

with a BMI greater than 30 have HDL-C levels less than 35 mg per dL. Body fat distribution, as measured by computed tomography scan or bone densitometry (Hologic) can distinguish visceral adiposity ("apple") in subcutaneous fat ("pear"). High visceral fat in both men and women better predicts a low HDL than BMI.

There is also significant clinical evidence that weight loss improves HDL-C levels. A metaanalysis of more than 70 studies found that, in general, HDL-C decreases during active weight loss (most likely due to fat restriction) but increases again when weight stabilizes at a lower level. Multiple regression analysis showed that for every 4.5 kg reduction in weight, LDL-C decreased by 4 mg per dL and HDL increased by approximately 2 mg per dL.

Low-fat diets decrease HDL. Orlistat, a pancreatic lipase inhibitor that blocks fat absorption, also lowers HDL slightly initially. Saturated fats raise HDL, possibly by inhibiting cholesterol ester transfer protein; polyunsaturated fats (omega-6) lower HDL-C; and monounsaturated fats are relatively neutral on HDL levels. Because weight loss diets mostly focus on saturated fat reduction, this may explain the initial decline in HDL during the weight loss phase. Once the weight loss has stabilized, other factors, such as reduced visceral adiposity, lead to an increase in HDL.

Perhaps the worst fat from a total lipid perspective are transfatty acids that raise LDL-C similar to a saturated fat but also lower HDL-C equal to a polyunsaturated fat. Transfatty acids are formed during the hydrogenation process of unsaturated fats to produce margarine or vegetable shortening. Hydrogens break the double bonds of the polyunsaturated fats (to saturate the carbons with hydrogen), and, in the process, transfatty acids are formed. Semiliquid margarine (liquid oil as the first ingredient on the label), soft margarine, shortening, and stick margarine have, respectively, less than 0.5 g, 7.4 g, 9.9 g, and 20.1 g of transfatty acids per 100 g. Therefore, stick margarine may be no better than butter from an LDL or HDL perspective. Higher intakes of margarine were also associated with a higher mortality rate in the Nurses' Health Study.

Many patients with low HDL who are overweight also have HTG. By lowering the triglyceride levels, the HDL-C rises. Low-carbohydrate diets that lower triglyceride levels generally also increase HDL-C (see High Triglycerides or Metabolic Syndrome). If triglycerides are not elevated and an obese patient has low HDL, caloric restriction along with an exercise program will most likely promote weight loss and raise HDL-C.

Caloric restriction requires significant patient education and motivation. Because fat is the most calorically dense food (9 kcal per gram versus 4 kcal per gram for protein and carbohydrates), avoiding fat should significantly reduce total caloric intake. This hypothesis only holds true if an individual does not totally compensate for fat caloric reduction by increasing the intake of carbohydrates. Dr. Dean Ornish's book *Eat More, Weigh Less* advocates a fat-restrictive diet while providing for relatively unlimited intake of complex carbohydrates to promote satiety. His book also incorporates advice regarding stress reduction through meditation. For most Americans, the Ornish diet represents a radical change from their standard diet. Ornish believes that comprehensive dietary changes rather than moderate steps toward a lower-fat diet are more effective. He argues that only moderate changes that do not provide for a low-fat, high-complex-carbohydrate diet relatively quickly will not benefit from the sense of well-being and lack of hunger the diet provides, and, therefore, compliance will be lost.

Rather than exclude specific food groups (i.e., fats), other weight loss programs recommend portion control on the basis of weight loss. The abundance of high caloric foods and large portion sizes most likely explains the high rate of obesity in the United States. Although airline food is notoriously disliked by passengers, the portions provided generally represent the meal size most Americans should consume. The Weight Watchers diet is built on calorie counting and portion control. Other popular diets, such as Jenny Craig, provide members with portion-controlled meals. Slim Fast is a nutritionally balanced beverage that is used as a meal substitute, thereby providing portion control. The major challenge with these diets is maintaining compliance in a culture in which food is so generously provided, and, often, the least expensive or most available are the most calorically dense.

The Mobile Lipid Clinic™ program provides the ability to print out menu or diet plans for the patient. These different diet plans give the physician or health professional the flexibility to choose the diet program that best suits the needs of each patient.

Exercise

Exercise promotes weight loss but also appears to raise HDL-C independently of the reduction in body weight. The impact of a 12-month exercise program was assessed in men with low to normal HDL-C. Exercise consisted of four supervised sessions per week of walking, jogging, or cycling to elicit 60% to 80% of maximal heart rate, and weight was stabilized with personalized diets. There were significant improvements in HDL-C, apolipoprotein AI, and apolipoprotein B in the patients with normal baseline HDL-C levels (mean, 43.3), but little effect on those with low HDL-C (mean, 32.4). This study suggests that genetically low levels of HDL do not respond to exercise. However, intense exercise may raise HDL in most people. In the U.S. National Runner Health Study, the distance run was the most important predictor of HDL-C levels. This study estimated that for every kilometer habitually run per week, there was a corresponding 0.2 mg per dL increase in HDL-C and a 0.1 mg per dL decrease in LDL.

Motivating patients to exercise is a difficult challenge for most physicians. For most patients older than 40 years, walking is probably the preferred program for long-term compliance. Walking with a spouse or friend may additionally improve compliance. The Mobile Lipid Clinic™ software program prints out the American Health Association sample walking or jogging program for the patient (Tables 3.7 and 3.8).

Cigarette Smoking Cessation

According to the Framingham Offspring Study (n = 4,107), cigarette smoking was significantly associated with a 4 mg per dL decrease of HDL in men and a 6 mg per dL in women. The 6 mg per dL decrease

Table 3.7. Sample Walking Program

	Warm up	Target zone exercising	Cool down	Total time
Week 1				
Session A	Walk 5 min	Then walk briskly 5 min	Then walk more slowly 5 min	15 min
Session B	Repeat above pattern			
Session C	Repeat above pattern			
Week 2	Walk 5 min	Walk briskly 7 min	Walk 5 min	17 min
Week 3	Walk 5 min	Walk briskly 9 min	Walk 5 min	19 min
Week 4	Walk 5 min	Walk briskly 11 min	Walk 5 min	21 min
Week 5	Walk 5 min	Walk briskly 13 min	Walk 5 min	23 min
Week 6	Walk 5 min	Walk briskly 15 min	Walk 5 min	25 min
Week 7	Walk 5 min	Walk briskly 18 min	Walk 5 min	28 min
Week 8	Walk 5 min	Walk briskly 20 min	Walk 5 min	30 min
Week 9	Walk 5 min	Walk briskly 23 min	Walk 5 min	33 min
Week 10	Walk 5 min	Walk briskly 26 min	Walk 5 min	36 min
Week 11	Walk 5 min	Walk briskly 28 min	Walk 5 min	38 min
Week 12	Walk 5 min	Walk briskly 30 min	Walk 5 min	40 min

Week 13 on:

Check your pulse periodically to see if you are exercising within your target zone. As you become more fit, try exercising within the upper range of your target zone. Gradually increase your brisk walking time from 30 to 60 min, three or four times a week. Remember that your goal is to get the benefits you are seeking and enjoy your activity.

Table 3.8. Sample Jogging Program

	Warm up	Target zone exercising	Cool down	Total time
Week 1				
Session A	Walk 5 min, then stretch and limber up	Then walk 10 min and try not to stop	Then walk more slowly 3 min and stretch 2 min	20 min
Session B	Repeat above pattern			
Session C	Repeat above pattern			
Continue with at least three exercise sessions during each week of the program.				
Week 2	Walk 5 min, then stretch and limber up	Walk 5 min, jog 1 min, walk 5 min, jog 1 min	Walk 3 min, stretch 2 min	22 min
Week 3	Walk 5 min, then stretch and limber up	Walk 5 min, jog 3 min, walk 5 min, jog 3 min	Walk 3 min, stretch 2 min	26 min
Week 4	Walk 5 min, then stretch and limber up	Walk 4 min, jog 5 min, walk 4 min, jog 5 min	Walk 3 min, stretch 2 min	28 min
Week 5	Walk 5 min, then stretch and limber up	Walk 4 min, jog 5 min, walk 4 min, jog 5 min	Walk 3 min, stretch 2 min	28 min
Week 6	Walk 5 min, then stretch and limber up	Walk 4 min, jog 6 min, walk 4 min, jog 6 min	Walk 3 min, stretch 2 min	30 min
Week 7	Walk 5 min, then stretch and limber up	Walk 4 min, jog 7 min, walk 4 min, jog 7 min	Walk 3 min, stretch 2 min	32 min
Week 8	Walk 5 min, then stretch and limber up	Walk 4 min, jog 8 min, walk 4 min, jog 8 min	Walk 3 min, stretch 2 min	34 min
Week 9	Walk 5 min, then stretch and limber up	Walk 4 min, jog 9 min, walk 4 min, jog 9 min	Walk 3 min, stretch 2 min	36 min
Week 10	Walk 5 min, then stretch and limber up	Walk 4 min, jog 13 min	Walk 3 min, stretch 2 min	27 min
Week 11	Walk 5 min, then stretch and limber up	Walk 5 min, jog 15 min	Walk 3 min, stretch 2 min	29 min
Week 12	Walk 5 min, then stretch and limber up	Walk 4 min, jog 17 min	Walk 3 min, stretch 2 min	31 min
Week 13	Walk 5 min, then stretch and limber up	Walk 2 min, jog slowly 2 min, jog 17 min	Walk 3 min, stretch 2 min	31 min

continued

Table 3.8. *Continued*

	Warm up	Target zone exercising	Cool down	Total time
Week 14	Walk 5 min, then stretch and limber up	Walk 1 min, jog slowly 13 min, jog 17 min	Walk 3 min, stretch 2 min	31 min
Week 15	Walk 5 min, then stretch and limber up	Jog slowly 3 min, jog 17 min	Walk 3 min, stretch 2 min	30 min

Week 16 on:

Check your pulse periodically to see if you are exercising within your target zone. As you become more fit, try exercising within the upper range of your target zone. Gradually increase your jogging time from 20 to 30 min (or more, up to 60 min), three or four times a week. Remember that your goal is to get the benefits you are seeking and enjoy your activity.

The exercise patterns for both of the walking and jogging programs are suggested guidelines. Listen to your body and build up less quickly, if needed.

Note: If you are older than 40 years and have not been active, you should not begin with a program as strenuous as jogging. Begin with the walking program instead (see Table 3.7). After completing the walking program, you can start with week 3 of the jogging program.

in HDL-C in women may explain the reason that cigarette-smoking women lose much of their 10-year advantage over men in CHD risk. Cigar and pipe smokers and cigarette smokers who quit at least 1 year previously have the same HDL-C as nonsmokers (see Chapter 6).

Moderate Alcohol Consumption

Alcohol consumption raises HDL-C, and many studies have documented a link between moderate alcohol consumption and a reduction in coronary artery disease. The inverse association between alcohol and CHD has been consistently reported in cross-cultural, case-controlled, and cohort studies. Wine consumption is the alcoholic beverage most clearly linked to CHD risk reduction by evaluating both mortality rates per 100,000 by amount of wine consumption (Fig. 3.6) and by comparing CHD rates in different countries compared to total wine consumption. Some studies suggest that red wine is more cardioprotective than white wine, hypothetically due to the increased content of the flavonoid antioxidants found in red wine. In countries where wine consumption is relatively low but beer and spirit consumption is high, there remains a decreased CHD rate among moderate alcohol consumers compared to nondrinkers. The CHD risk benefit of moderate alcohol consumption must also be evaluated in the context that

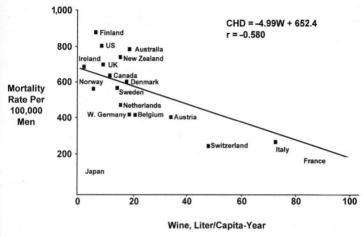

$$CHD = -4.99W + 652.4$$
$$r = -0.580$$

Figure 3.6. Wine consumption and coronary heart disease (CHD). (From Hegsted, Ausman. *J Nutr* 1988;118:1184, with permission.)

heavy alcohol consumption is associated with hypertension, arrhythmias, and increased mortality due to accidental death and liver disease.

Alcohol appears to increase HDL-C by inhibiting cholesterol ester transfer protein. On average, HDL-C increases by 4 mg per dL for a 30 g (two drinks) daily increase in alcohol. Based on the Physician's Health Study or Lipids Research Clinics Study, this would result in an approximate 17% reduction in CHD rates. However, the observational trials suggest that reduction in CHD rates is approximately 25%. Other possible benefits of alcohol on CHD risk reduction include decreases in circulating clotting proteins and platelet aggregability and increases in fibrinolytic activity and insulin sensitivity.

Diabetics also appear to benefit from moderate alcohol consumption. For diabetics who had, on average, one drink per day (14 g of alcohol per day), the relative risk of mortality was 0.21 compared to nondrinkers. Even diabetics who drink occasionally (less than one drink per week) had a risk of mortality of 0.54 compared with those who had never consumed alcohol.

Although nonconclusive, "binge" drinking does not appear to have as much cardioprotective effect. The national guidelines also recommend drinking alcohol with a meal rather than on an empty stomach because a meal diminishes the blood alcohol level somewhat. Drinking with meals does not seem to change the relationship between average

Table 3.9. Nonpharmacologic Therapies to Raise High-Density Lipoprotein (HDL)

Therapy	Expected HDL increase (mg/dL)
Smoking cessation	5
Alcohol intake	4
4.5 kg of sustained weight loss	2
Exercise (running 10 km/wk)	2
Total	**13**

intake and HDL-C, but postprandial triglycerides are higher, and LDL-C is lower. Because the HDL-C and LDL-C effects persist after the transitory increase in triglycerides, the overall effect of alcohol given with a meal suggests an antiatherogenic effect.

Although the benefits of alcohol on HDL-C and CHD mortality are well documented, clinical advice to abstainers to start consuming alcohol for cardioprotective purposes has not yet been substantiated in clinical trials. Therefore, because alcohol abuse is a serious health problem, caution must be advised on an individual basis regarding whether to recommend that a patient initiate drinking to raise HDL-C and potentially reduce CHD risk. Table 3.9 lists the potential cumulative effects of nonpharmacologic therapies to raise HDL.

FUNCTIONAL FOODS

The definition of *functional food*, according to the International Life Science Institute, is food that, by virtue of physiologically active food components, provides health benefits beyond basic nutrition. The American Dietetic Association emphasizes that functional foods have "a potentially beneficial effect on health when consumed as part of a varied diet on a regular basis at effective levels." Many Americans have the misconception that eating a healthy functional food can offset the harmful effects of poor dietary habits. Therefore, there is a danger of overemphasis on the benefits of individual foods or dietary supplements instead of the total diet. Nonetheless, as long as functional food and dietary supplements are advised in the context of a total healthy diet, these nonpharmacologic therapies may provide significant clinical benefits.

Soluble Viscous Fiber

The FDA has approved two viscous-soluble fibers, oat β-glucan and psyllium seed husk, for the food-specific health claim for reducing the risk of heart disease. The mechanism by which viscous-soluble fibers lower LDL-C is not completely understood but probably relates to their ability to either reduce the absorption of cholesterol bile acids or delay lipid digestion. The higher the viscosity of the fiber, the greater the LDL-C reduction. A metaanalysis of studies has determined that 3 g per day of β-glucan or approximately 7 g per day of psyllium lowers LDL by 4% to 5%. Higher doses of viscous-soluble fiber may provide greater LDL-C reduction, especially in patients with hypercholesterolemia. Psyllium can also be consumed as bulk laxative to lower cholesterol. Although other viscous-soluble fibers, such as pectin or guar gum, are available as dietary supplements, these fibers do not have FDA-approved health claims, and there is not the plethora of data available regarding cholesterol lowering compared to oat β-glucan or psyllium.

Plant Sterols and Stanol Esters

Plant sterols are natural components of vegetable oils and pine trees that inhibit intestinal cholesterol absorption. Plant stanols, the derivatives of sterols, may have a greater cholesterol lowering effect than plant sterols. Both the plant sterols and stanols put in a fat medium such as margarine have been shown to lower LDL by 7% to 14%. The fat medium appears necessary to disperse the plant sterol or stanol in the intestinal lumen to prevent cholesterol absorption. The data regarding using sterol capsules to lower cholesterol are not as well established. Two margarines—Benecol, containing plant stanols, and Take Control, containing plant sterols—are FDA approved to claim reductions in serum cholesterol. The NCEP ATP III advocates adding 2 g per day of plant sterols or stanols to the diet if a low-saturated-fat intake inadequately lowers the LDL-C to goal (Table 3.10). Adding 2 g per day equates to approximately two servings (tablespoons) of Benecol or Take Control per day. These margarines are relatively expensive, ranging in price from $5.00 per week for Benecol to $2.50 per week for Take Control. Most patients enjoy the taste, and a 7% to 14% additional LDL-C reduction may obviate the need for drug therapy or decrease the dose of statin required to achieve goal. Plant stanol capsules are probably less effective unless consumed with a meal containing fat.

Soy Protein

Soy protein has been demonstrated and approved by the FDA to have an effect on lowering cholesterol in patients who consume at least 25 g of soy protein daily. The FDA concluded that the effect of soy products

Table 3.10. Summary of American Heart Association (AHA) and National Cholesterol Education Program Adult Treatment Panel III (NCEP ATP III) Nutrition Recommendations

Dietary recommendation	Details
Exclusionary	Saturated fatty acids: <7% total kcals[a]
	Cholesterol: <300 mg/day in general healthy population[b]; <200 mg/day in those with multiple risk factors or documented disease[a]
	Trans fat: should be classified as saturated fat[c]
	Salt: <6 g/day; sodium: <2.4 g/day[c]
Intermediate	Polyunsaturated fatty acids: up to 10% total kcals[a]
	Total fat: <30% of total kcals; 25–35% of total kcals[c]
	Balance total calories to achieve or maintain a desirable body weight[a]
	Alcohol: 0–1 drinks/day for women and 0–2 drinks/day for men[c]
Inclusive	Monounsaturated fatty acids: up to 20% total kcals[c]
	Omega-3 fatty acids from fish or vegetable oils: approximately 900 mg/day[c]; >2 servings of fish/week[b]
	Folate: 400–1,000 µg/day[c]
	Potassium: approximately 2,000 mg/day via diet[c]
	Calcium: intake for general health[c]
	Antioxidant rich foods, fruits, vegetables, and grains[b]
	Soy protein: approximately 25 g/day via food sources; to replace animal protein[c]
	Soluble fiber: 10–25 g/day[c]
	Stanols/sterols: 2–3 g/day[c]
	Dietary fiber: >25 g/day; 20–30 g/day[c]

[a]Recommendations are identical for both AHA and NCEP ATP III.
[b]Recommendations from the AHA.
[c]Recommendations from NCEP ATP III.
Note: Exclusionary refers to recommendations that involve the exclusion or restriction of a food or food components; intermediate refers to recommendations that do not fully fit the definition of inclusive or exclusionary; and inclusive refers to recommendations that involve inclusion of foods or food components.

on blood lipids is due to the protein component and not necessarily the isoflavones, such as genistein and daidzen. Isoflavones are often sold as dietary supplements, and the data supporting their hypocholesterolemic effects are not as convincing as the total soy protein. Isoflavones, which are phytoestrogens, have also been touted to reduce hot flashes in postmenopausal women and improve bone density, but conclusive data are lacking.

To reach 25 g of soy protein daily is challenging because food products containing adequate amounts of soy protein are not widely available or require an acquired taste.

Nuts

Several observational studies have suggested that the frequent consumption of nuts may be protective against CHD. Nuts, due to their high fat content, have been perceived as unhealthy foods. However, five large prospective cohort trials [The Adventist Health Study, the Iowa Women's Health Study, the Nurses' Health Study, the Physician's Health Study, and the Cholesterol and Recurrent Events (CARE) Study] have consistently found an inverse association between nut consumption and the risk of CHD (Table 3.11 and Fig. 3.7). Several studies have also shown that nuts, especially walnuts and almonds, lower LDL-C. The potential benefits of nuts on CHD risk underscore the importance of distinguishing different types of fat. Most fats in nuts are mono- or polyunsaturated fats that lower LDL-C (Table 3.12). Nuts also reduce the glycemic load of the diet and, therefore, may reduce insulin secretion and improve satiety. Nuts are also rich in the amino acid arginine, which is the precursor of nitric oxide that promotes vasodilation. Therefore, nuts may represent a reasonable snack food, as opposed to candy bars or other high simple carbohydrate foods, as part of a total diet low in saturated fat and cholesterol.

DIETARY SUPPLEMENTS

The 1994 Dietary Supplement Health and Education Act (DSHEA) defines *dietary supplement* as any product (other than tobacco) intended for ingestion as a supplement to the diet that contains the following ingredients: vitamins, minerals, amino acids, herbs, botanicals, concentrates, metabolites, constituents, and extracts of these substances. More than 100 million Americans (over 50% of the U.S. population) report using dietary supplements, and it is estimated that more than $17 billion dollars in the United States and $43 billion dollars worldwide are spent on them each year (Fig. 3.8). Most people are under the impression that these supplements offer health benefits and are closely regulated to ensure safety and efficacy. Unfortunately, however, the DSHEA allows for the promotion of dietary supplements without FDA review. Therefore, the FDA is not responsible for approving supplement ingredients or products before marketing. It is only after a dietary supplement is marketed that the FDA has the responsibility to show that the product is unsafe and take action to restrict its use. The manufacturers of dietary supplements are, thus, held directly accountable for product safety and label accuracy; they cannot make the health claim that a product is intended to diagnose, treat, cure, or even prevent disease. With a myriad of dietary supplements available over the counter, it is important to evaluate their efficacy and safety (Table

Table 3.11 Review of Prospective Cohort Studies on Nut Consumption and Risk of Coronary Heart Disease (CHD)

Author	Study	Sample	No. yr of follow-up	No. CHD cases	Main results
Fraser et al.	The Adventist Health Study	31,208 men and women, white	6 (1977–1982)	134 nonfatal MI and 463 fatal CHD	Multivariate RR = 0.52 for nonfatal MI and 0.62 for fatal CHD Comparison: ≥5 times/wk vs. <1/wk
Fraser et al.	The Adventist Health Study	1,668 men and women, black	9 (1977–1985)	153 deaths due to all causes	Multivariate RR = 0.60 Comparison: ≥5 times/wk vs. <1/wk
Prineas et al.	Iowa Women's Health Study	41,837 women, white	5 (1986–1990)	154 fatal CHD	Multivariate RR = 0.43 Comparison: 2–4 times/wk vs. 0/wk
Kushi et al.	Iowa Women's Health Study	34,486 women, white	7 (1986–1992)	242 fatal CHD	Multivariate RR = 0.60 Comparison: >4 times/wk vs. 0/wk
Hu et al.	Nurses' Health Study	86,016 women, white	14 (1980–1994)	861 nonfatal MI and 394 fatal CHD	Multivariate RR = 0.65 for total CHD, 0.61 for fatal CHD, and 0.68 for nonfatal MI Comparison: ≥5 times/wk vs. almost never
Albert et al., unpublished data	Physicians' Health Study	22,071 men, white	11	449 cardiac deaths, 122 sudden deaths	Inverse linear relationship between nut consumption and total and sudden cardiac death (RRs not provided)
Brown et al., unpublished data	CARE study	3,575 with existing MI	4.2	323 recurrent MIs	Multivariate RR ≥0.75 Comparison: ≥2 times/wk vs. never or less than once a month

CARE, Cholesterol and Recurrent Events; MI, myocardial infarction; RR, relative risk.

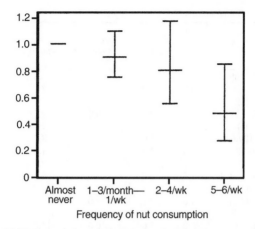

Figure 3.7. Multivariate relative risk of cardiovascular heart disease according to frequency of nut consumption among nonsmokers and occasional or nondrinkers (one drink per week or less) in the Nurses' Health Study. Adjusted for: age (5-year category); time period (7 periods); body mass index (five categories); history of hypertension; history of diabetes; history of hypercholesterolemia; menopausal status (premenopausal, postmenopausal without hormone replacement), postmenopausal with past hormone replacement, postmenopausal with current hormone replacement; parental history of myocardial infarction before 60 years of age; multiple vitamin use; aspirin use (nonuser, one to six tablets per week, seven+ per wk, and dose unknown); vigorous exercise once a week or more; and total energy intake.

3.13). There is strong scientific evidence supporting the use of plant sterols/stanols, omega-3 fatty acids, niacin, folate, vitamin B_6/B_{12}, and tree nuts. There is potential evidence with soy protein, tea extracts, policosanol, guggulipids, coenzyme Q10, and L-arginine. There has been a lack of evidence with garlic and antioxidants.

Dietary Supplements Supported by the National Cholesterol Education Program Adult Treatment Panel III

Omega-3 Fatty Acids

The omega-3 fatty acids, eicosapentaenoic acid (EPA) and docosahexanoic acid (DHA), are found predominantly in fatty fish (salmon, tuna, mackerel, sardines, and herring) and fish oils. Dietary intake of omega-3 fatty acids reduces plasma concentrations of triglycerides by decreasing hepatic secretion of VLDL and by increasing chylomicron catabolism. Either fatty fish consumption or gelatin capsules contain-

Table 3.12. Fat Composition of Nuts[a]

	Total fat (g)	Saturated fat (g)	Monoun-saturated fat (g)	Polyun-saturated fat (g)	Ratio of unsaturated to saturated fat (g)
Almonds (~24 nuts)	14.5	1.5	10.0	3.0	8.7
Brazil nuts (8 medium nuts)	19.0	5.0	7.0	7.0	2.8
Cashews (18 medium nuts)	13.0	2.5	8.0	2.5	4.2
Hazelnuts (~12 nuts)	18.0	1.0	15.0	2.0	17.0
Macadamia (~12 nuts)	20.0	2.5	16.5	1.0	7.0
Peanuts (~35 pieces)	13.5	2.0	7.0	4.5	5.8
Pecans (~15 halves)	19.0	2.0	12.0	5.0	8.5
Pistachios (~47 nuts)	14.0	2.0	8.0	4.0	6.0
Walnuts, English (~14 halves)	18.0	2.0	5.0	11.0	8.0
Average	16.6	2.3	9.8	4.4	6.2

[a]All values for dried or dry-roasted nuts.
Adapted from Dreher, et al. (1996).

ing EPA and DHA have been shown to significantly lower triglyceride levels with variable effects on LDL and HDL. Many trials have linked fish consumption with a decrease in CHD risk in both primary and secondary prevention trials. The Diet and Reinfarction trial (DART)

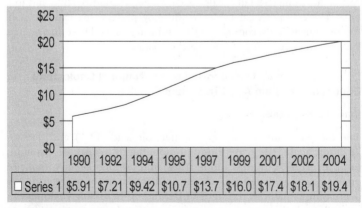

	1990	1992	1994	1995	1997	1999	2001	2002	2004
☐ Series 1	$5.91	$7.21	$9.42	$10.7	$13.7	$16.0	$17.4	$18.1	$19.4

Figure 3.8. Dollars spent on dietary supplements.

Table 3.13. Scientific Evidence for Dietary Supplements

Supported by the National Cholesterol Education Program Adult Treatment Panel III
  Plant sterols/stanols
  Omega-3 fatty acids
  Niacin
  Folate, vitamin B_6, vitamin B_{12}
  Tree nuts
Potential evidence
  Soy protein/isoflavone
  Tea extracts
  Policosanol
  Guggulipid
  Coenzyme Q10
  L-Arginine
Lack of evidence
  Antioxidants/vitamin E
  Garlic

found a fish diet superior to a high-fiber and low-fat diet in reducing cardiovascular events in patients with CHD. Fish oil concentrates have been found to decrease morbidity and mortality. Several of these studies used supplements containing long-chain omega-3 fatty acids (EPA and DHA) at doses ranging from 850 mg to 2.9 g per day. Other studies have shown that higher doses (3 to 4 g per day) provided as supplements can reduce plasma triglyceride levels in patients with HTG.

The largest clinical trial, the Italian Gruppo Italiano Per lo Studio Della Streptokinase Nell'Infarto Miocardio (GISSI) Prevention trial, administered fish oil supplements to 2,836 patients with preexisting coronary disease compared to 2,828 patients receiving placebo. The group who received the fish oil supplements (1 g per day of omega-3 fatty acids, 70% DHA) had a 14% reduction in total deaths and a 17% reduction in cardiovascular deaths. Based on the results of the GISSI trial, the American Heart Association has included eating more fish or supplementing the diet with 1 g of omega-3 fatty acids per day as part of its secondary prevention guidelines.

Omega-3 fatty acid capsules can be combined with statins to further lower triglycerides in patients with combined hyperlipidemia. The combination of a statin plus omega-3 fatty acids may be used to treat combined hyperlipidemia because other combination therapies, such as a statin/fibrate or statin/niacin, have a higher incidence of side effects. However, omega-3 fatty acids are not as potent at lowering triglycerides as niacin or fibrates and do not raise HDL.

Generally, 2 to 3 g of pure EPA or DHA, or both, is necessary to lower triglycerides by 30% or more, but lower doses used chronically may lower triglycerides by 10% to 20%. The side effects of high-dose fish oil include nausea, abdominal bloating, flatulence, and a fishy aftertaste.

Niacin

Nicotinic acid or niacin is a soluble B vitamin that has favorable effects on all of the lipid subfractions. Niacin lowers the hepatic production of VLDL and LDL through the reduction of apolipoprotein B secretion. It increases HDL by reducing the hepatic uptake of apolipoprotein AI, which delays HDL catabolism. Niacin also lowers lipoprotein(a) and fibrinogen levels. Niacin is the most potent drug to raise HDL and the only known approved lipid-altering drug (with the exception of estrogen) that lowers lipoprotein(a). On average, niacin lowers LDL by 10% to 20%, triglycerides by 20% to 40%, and lipoprotein(a) by 10% to 30% and raises HDL by 15% to 30%.

Niacin has been proven to raise HDL-C and lower triglycerides at low doses (500 to 1,000 mg per day). It decreases LDL modestly at higher doses (1,000 to 3,000 mg per day). Slo-Niacin is the only over-the-counter, sustained-release niacin that has been tested in clinical trials. Niacin independently has been demonstrated to reduce cardio-vascular morbidity and mortality. Clinical trials have demonstrated a reduction in atherosclerotic development if used in conjunction with a statin. Moreover, niacin is effective in patients with hypercholesterol-emia and in combined hyperlipidemia associated with normal and low levels of HDL cholesterol.

The use of niacin is often limited by poor tolerability. The most common side effect is cutaneous flushing and pruritus. Flushing can be effectively reduced by instructing the patient to take niacin with a meal and avoid concomitant intake of alcohol, spicy food, and hot liquids. Daily aspirin can reduce the flushing and pruritus. Taking one package of supplements in the morning with breakfast and the second packet in the evening with dinner can also minimize the potential for a niacin flush. Niacin can precipitate gout through ele-vated uric acid levels; it can also worsen insulin resistance and raise plasma homocysteine levels. Niacin should be discontinued if liver enzymes (serum glutamic-oxaloacetic transaminase and serum glutamic-pyruvic transaminase) exceed three times the upper limit of normal. Many over-the-counter niacin supplements may not be labeled as sus-tained release, but if niacin is combined with a fiber, such as oat or rice bran, this can cause a sustained release and adversely affect the liver enzymes.

To make nicotinic acid therapy more tolerable, researchers have studied the effect of several synthetic prodrug esters of nicotinic acid in humans, albeit with discouraging results. It was hoped that these intact esters would be absorbed into the bloodstream and then slowly hydrolyze, releasing enough free nicotinic acid to reduce lipid levels without causing flushing. One such ester is inositol hexaniacinate, a chemical containing six molecules of nicotinic acid esterified to one molecule of the inositol. Although treatment with inositol hexaniacinate showed promising lipid-lowering effects in a rabbit model of hyperlipidemia, this agent has little, if any, effect on lipid levels in humans. No randomized, placebo-controlled trials have shown the efficacy of inositol hexaniacinate in lowering lipid levels, and several studies suggest the treatment has no effect on lipoprotein levels. Nicotinamide does not cause flushing but has no lipid effects.

In 1998, the FDA approved the first extended-release prescription form of nicotinic acid for the treatment of dyslipidemia—Niaspan (Kos Pharmaceuticals, Miami, FL). This formulation has proven to be safe and effective in several patient populations, including those with type 2 diabetes. Niaspan appears as effective as immediate-release niacin on a gram-for-gram basis, with fewer flushing episodes.

A more successful strategy for improving the tolerability of nicotinic acid has come with the development of sustained-release formulations, which appear to cause less flushing and have higher adherence rates than immediate-release niacin. However, several sustained-release niacin preparations have been shown to be more hepatotoxic than immediate-release niacin, and the use of some preparations has resulted in fulminant hepatic failure. Because of this danger, the use of over-the-counter sustained-release niacin should be limited to products that have been objectively shown to be safe and effective.

Folic Acid and Vitamins B_6 and B_{12}

Studies have shown that elevated homocysteine levels are a risk factor for cardiovascular disease. Homocysteine causes endothelial injury and dysfunction, leading to thrombosis. The normal metabolism of homocysteine requires an adequate supply of folate, vitamin B_6, vitamin B_{12}, and riboflavin (Fig. 3.9). Folic acid, vitamin B_6, and vitamin B_{12} lower homocysteine levels and have been shown to reduce endothelial dys-

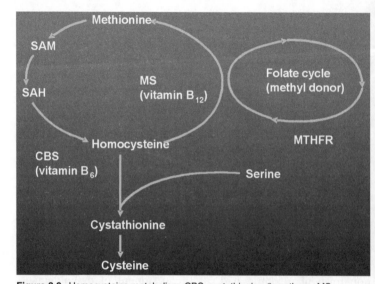

Figure 3.9. Homocysteine metabolism. CBS, cystathionine β-synthase; MS, methionine synthase; MTHFR, methylene tetrahydrofolate reductase; SAH, *S*-adenosyl homocysteine; SAM, *S*-adenosyl methionine. (From Fallest-Strobl, et al. *Am Fam Physician* 1997;56:1607, with permission.)

function. A metaanalysis study showed that as much as 10% of coronary artery disease risk was attributed to hyperhomocystinemia. An increase in homocysteine of 5 μmol per L could increase coronary risk similar to an increase of 20 mg per dL in serum cholesterol. The most effective therapy for lowering homocysteine is the administration of folate (1 to 2 mg daily). In addition, supplemental therapy should include pyridoxine (10 to 25 mg daily) and vitamin B_{12} (400 μg orally daily).

Dietary Supplements with Potential Evidence of Health Benefits

Tea Extracts/Flavonoids

Flavonoids are chemicals found in plants and act as potent antioxidants. In the human diet, they are mostly consumed in both green and black tea. They are also found in grape juice and wine. There is emerging evidence that tea may reduce the risk of CHD. Three observational trials, the Zutphen Elderly Study, the Boston Area Health Study, and the Scottish Heart Healthy Study, all found significant reductions in cardiovascular events among the heaviest tea consumers. In the Zutphen Elderly Study, a prospective study of 806 men aged 65 to 84 years, catechin intake (which belongs to the flavonoid family) was inversely associated with ischemic heart disease mortality; the multivariate-adjusted risk ratio in the highest tertile of intake was 0.49. In the Boston Health Study, one cup of tea per day was associated with a 44% reduction in MI risk compared to non-tea drinkers. Grape juice has also been shown to reduce LDL oxidation, improve endothelial function, and reduce platelet aggregability. Therefore, increasing flavonoid intake via tea, grape juice, or wine may reduce LDL oxidation and platelet aggregation, which may potentially reduce CHD risk.

Policosanol

Policosanol is a mixture of fatty alcohols (octacosanol, hexacosanol, and triacontanol) derived from the wax of honeybees. Policosanol reduces cholesterol and platelet aggregation and is believed to inhibit the oxidation of LDL. Efficacy and safety have been proven in a few clinical trials. In a randomized, double-blind study, the efficacy and tolerability of policosanol at doses of 20 mg per day and 40 mg per day were compared with placebo. After 24 weeks, policosanol at 20 and 40 mg per day lowered LDL cholesterol by 27.4% and 28.1%, respectively, whereas total cholesterol was reduced by 15.6% and 17.3%, respectively. HDL was increased by 17.6% in the 20-mg-per-day and 17% in the 40-mg-per-day policosanol groups. There were no significant changes in the placebo group. In a double-blind, multicenter, placebo-controlled trial, the effects of policosanol were measured in menopausal women. Patients were randomized to receive placebo or policosanol, 5 mg per day, for 8 weeks, and the dose was doubled to 20 mg per day for the next 8 weeks. Policosanol (5 and 10 mg per day) decreased LDL cholesterol by 17.3% and 26.7%, respectively. HDL levels were raised by 7.4% at study completion.

Guggulipid/Guggul/Commiphora Mukul

Guggul is a botanical extract found in India from the mukul myrrh tree (*Commiphora mukul*). Guggul extract isolates the ketonic steroid compounds from the plant. A number of small studies have shown guggul to lower cholesterol and triglycerides. Guggulipid lowers VLDL cholesterol and LDL cholesterol while elevating HDL cholesterol. The mechanism of action is thought to be through the increased liver metabolism of LDL. It is also believed to inhibit platelet aggregation and to act as an antioxidant. In a double-blind, placebo-controlled study of guggul, 61 patients were followed for 24 weeks. The guggulipid subjects (25 mg three times per day) had an 11.7% reduction in total cholesterol, 12.7% decrease in LDL, and 12% decrease in triglycerides. In another recent double-blind trial in 100 patients, guggulipid, at a standard and high dose, did not lower LDL compared to placebo. Safety of use beyond 6 months has not been studied.

Coenzyme Q10 (Ubiquinone)

Coenzyme Q10, or ubiquinone, is a potent antioxidant that is produced during the synthesis of cholesterol. Controlled clinical trials conducted in Europe and Japan support the contention that coenzyme Q10 might improve congestive heart failure. However, two recent studies—one from Australia and the other from the University of Maryland—found that, compared with placebo, coenzyme Q10 did not improve morbidity or mortality. Although the data are limited, there is a theoretical benefit of coenzyme Q10 (50 to 60 mg per day) in reducing the risk of myopathy associated with statins. Statins, by inhibiting the hepatic synthesis of cholesterol, reduce plasma ubiquinone levels. The statin-induced decrease in ubiquinone levels is considered one of the potential causes of muscle toxicity (myopathy) associated with statin use. Coenzyme Q10 might be justified to enhance the safety of statin therapy. Currently, the American Heart Association does not recommend using antioxidant vitamin supplementation until more complete data are available.

L-Arginine

L-Arginine is the substrate for nitric oxide production. It is converted to nitric oxide by nitric oxide synthase in the endothelial cells. Endothelium dysfunction could be attributed to L-arginine deficiency. This hypothesis has led some to believe that L-arginine deficiency leads to coronary artery disease. Dietary supplement with L-arginine has been shown to improve endothelial function. A medical food bar enriched with L-arginine (Heart Bar) has been tested in placebo-controlled trials for claudication and demonstrated a beneficial improvement in walking time. Most published human studies are small. Larger, well-designed studies are needed before L-arginine can be recommended.

Dietary Supplements with a Lack of Evidence of Health Benefits

Antioxidants/Vitamin E

Vitamin E occurs in at least eight naturally occurring compounds, with alpha-tocopherol being the most active compound. A large body of experimental evidence supports the hypothesis that oxidation of LDL plays an important role in the process of atherosclerosis. In several mouse studies, antioxidants, such as vitamin E, have been effective in reducing atherosclerosis. However, the results of antioxidant trials to prevent CHD have been mixed, with most being disappointing.

The beneficial effects of vitamin E supplementation have been demonstrated in the Nurse's Health Study. This large prospective study with up to 8 years of follow-up demonstrated that women given vitamin E supplements (median dose, 208 IU per day) had a lower risk of coronary artery disease. Large, double-blind, placebo-controlled trials such as the Cambridge Heart Antioxidant Study (CHAOS) have also shown that vitamin E supplementation is a safe and economical mechanism for reducing the risk of coronary artery disease. In the CHAOS study, 400 to 800 IU of vitamin E alone in more than 1,000 patients with documented CHD resulted in a 47% reduction in cardiovascular events.

Conversely, the three largest trials with vitamin E—the GISSI, the Canadian Heart Outcome Prevention Evaluation Study, and the Heart Protection Study—have all shown that, although there were no adverse effects of vitamin E, daily supplementation had no effect on cardiovascular outcomes. The Heart Protection Study, consisting of 20,536 UK adults 40 to 80 years old, demonstrated no benefit with vitamin E, C, or betacarotene. Moreover, the antioxidant vitamins studied did not appreciably modify the effects of simvastatin on plasma lipid concentrations or on vascular disease outcomes. The role of vitamin E or other antioxidants for the treatment of atherosclerosis remains uncertain.

Garlic

Garlic is ranked as the top herbal product used in the United States. The intact garlic bulb contains an odorless amino acid, alliin, which is converted enzymatically to allicin when the garlic cloves are crushed. Allicin is responsible for the characteristic odor of fresh garlic and is believed to be the component that exerts the cholesterol-lowering effect. A metaanalysis of selected trials found that garlic tablets reduced serum cholesterol concentrations by approximately 9%. How-

Table 3.14. Nutritional Intervention Trial: Expected Outcomes

Active compounds	Low-density lipoprotein	High-density lipoprotein	Triglycerides	Homocysteine
Plant sterols	5% to 15%	+0% to +3%	NC	NC
Niacin	NC	+5% to +10%	−0% to 10%	NC
Omega-3 fatty acids	NC	+0% to +5%	−10% to 20%	NC
Folic acid, vitamins B_6 and B_{12}	NC	NC	NC	−10% to 20%

NC, no change.

ever, many of the trials did not perform standard laboratory measurements and did not control or monitor dietary compliance. One study randomized 50 patients with hypercholesterolemia to placebo or garlic powder (300 mg orally three times per day). After a 12-month follow-up, there were no significant changes in lipids or lipoprotein concentrations in either group. The best placebo-controlled trials with garlic have failed to demonstrate a cholesterol-lowering effect.

Conclusions

Although the individual effects of the various dietary supplements may provide only modest benefit, in combination, certain supplements may provide significant risk factor modification (Table 3.14). Even though DSHEA allows for the promotion of dietary supplements without FDA review, it is important for consumers to realize that some of these products may not be efficacious and some may be harmful. Consumers who decide to use dietary supplements should do so with care, making sure they have the necessary information. Only through scientific evidence can a dietary supplement be deemed safe and efficacious. Dietary supplements should only be recommended if they fulfill at least one of the following criteria: (a) proven clinical trial evidence demonstrating the beneficial effects on cardiovascular risk factors; (b) clinically proven evidence to reduce cardiovascular events (MI, total CVD, or strokes); or (c) national guidelines recommending the nutritional product to reduce the risk of CVD.

SELECTED READING

Alpha-Tocopherol, Beta Carotene Cancer Prevention Study Group. The effect of vitamin E and beta carotene on the incidence of lung cancer and other cancers in male smokers. *N Engl J Med* 1994;330:1029–1035.

Albert CM, Hennekens CH, O'Donnell CJ, et al. Fish consumption and risk of sudden cardiac death. *JAMA* 1998;279:23–28.

Anderson JW. Dietary fibre, complex carbohydrate and coronary artery disease. *Can J Cardiol* 1995;11[Suppl G]:55G–62G.

Appel LJ, Moore FJ, Obarzanek E, et al. A clinical trial of the effects of dietary patterns on blood pressure. *N Engl J Med* 1997;336;1117–1124.

Blackburn H. The public health view of the diet and mass hyperlipidemia. *Cardiovasc Rev Rep* 1990;11:25–32.

Clinical guidelines on the identification, evaluation, and treatment of overweight and obesity in adults: the evidence report. *Obes Res* 1998;6[Suppl]:51S–210S.

Clinical guidelines on the identification, evaluation and treatment of overweight and obesity in adults: the evidence report. Bethesda, MD: National Heart, Lung and Blood Institute, 1998: NIH publication 98-4083.

Course JR III, Morgan T, Terry JG, et al. A randomized trial comparing the effects of soy protein containing varying amounts of isoflavones on plasma concentrations of lipids and lipoproteins. *Arch Intern Med* 1999;159:2070–2076.

Criqui MH. Alcohol in the myocardial infarction patient. *Lancet* 1998;352:1873 [letter].

Davidson MH, Dugan LD, Burns JH, et al. The hypocholesterolemic effects of beta-glucan in oatmeal and oat bran: a dose-controlled study. *JAMA* 1991;265:1833–1839.

DeBusk RM. Dietary supplements and cardiovascular disease. *Curr Atheroscler Rep* 2000;2:508–514.

Devaraj S, Jialal I. Antioxidants and vitamins to reduce cardiovascular disease. *Curr Atheroscler Rep* 2000;2:342–351.

Ginsberg HN, Kris-Etherton P, Dennis B, et al., for the Delta Research Group. Effects of reducing dietary saturated fatty acids on plasma lipids and lipoproteins in healthy subjects. The Delta Study, Protocol 1. *Arterioscler Thromb Vasc Biol* 1998;18:441–449.

GISSI-Prevenzione Investigators. Dietary supplementation with n-3 polyunsaturated fatty acids and vitamin E after myocardial infarction: results of the GISSI-Prevenzione trial. *Lancet* 1999;534:447–455.

Grundy SM. Comparison of monounsaturated fatty acids and carbohydrates for lowering plasma cholesterol. *N Engl J Med* 1986;314:745–748.

Grundy SM, Barrett-Connor E, Rudel LL, et al. Workshop on the impact of dietary cholesterol on plasma lipoproteins and atherogenesis. *Arteriosclerosis* 1988;8:95–101.

Hasler CM, Kundrat S, Wool D. Functional foods and cardiovascular disease. *Curr Atheroscler Rep* 2000;2:467–475.

Hennekens CH, Buring JE, Manson JE, et al. Lack of effect of long-term supplementation with beta-carotene on the incidence of malignant neoplasms and cardiovascular disease. *N Engl J Med* 1996;334:1145–1149.

HOPE (The Heart Outcomes Prevention Evaluation Study Investigators). Vitamin E supplementation and cardiovascular events in high-risk patients. *N Engl J Med* 2000;342:154–160.

Hopkins PN. Effects of dietary cholesterol: a meta-analysis and review. *Am J Clin Nutr* 1992;55:1060–1070.

Jones PH. Diet and pharmacologic therapy of obesity to modify atherosclerosis. *Curr Atheroscler Rep* 2000;2:314–320.

Keebler ME, De Souza C, Fonseca V. Diagnosis and treatment of hyperhomocysteinemia. *Curr Atheroscler Rep* 2000;3:54–63.

Keys A, Aravanis C, Blackburn H. *Seven countries: a multivariate analysis on death and coronary heart disease.* Cambridge, MA: Harvard University Press, 1980;132.

Kris-Etherton PM, Person TA, Wan Y, et al. High-monounsaturated fatty acid diets lower both plasma cholesterol and triacylglycerol concentrations. *Am J Clin Nutr* 1999;70:1009–1015.

Kromhout D, Bloemberg BPM, Feskens EJM, et al. Alcohol, fish, fibre and antioxidant vitamin intake do not explain population differences in coronary heart disease mortality. *Int J Epidemiol* 1996:25: 753–759.

Kromhout D, Coulander CDL. Diet, prevalence, and 10-year mortality from coronary heart disease in 871 middle-aged men: the Zutphen Study. *Am J Epidemiol* 1984;119:733–741.

Kromhout D, Menotti A, Bloemberg B, et al. Dietary saturated and trans fatty acids and cholesterol and 25-year mortality from coronary heart disease: The Seven Countries Study. *Prev Med* 1995;24: 308–315.

Law MR. Plant sterol and stanol margarines and health. *West J Med* 2000;173:43–47.

Nestel P. Effects of fish oils and fish on cardiovascular disease. *Curr Atheroscler Rep* 2000;3:68–73.

Rimm E. Alcohol and cardiovascular disease. *Curr Atheroscler Rep* 2000; 2:529–535.

Sirtori CR, Lovati MR. Soy proteins and cardiovascular disease. *Curr Atheroscler Rep* 2000;3:47–53.

Stampfer MJ, Hennekens CH, Manson JE, et al. Vitamin E consumption and the risk of coronary disease in women. *N Engl J Med* 1993;328:1444–1449.

Van Horn L, Liu K, Parker D, et al. Serum lipid response to oat product intake with a fat modified diet. *JADA* 1986;86:759–776.

Chapter 4

Drug Therapy for Dyslipidemia

Lipid-lowering drugs are among the most prescribed medications in the world, with more than 20 million people prescribed this class of drugs. Since the U.S. Food and Drug Administration (FDA) approval of lovastatin in 1987, statins have been the most widely used for the treatment of dyslipidemia to reduce the risk of cardiovascular disease. There has been considerable debate in the medical community regarding the clinical significance of the potential differences between the drugs in this class. Statins are structural inhibitors of 3-hydroxy-3-methylglutaryl coenzyme A (HMG-CoA) reductase, the rate-limiting enzyme for hepatic cholesterol biosynthesis resulting in the upregulation of the low-density lipoprotein (LDL) receptor and the lowering of LDL cholesterol (LDL-C) in the blood. Therefore, all statins share a similar structure (the *pharmaphore*) that inhibits the enzyme. The fungally derived statins (lovastatin, simvastatin, and pravastatin) have other structural similarities, and the synthetic statins (cerivastatin, fluvastatin, atorvastatin, rosuvastatin, and pravastatin) also have clinical structures in common (Fig. 4.1). Therefore, classifying statins as fungal metabolites (natural statins) versus synthetic statins has, historically, been a way to differentiate the two types. Another classification involves defining statins by their solubility in octanol (lipophilicity) or water (hydrophilicity). Pravastatin, rosuvastatin, and, to a much lesser degree, fluvastatin, are considered hydrophilic statins, and the other statins are considered lipophilic statins (Fig. 4.2). This chapter highlights the clinical significance of the differences between the statins and how these differences may affect patient care. Other

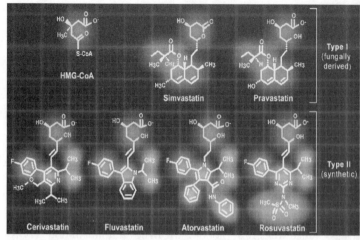

Figure 4.1. Two-dimensional chemical structures of statins. HMG-CoA, 3-hydroxy-3-methylglutaryl coenzyme A. (Reprinted with permission from Istvan and Deisenhofer.)

widely used lipid-altering drugs include fibrates, niacin, and intestinally active drugs, such as ezetimibe and colesevelam. This chapter also focuses on the clinical difference between the other lipid-altering drugs and the impact on patient outcomes.

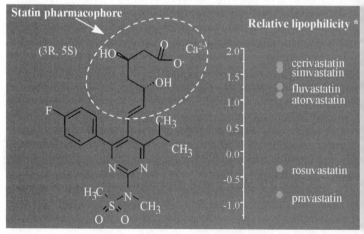

Figure 4.2. Properties of rosuvastatin. *Log D at pH 7.4. (From Davidson MH, Toth PP. *Prog Cardiovas Dis* 2004;47:73–104, with permission.)

STATINS

Statins have clinically relevant differences in efficacy, pharmacokinetics, and safety profiles. However, much attention regarding differences in the statin class of drugs has focused on the pleiotropic or non–lipid-mediated effects. Virtually all cells possess the mevalonate pathway that is affected by statin therapy. It is not surprising, therefore, that the influence of statins may not be limited to the cardiovascular system. In addition to cholesterol, the mevalonate pathway leads to the formation of dolichols; ubiquinones involved in election transport; and isoprenoids, which take part in the posttranslational modification of many proteins, including those needed for cell proliferation, and has an essential role in lipoprotein synthesis. Although a wide range of pleiotropic effects, such as vasodilation; antithrombosis, antioxidant, antiproliferative, and antiinflammatory effects; and plaque stabilization, have been reported for statins, the difficulty is to determine which have clinical and practical relevance beyond those associated with lipoprotein changes. In addition, at the present time, little is known regarding whether these effects are dose-dependent, which part of the molecular structure they can be attributed to, and to what extent they contribute to clinical outcomes independent of reduction in the known coronary artery disease risk factors. The arguments in favor of pleiotropic effects for statins that may influence outcomes include the early separation of the survival curves in the placebo and treatment groups in the Scandinavian Simvastatin Survival Study (4S), West of Scotland Coronary Prevention Study (WOSCOPS), Air Force/Texas Coronary Atherosclerosis Prevention Study (AFCAPS/TexCAPS), and Heart Protection Study (HPS) trials that is difficult to explain on the basis of changes in atheromatous plaque burden alone. In addition, in the Myocardial Ischemia Reduction with Acute Cholesterol Lowering (MIRACL) trial, atorvastatin, 80 mg, was associated with a significant decrease in the rehospitalization rate for ischemia in patients with unstable angina within 16 weeks. Positron emission tomography scanning has demonstrated that myocardial perfusion can be improved within as little as 90 days in patients with hypercholesterolemia after short-term aggressive lipid-lowering with a statin combined with cholestyramine and dietary management. In the WOSCOPS trial, the Framingham risk equation predicted very closely the observed risk reduction; however, in the pravastatin-treated cohort, there was a lower rate than predicted (24% predicted vs. 35% achieved).

Similarly, post-hoc overlap analysis of WOSCOPS indicated that patients who had achieved similar on-treatment LDL-C levels with pravastatin had a lower coronary heart disease (CHD) event rate than those

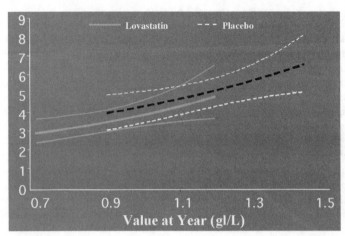

Figure 4.3. Relation of year 1 apolipoprotein B with acute major coronary events (with 95% confidence interval). Logistical regression models adjusted for age, sex, marital status, hypertension, smoking, and family history. (From Gotto AM Jr, et al. *Circulation* 2000;101:477–484, with permission.)

who received placebo (6.3% vs. 9.6%; a 36% difference). This suggested some added effects, or pleiotropic effects, of statins that may reduce events. Because the Framingham equation does not include triglycerides (TGs) or use apolipoprotein B (Apo B), the possibility exists that at least part of this added benefit may be due to the statins' effects on lowering TGs. The predominant benefits of statins on CHD risk reduction are due to their effects on LDL, but the effects that statins have on TGs and HDL may also contribute to the risk reduction. In the 4S and AFCAPS/TexCAPS trial, Apo B, rather than LDL, was a better predictor of event reduction (Figs. 4.3 and 4.4). Because Apo B is contained in LDL, intermediate-density lipoprotein, and very-low-density lipoprotein (VLDL) [or the non–high-density lipoprotein (HDL)], the statin impact on the TG-containing intermediate-density lipoprotein and VLDL may contribute to the risk-modifying benefits. The AFCAPS/TexCAPS trial also demonstrates that the best overall predictor of events on treatment is Apo B/Apo AI, which supports the concept that raising HDL (the Apo AI–containing particles) also contributes to risk reduction. Therefore, the lipid changes appear to explain all the expected outcome benefits of statin therapy. In fact, all the major statin trials are remarkably consistent in that the LDL reduction correlates with the event reduction in a linear fashion (Fig. 4.5). Although statins have demonstrated pleiotropic effects,

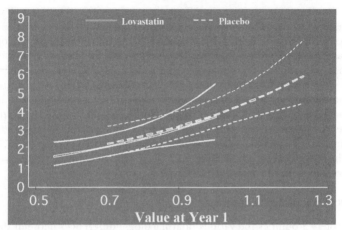

Figure 4.4. Relation of year 1 apolipoprotein B/A1 with acute major coronary events (with 95% confidence interval). Logistical regression models adjusted for age, sex, marital status, hypertension, smoking, and family history. (From Gotto AM Jr, et al. *Circulation* 2000;101:477–484, with permission.)

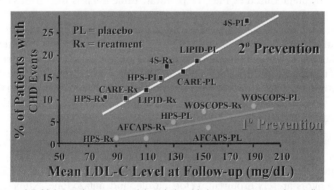

Figure 4.5. Major statin outcome trials: relationship between coronary heart disease (CHD) and low-density lipoprotein cholesterol (LDL-C). 4S, Scandinavian Simvastatin Survival Study; AFCAPS, Air Force Coronary Atherosclerosis Prevention Study; CARE, Cholesterol and Related Events; HPS, Heart Protection Study; LIPID, Long-term Intervention with Pravastatin in Ischaemic Disease; WOSCOPS, West of Scotland Coronary Prevention Study. (From Yusuf S, et al. *Circulation* 1996;93:1774–1776, with permission.)

these effects do not appear to differentiate statins within the class itself as multiple statins, both fungal metabolites and synthetic or hydrophilic and lipophilic, have been shown to reduce CHD events in a similar fashion based on their efficacy in modifying lipoproteins. In addition, nonstatin therapies, such as fibrates and niacin, reduce CHD events to a similar degree as statins with less potent effects on reducing LDL-C. One of the most important clinical trials to refute a special benefit of statin beyond the lipid changes is the Program on the Surgical Control of the Hyperlipidemias (POSCH) trial, which demonstrated that partial ileal bypass surgery, which lowered LDL by 38%, reduced major CHD events by 35%. This surgical treatment for lowering LDL was almost identical to statins in lowering LDL and decreasing CHD events (Table 4.1).

Pharmacologic Differences

Table 4.2 outlines the various pharmacologic differences between the statins. Table 4.3 lists the important drug interactions.

Lovastatin, simvastatin, and atorvastatin are metabolized via the cytochrome P450 3A4 (CYP3A4) pathway. Fluvastatin is metabolized by the CYP2C9 pathway, and cerivastatin is metabolized by dual CYP2C9 (or 2C8) and 3A4 pathways. Pravastatin and rosuvastatin are not significantly metabolized by the CYP pathway. Table 4.4 lists the various CYP isoenzymes known to oxidize clinically used drugs. This table illustrates the wide variety of potential drug interactions that may occur with statins that are metabolized by the CYP3A4 pathway. Pharmacokinetic clinical trials have documented that, if concomitantly used, two drugs that are both metabolized via the CYP3A4 pathway compete for the pathway, resulting in increased serum concentrations for both drugs.

Potent CYP3A4 Inhibitors

In addition to cyclosporine, drugs that significantly inhibit the CYP3A4 pathway are of most concern regarding combination therapy with lovastatin, simvastatin, and atorvastatin. The most commonly used CYP3A4 inhibitors are erythromycin, ketoconazole, and nefazodone. Numerous case reports have described the development of rhabdomyolysis when lovastatin was combined with erythromycin. Erythromycin alone can cause QT prolongation. Therefore, special caution should be considered for patients with a history of arrhythmias when combining a CYP3A4 statin with erythromycin. Erythromycin also affects the metabolism of calcium channel blockers that use the CYP3A4 pathway (i.e., felodipine, nisoldipine, and nifedipine). Patients should be monitored carefully and the

Table 4.1. Outcomes Studies of Statin Medications

Study	Design	Patient characteristics	Treatment groups	Results
Primary prevention				
Air Force/Texas Coronary Atherosclerosis Prevention Study (AFCAPS/TexCAPS)	Multicenter, double-blind, placebo-controlled; 5.6-yr follow-up	6,605 men and women; LDL, 151 mg/dL; age, 58 yr	Diet with placebo or lovastatin, 20–40 mg/day	36% reduction in first major coronary event; 33% reduction in PTCA and CABG
West of Scotland Coronary Prevention Study (WOSCOPS)	Multicenter, double-blind, placebo-controlled; 5-yr follow-up	6,595 men; no history of MI; LDL, 192 mg/dL; age, 55 yr	Diet with placebo or pravastatin, 40 mg/day	30% reduction in nonfatal MI or CHD death; 22% reduction in death from any cause
Secondary prevention				
Scandinavian Simvastatin Survival Study (4S)	Multicenter, double-blind, placebo-controlled; 5.4-yr follow-up	4,444 men and women; angina or previous MI; cholesterol 261 mg/dL; LDL 187 mg/dL; age 60 yr	Diet with placebo or simvastatin, 40 mg/day	Reduction in total mortality; 34% reduction in fatal/nonfatal MI and sudden cardiac death; 37% reduction in any coronary event
Anglo-Scandinavian Cardiac Outcomes Trial—Lipid Lowering Arm (ASCOT-LLA)	Multicenter, double-blind, placebo-controlled; 3.36-year follow-up	10,305 men and women; ≥3 additional CV risk factors, no h/o CHD; median LDL, 131 mg/dL; median age, 63 yr	Diet with placebo or atorvastatin, 10 mg/day	36% reduction in nonfatal MI and fatal CHD; 27% reduction in fatal and nonfatal stroke; 21% reduction in total cardiovascular events; 29% reduction in total coronary events

continued

Table 4.1. *Continued*

Study	Design	Patient characteristics	Treatment groups	Results
Cholesterol and Related Events (CARE)	Multicenter, double-blind, placebo-controlled; 5-yr follow-up	4,159 men and women; previous MI; mean LDL, 139 mg/dL; age, 59 yr	Diet with placebo or pravastatin, 40 mg/day	
Heart Protection Study (HPS)	Multicenter, double-blind, placebo-controlled; 5-yr follow-up	20,536 adults; coronary disease, other occlusive arterial disease, diabetes, or hypertension	Diet with placebo or simvastatin, 40 mg/day	
Long-term Intervention with Pravastatin in Ischaemic Disease (LIPID)	Multicenter, double-blind, placebo-controlled; 6.1-yr follow-up	9,014 men and women; angina or previous MI; median LDL, 150 mg/dL; age, 62 yr	Diet with placebo or pravastatin, 40 mg/day	

CABG, coronary artery bypass grafting; CHD, coronary heart disease; CV, cardiovascular; h/o, history of; LDL, low-density lipoprotein; MI, myocardial infarction; PTCA, percutaneous transluminal coronary angioplasty.

Table 4.2. Summary of the Comparative Pharmacokinetics of Statins in Healthy Volunteers

Variable	Atorvastatin	Fluvastatin	Lovastatin	Pravastatin	Rosuvastatin	Simvastatin
Prodrug	No	No	Yes	No	No	Yes
Lipophilicity (logP)	4.06	3.24	4.30	−0.23	−0.33	4.68
Affinity for Pgp transporter	Yes	No	Yes	Yes	No	Yes
t_{max} (h)	1.0–2.0	0.5–1.0	2.0–4.0	1.0–1.5	3.0–5.0	1.3–3.0
Absorption (%)	30	98	30–31	34	40–60	60–80
Hepatic first-pass metabolism (%)	20–30	40–70	40–70	50–70	50–70	50–80
Bioavailability (%)	12–14	29	<5	18	20	<5
Protein binding (%)	>98	>98	>95	43–54	88	95
Major metabolic enzyme	CYP3A4	CYP2C9	CYP3A4	Enzymatic and nonenzymatic	Minimal CYP450	CYP3A4
Systemic active metabolites (no.)	Yes (2)	No	Yes (3)	No	Minimal	Yes (3)
Renal excretion(%)	≤2	<6	≥10	20	10	13
$t_{1/2}$ (h)	14–15	3.0	2.0	2.0	20	1.4–3.0

CYP450, cytochrome P450; Pgp, P-glycoprotein; t_{max}, time of maximum circulating concentration; $t_{1/2}$, half-life.

Table 4.3. Clinically Relevant Statin Drug Interactions

Drug	Atorvastatin	Fluvastatin	Lovastatin	Pravastatin	Rosuvastatin	Simvastatin
Azole antifungals	+	–	+	–	–	+
CCBs	–	–	+	–	–	+
Cyclosporine	+	–	+	+	+	+
Erythromycin	+	–	+	–	–	+
Gemfibrozil	NA	–	+	+	+	+
Fenofibrate	NA	NA	NA	–	–	–
HIV PIs	+	–	+	–	–	+
Warfarin	+	+	+	+	+	+

+, interaction reported; –, no interaction reported; CCB, calcium channel blocker (i.e., diltiazem, verapamil); HIV, human immunodeficiency virus; PI, protease inhibitor; NA, not available.

Table 4.4. Human Cytochrome P450 (CYP) Isoenzymes Known to Oxidize Clinically Used Drugs

CYP2C9	CYP2C19	CYP2D6	CYP3A4
Alprenolol	Diazepam	Amitriptyline	**Atorvastatin**
Diclofenac	Ibuprofen	Bufarol	**Cerivastatin**
Fluvastatin	Mephenytoin	Codeine	Cyclosporine
Hexobarbital	Methylphenobarbital	Debrisoquine	Erythromycin
N-desmethyl-diazepam	Omeprazole	Desipramine	Felodipine
Tolbutamide	Proguanil	Dextromethorphan	Lidocaine
Warfarin	Phenytoin	Encainide	**Lovastatin**
		Flecainide	Mibefradil
		Imipramine	Midazolam
		Metoprolol	Nifedipine
		Nortriptyline	Quinidine
		Perhexiline	**Simvastatin**
		Perphenazine	Terbinafine
		Propafenone	Triazolam
		Propanolol	Verapamil
		Sparteine	Warfarin
		Thioridazine	
		Timolol	

Note: Statins in bold.

dosage of calcium channel blocker decreased if necessary when erythromycin is added. Concern should be especially heightened if a patient is also taking a CYP3A4 statin. If a short course of macrolide antibiotics is required, the safest strategy for patients taking a CYP3A4 statin is that treatment should be suspended for the duration of the antibiotic treatment. Alternatively, azithromycin, which does not significantly affect the CYP3A4 pathway, can be considered, especially if several courses of antimicrobial therapy are contemplated. Erythromycin does not appear to significantly affect the pharmacokinetics of pravastatin, fluvastatin, or rosuvastatin. Similar drug interactions may exist with ketoconazole and itraconazole, and there have been a number of reports of myopathy when these antifungals have been combined with lovastatin. Neither pravastatin nor rosuvastatin appears to affect itraconazole levels. Fluconazole does not inhibit the CYP3A4 pathway and can be a safer alternative to combine with lovastatin, simvastatin, or atorvastatin, if necessary.

The antidepressant drugs fluoxetine, fluvoxamine, nefazodone, and sertraline also inhibit CYP3A4 statins and should be used cautiously with the CYP3A4 statins. There have been two reports of nefazodone combined with simvastatin causing myopathy. Alternatives for the treatment of depression are paroxetine and venlafaxine, which do not inhibit the CYP3A4 pathway.

The protease inhibitors (indinavir, nelfinavir, ritonavir, and saquinavir) inhibit CYP3A4 metabolism. These drugs also may induce dyslipidemia. There are few data regarding the coadministration of these drugs with CYP3A4 statins; thus, caution is required. Until more data are available, pravastatin, rosuvastatin, and fluvastatin are the preferred statins to initiate in patients taking protease inhibitors. Indinavir appears to be a less potent inhibitor of CYP3A4 and may be the option to consider if initiating a protease inhibitor to patients taking a CYP3A4 statin. Amiodarone appears to be a potent CYP3A4 inhibitor and, therefore, should be used with caution for patients taking these statins. With simvastatin, 80 mg, in combination with amiodarone, the myopathy rate was 6% (vs. 0.06% overall). For patients taking amiodarone, the dose of simvastatin should not exceed 20 mg.

Calcium Channel Blockers

Calcium channel blockers are the most common chronic drugs used in combination with statins. Mibefradil, a novel calcium channel blocker, is a strong inhibitor of CYP3A4 and was removed from the market after several cases of rhabdomyolysis when combined with simvastatin. However, other calcium channel blockers are substrates and, therefore, weak inhibitors of CYP3A4 metabolism. Concomitant use of diltiazem and simvastatin does cause modest increases in serum concentrations for both drugs. Alternatively, pravastatin does not impact diltiazem pharmacokinetics. Despite the effects of calcium channel blockers on CYP3A4 statin pharmacokinetics, there is little evidence of clinically significant drug interactions. Post-marketing adverse experiences and data from mega-trials do not raise concern regarding the concomitant use of calcium channel blockers and CYP3A4 statins. In the 4S and ongoing HPS trials, there were only rare cases of myopathy reported, including a large number of patients taking calcium channel blockers. In the HPS, there were more than 3,000 patients taking calcium channel blockers at randomization and more than 10,000 patients in the simvastatin-treated cohort. Of the two cases of myopathy while taking simvastatin (compared with one with placebo), 40 mg, neither patient was on a calcium channel blocker (one patient's myopathy was apparently precipitated by erythromycin). However, in the Study of the Effectiveness of Additional Reductions in Cholesterol and Homocysteine (SEARCH) trial with 80 mg of simvastatin, 0.6% of patients taking verapamil developed myopathy compared to 0.06% (a tenfold increase) for patients not on calcium channel blockers. These data support the safe use of CYP3A4 statins up to the 40-mg dose. However, for patients taking 80 mg of a CYP3A4 metabolized statin, caution is necessary and use with calcium channel blockers and other CYP3A4-substrated drugs should be avoided if possible.

Conjugated estrogen is also metabolized via CYP3A4 but has not been associated with a higher incidence of myopathy when combined with CYP3A4 statins. However, when combining multiple CYP3A4 drugs together with a CYP3A4 statin, caution is advised. For example, an elderly female on diltiazem, hormone replacement therapy, and fluoxetine may be at increased risk for myopathy if simvastatin or atorvastatin is initiated or the dose is escalated.

Grapefruit Juice

Fresh or frozen grapefruit inhibits intestinal CYP3A4 but appears to have minimal effects on hepatic CYP3A4. Therefore, grapefruit juice (at least 200 mL) can increase serum concentrations of numerous CYP3A4 substrate drugs that undergo intestinal first-pass metabolism via this enzyme. Grapefruit juice was reported to significantly increase serum concentrations of the calcium channel blocker felodipine and simvastatin. Neither pravastatin nor rosuvastatin pharmacokinetics are affected by grapefruit juice. The primary substance responsible for inhibition was identified *in vitro* to be a furanocoumarin compound widely found in nature—6,7-dihydroxybergamuttin. This inhibitory substance is less potent than known CYP3A4 inhibitors such as ketoconazole, and published reports of myopathy due to grapefruit juice and CYP3A4 statins are lacking. Nevertheless, it is probably advisable to separate by 2 hours the dosing of CYP3A4 statins and consumption of grapefruit juice. Orange juice, which lacks 6,7-dihydroxybergamuttin, does not inhibit CYP3A4. Little is known about the effects of other citrus fruits on CYP enzymes.

Warfarin

Warfarin is given as a racemic mixture. The relatively weak anticoagulant R-warfarin is metabolized primarily by CYP1A2, and the more potent S-warfarin is metabolized by CYP2C9. The protein binding of the various statins may affect warfarin levels by mutual displacement from plasma protein-binding sites, but these effects are not mediated by the CYP enzymes and are generally not clinically significant. All statins are listed in the *Physicians' Desk Reference* as drugs that may affect the international normalized ratio for patients on warfarin. Atorvastatin did not significantly affect prothrombin time for patients in the preapproval clinical development program, but a formal interaction clinical trial has not been reported.

Cyclosporine

Cyclosporine is metabolized via the CYP3A4 pathway. Although substrates are not inhibitors of the CYP3A4 pathway, statins such as lovastatin, simvastatin, and atorvastatin may significantly increase cyclosporine levels, and cyclosporine may markedly increase statin levels. Cyclosporine is an inhibitor of both the CYP3A4 metabolic pathway and the intestinal P-glycoprotein drug efflux pump system. Cyclosporine appears to significantly increase the area under the curve (AUC) for all statins, including pravastatin and rosuvastatin (Fig. 4.6). This suggests another mechanism by which cyclosporine significantly increases statin blood levels. *In vitro* studies with cells transfected with the hepatic influx organic anion transporter C have demonstrated that cyclosporine competitively inhibits rosuvastatin uptake of these cells. All statins are ligands for this transporter. Inhibition of this transporter by cyclosporine may make an important contribution to the cyclosporine-statin interaction. Numerous cases of myopathy have been reported with cyclosporine and statin combination therapy. The frequency of myopathy with this combination is perhaps higher than anticipated based on CYP metabolism alone. Pravastatin and fluvastatin (which is metabo-

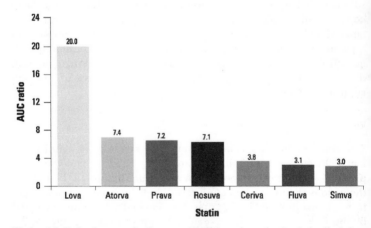

Figure 4.6. Ratio of area under the curve (AUC) in cyclosporine-treated patients to AUC in historical control patients. (From Davidson MH, Toth PP. *Prog Cardiovas Dis* 2004;47:73–104, with permission.)

lized via CYP2C9) are believed to have a lower propensity for myopathy in cyclosporine-treated patients. However, Gruer et al. compared the incidence of myopathy, myositis, and rhabdomyolysis in patients taking cyclosporine and simvastatin or pravastatin in a report with the FDA. Although not a controlled trial, the proportional concomitant use ratio of serious muscle abnormalities was similar for both simvastatin and pravastatin. These data may be biased against pravastatin because of the more frequent use of this statin in posttransplant patients. Nevertheless, pravastatin must also be used cautiously in patients taking cyclosporine. The safety of combining low dosages of simvastatin (10 mg per day) and pravastatin with cyclosporine has been documented in controlled trials, but these trials, due to the intensive monitoring of laboratory data, may underestimate the propensity for significant adverse drug reactions. Fluvastatin has been studied in post–renal transplant patients taking concomitant cyclosporine. In these controlled studies, there was an absence of reports of myopathy or rhabdomyolysis. In the Assessment of Lescol in Renal Transplant (ALERT) trial, approximately 2,000 post–renal transplant patients taking cyclosporine were randomized to fluvastatin or placebo. None of the approximately 1,000 patients taking concomitant fluvastatin and cyclosporine has developed significant myositis. Therefore, fluvastatin may be the preferred statin in posttransplant patients. In regards to statin interaction with fibrates, there appear to be significant differences between gemfibrozil and fenofibrate. Gemfibrozil inhibits the glucuronidation of statins by uridine diphosphate–glucuronosyltransferase (UGT 1A1, UGT A3), which promotes this clearance or lactonization to inactive forms. Fenofibrate appears to be a weaker inhibitor of glucuronidation of statins than gemfibrozil (Fig. 4.7). This difference appears to explain the statin interaction profile of gemfibrozil compared to fenofibrate. Gemfibrozil increases the AUC of all the statins evaluated (atorvastatin has not been evaluated). However, fenofibrate does not significantly increase the AUC of simvastatin, cerivastatin, pravastatin, or rosuvastatin.

Clinically Relevant Differences Among the Statins

Table 4.5 lists the labeled indications for the statins, and Table 4.1 lists the statin outcome trials. An objective synthesis of all the available statin data that includes efficacy, safety, pharmacokinetic interactions, and outcome trials can provide potential differentiating factors of each statin and the clinical relevance of these differences.

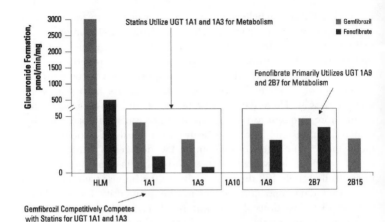

Figure 4.7. The glucuronidation of the fibrate fenofibrate utilizes a different family of enzymes than the glucuronidation of the fibrate gemfibrozil. Gemfibrozil utilizes the same enzymes as most statins. (From Davidson MH, Toth PP. *Prog Cardiovas Dis* 2004; 47:73–104, with permission.)

Lovastatin

Lovastatin is a short-half-life prodrug that is lipophilic and metabolized by the CYP3A4 pathway. The immediate-release formulation should be administered with a meal, but the extended-release formulation (Altocor) can be administered apart from food. Lovastatin has proven outcome benefits in primary prevention, as demonstrated in the AFCAPS/TexCAPS trial. Lovastatin is the only generic statin in the United States until 2006, when pravastatin and simvastatin go off patent. Therefore, if cost is an overriding issue for a patient, generic lovastatin would most likely provide the greatest LDL reduction (up to the limit of an approximately 40% decrease) for the cost.

Pravastatin

Pravastatin is a short-half-life hydrophilic statin that is not affected by food intake. It is available at doses of 10 to 80 mg and provides LDL reductions of 25% to 40%. Pravastatin has the best profile among the statins in regards to outcome trials. It has shown cardiovascular benefits in patients with coronary disease [Cholesterol and Related Events (CARE) and Long-Term Intervention with Pravastatin in Ischaemic Disease (LIPID)], in high-risk primary prevention (WOSCOPS), and in the elderly [Prospective Study of Pravastatin in the Elderly at Risk (PROSPER)].

Table 4.5. HMG-CoA Reductase Inhibitor U.S. Food and Drug Administration–Approved Indications

Indication	HMG-CoA reductase inhibitors					
	Atorvastatin (Lipitor)	Fluvastatin (Lescol/XL)	Lovastatin (Altocor/Mevacor)	Pravastatin (Pravachol)	Rosuvastatin (Crestor)	Simvastatin (Zocor)
Primary hypercholesterolemia	√[a]	√[a]	√[a]	√[a]	√[a]	√[a]
Mixed dyslipidemia	√[b]	√[b]	—	√[b]	√[b]	√[b]
Hypertriglyceridemia	√[c]	—	—	√[c]	√[c]	√[c]
Primary dysbetalipoproteinemia	√[d]	—	—	√[d]	—	√[d]
Homozygous familial hyperlipidemia	√	—	—	—	√	√
Primary prevention coronary events	—	—	√	√	—	—
Secondary prevention cardiovascular event(s)	—	√	√	√	—	√

HMG-CoA, 3-hydroxy-3-methylglutaryl coenzyme A.
[a]Includes heterozygous familial and nonfamilial hypercholesterolemia.
[b]Includes Fredrickson types IIa and IIb.
[c]Includes Fredrickson type IV.
[d]Includes Fredrickson type III.

Simvastatin

Simvastatin is a short-half-life prodrug. It is lipophilic and metabolized by CYP3A4. The drug may be administered without regard to food. Simvastatin, at doses of 5 to 80 mg, provides LDL reductions of 25% to 50%. For patients taking potent CYP3A4 inhibitors gemfibrozil or cyclosporine, the dose should not exceed 10 mg per day. For patients taking verapamil or amiodarone (less potent CYP3A4 inhibitors), the dose of simvastatin should not exceed 20 mg per day. Simvastatin is the only statin to show a reduction in total mortality in both the 4S and HPS trials. Based on these outcome trials, simvastatin, 40 mg, is an approved starting dose for all high-risk patients (including diabetic patients) regardless of the baseline LDL level, and this is a unique indication among all the statins.

Fluvastatin

Fluvastatin is a short-half-life synthetic, racemic mixture metabolized by CYP2C9. A new modified-release formulation of fluvastatin, 80 mg fluvastatin XL, provides enhanced efficacy and safety compared to the immediate-release dose. Because fluvastatin is metabolized by 2C9, there are significantly less drug interactions, except for fluconazole (a 2C9 inhibitor) and warfarin. Fluvastatin XL, 80 mg, lowers LDL by approximately 35%, which is similar to atorvastatin, 10 mg, or simvastatin, 20 mg, with a reduced cost. Fluvastatin is the only statin that has been shown not to be affected by gemfibrozil and, therefore, is probably the statin of choice to combine with this fibrate. Although fluvastatin is probably affected by concomitant cyclosporine, in the ALERT trial, post–renal transplant patients had a reduced incidence of cardiovascular events while taking fluvastatin, and no patients developed rhabdomyolysis. Therefore, the ALERT trial indicates that for post–renal transplant patients on cyclosporine, fluvastatin is probably the statin of choice.

Atorvastatin

Atorvastatin is a long-half-life lipophilic statin that is metabolized by CYP3A4. Atorvastatin at doses of 10 to 80 mg is the leading prescribed statin in the world, providing LDL reduction at 38% to 55%. Although the usual cautionary drug interactions exist for atorvastatin similar to other CYP3A4-metabolized statins, atorvastatin, in the clinical trial program, has an extremely low rate of myopathy. In almost 10,000 patients on atorvastatin, there have been no cases of myopathy (creatine phosphokinase greater than ten times the upper limits of normal with symptoms). The 80-mg atorvastatin dose has an incidence of liver enzyme three times the upper limits of normal of approximately 2.5%, which is the highest of all the statins, but a low incidence of 0.5% for all the other doses. The Anglo-Scandinavian Cardiac Outcomes Trial (ASCOT) showed the benefits of atorvastatin, 10 mg, in hypertensive patients, and the CARDS trial demonstrated a benefit in diabetic patients.

Rosuvastatin

Rosuvastatin is the most recent FDA-approved statin (doses, 5 to 40 mg) for the treatment of dyslipidemia. Rosuvastatin, which has a structure similar to other synthetic statins (Fig. 4.1), has a long half-life (20 to 24 hours) similar to atorvastatin and hydrophilicity comparable to pravastatin. Consequently, rosuvastatin is minimally metabolized and has no significant CYP drug interactions. The efficacy of rosuvastatin is superior to that of other statins (Fig. 4.8). Compared to atorvastatin, rosuvastatin provides approximately 8% additional lowering of LDL on an equivalent dose level. This provides modestly more efficacy than a doubling of the dose of atorvastatin. Rosuvastatin also increases HDL slightly more than atorvastatin, especially at the highest doses (Fig. 4.9).

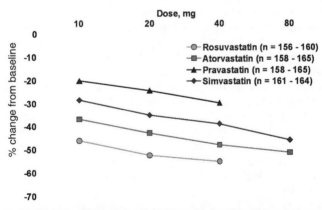

Figure 4.8. Trial 65—STELLAR (week 6). Rosuvastatin, 10 to 40 mg, versus comparators: percent low-density lipoprotein cholesterol change from baseline. *P* <.001 vs. comparators on a mg-to-mg basis. Data presented as means. (From Jones P, et al. *Am J Cardiol* 2003;92:152–160, with permission.)

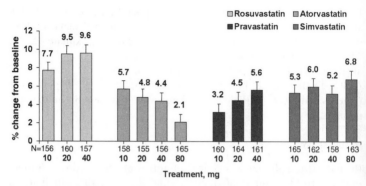

Figure 4.9. Trial 65—STELLAR (week 6). Rosuvastatin (RSV), 10 to 40 mg, versus comparators: percent high-density lipoprotein cholesterol change from baseline. *P* <.002 RS, 10 mg, vs. pravastatin (PRA), 10 mg. *P* <.002 RSV, 20 mg, vs. atorvastatin (ATV), 20 mg, 40 mg, 80 mg; PRA, 20 mg, 40 mg; simvastatin (SIM), 40 mg. *P* <.002 RSV, 40 mg, vs. ATV, 40 mg, 80 mg; PRA, 40 mg; SIM, 40 mg. Data presented as Least square means ± standard error. (From Jones P, et al. *Am J Cardiol* 2003;92:152–160, with permission.)

The safety of rosuvastatin at doses of 5 to 10 mg is comparable to other statins in regards to liver function abnormalities and myopathy rates, especially considering the efficacy of LDL reduction (Figs. 4.10 and 4.11). Proteinuria, as determined by urine dipstick, was also noted in 12% of patients taking the 80-mg dose. After an extensive accumulation of safety data on the 40-mg dose, the FDA approved rosuvastatin at the dose range of 5 to 40 mg. The proteinuria at the 40-mg dose of rosuvastatin does not appear to be significantly different than the comparator statins. For patients with dyslipidemia, titration to the 40-mg dose should be restricted to patients who are not at goal while taking the 20-mg dose. The starting dose range is 5 to 20 mg, in which the usual starting dose is 10 mg, but 5 mg should be considered for patients on potentially interacting drugs such as gemfibrozil and cyclosporin or with moderate to severe renal impairment (creatinine greater than 20 mg per dL), and the 20-mg starting dose should be considered for high-risk patients who require more than a 50% reduction in LDL.

The lack of CYP for rosuvastatin allows this therapy to be used without precautions in patients who are taking CYP3A4-inhibiting drugs, such as amiodarone, verapamil, or ketoconazole. As compared to gemfibrozil, rosuvastatin has been shown not to have a pharmacokinetic

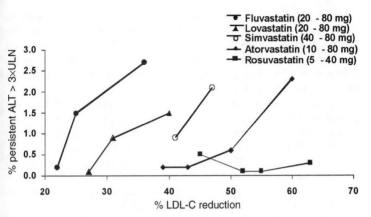

Figure 4.10. Relative safety of the statins based on frequency of alanine aminotransferase (ALT) greater than three times the upper limits of normal (ULN) by percent low-density lipoprotein cholesterol (LDL-C) reduction. (From Davidson MH. *Am J Cardiol* 2004;93(Suppl):3C–11C, with permission.)

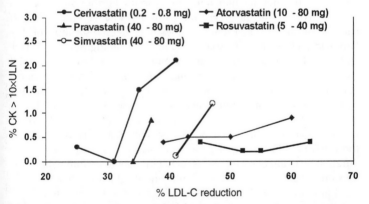

Figure 4.11. Relative safety of the statins based on frequency of creatine phosphokinase (CK) greater than ten times the upper limits of normal (ULN) by percent low-density lipoprotein cholesterol (LDL-C) reduction. (From Davidson MH. *Am J Cardiol* 2004;93(Suppl):3C–11C, with permission.)

interaction with fenofibrate. Therefore, the usual caution regarding the concomitant use of statin and fibrates may not apply without the combination of rosuvastatin and fenofibrate. Both gemfibrozil and cyclosporin significantly increase the AUC for rosuvastatin. In combination with these drugs, rosuvastatin should be initiated at the 5-mg dose and should not exceed 10 mg.

The flexible starting dose of rosuvastatin (5 to 20 mg), which is flat priced, provides an efficacious alternative to dose titration for other statins to achieve the National Cholesterol Education Program Adult Treatment Panel (NCEP ATP III) goals. In clinical practice, the dose titration of statins is underutilized and physicians are reluctant to titrate to the highest statin dose. Rosuvastatin, by providing increased efficacy at the usual starting dose, may obviate the need for more frequent dose titration to achieve the NCEP ATP III goals.

EZETIMIBE

Ezetimibe (Zetia) is the first of a new class of lipid-lowering drugs known as *cholesterol absorption inhibitors*. Ezetimibe localizes at the brush border of the small intestine and selectively inhibits the absorption of cholesterol from the intestinal lumen into enterocytes. Further investigation is needed to determine the precise mechanism by which ezetimibe inhibits cholesterol absorption. Ezetimibe does not affect absorption of TGs, fatty acids, bile acids, or fat-soluble vitamins, including vitamins A, D, E, and α- and β-carotenes. After oral administration, ezetimibe is rapidly glucuronidated in the intestines, and, once glucuronidated, it undergoes enterohepatic recirculation, thereby repeatedly delivering the drug to its site of action and minimizing systemic exposure. Notably, the glucuronide of ezetimibe is even more potent as a cholesterol absorption inhibitor than the parent compound, possibly due to its localization in the intestines. The enterohepatic recirculation may explain the long duration of action of ezetimibe; as such, its long elimination half-life permits once-daily dosing. Both ezetimibe and its glucuronide are recirculated enterohepatically and delivered back to the site of action in the intestine, resulting in multiple peaks of drug, accounting for a half-life of approximately 22 hours. The timing of dosing does not affect its activity, and food does not affect its bioavailability.

In animal models, ezetimibe decreased delivery of cholesterol from the intestine to the liver, reduced hepatic cholesterol stores, upregulated LDL-C receptors on liver cell membranes, and increased clearance of cholesterol from blood. In a 2-week, double-blind, placebo-controlled, crossover study of 18 hypercholesterolemic patients, ezetimibe, 10 mg once daily, inhibited intestinal cholesterol absorption by 54%, as compared with placebo (P <.001). Although hepatic cholesterol synthesis increased with ezetimibe, plasma LDL-C was reduced by 20% relative to placebo (P <.001).

Ezetimibe does not interact with drugs metabolized by CYP1A2, -2D6, -2C8, -2C9, or -3A4, suggesting that it has low potential for participating in drug–drug interactions. Importantly, ezetimibe does not interact with statins, including atorvastatin, simvastatin, lovastatin, and fluvastatin. Accordingly, ezetimibe can be taken at the same time as the statin during coadministration therapy. Moreover, clinically significant interactions were not observed when ezetimibe was administered in conjunction with caffeine, dextromethorphan, midazolam, tolbutamide, antacid, cimetidine, oral contraceptives, warfarin, digoxin, or glipizide. Concomitant administration of fenofibrate (200 mg once daily) increased the mean maximum plasma concentration and area under the time-versus-plasma concentration curve for total ezetimibe by approximately 64% and 48%, respectively; however, these effects were not clinically significant. The pharmacokinetics of fenofibrate were not significantly affected by ezetimibe (10 mg once daily). Thus, its pharmacokinetic profile and novel mechanism of action make ezetimibe an ideal drug for use in combination therapy for hypercholesterolemia.

Efficacy of Ezetimibe

Ezetimibe Monotherapy

Monotherapy with ezetimibe has been shown to effectively reduce LDL-C in patients with hypercholesterolemia. In two randomized, placebo-controlled phase III trials of 892 and 827 patients, 12 weeks of once-daily treatment with ezetimibe, 10 mg, decreased LDL-C by 17.7% and 18.2%, respectively, compared with placebo (P <.01), and increased HDL cholesterol by 1.3% and 1.0%, respectively, versus decreases of 1.6% and 1.3%, respectively, with placebo (all P <.01).

Ezetimibe Plus Statin Coadministration Therapy

Ezetimibe was coadministered with a statin in four randomized, double-blind, placebo-controlled, multicenter studies of patients with primary hypercholesterolemia. After patients were stabilized on the NCEP Step I diet (or stricter) and discontinued all previous lipid-lowering therapy, they entered a 4-week, single-blind, placebo run-in period. Patients with baseline LDL-C levels between 145 mg per dL

(3.35 mmol per L) and 250 mg per dL (6.48 mmol per L) and TGs less than or equal to 350 mg per dL (3.99 mmol per L) were then randomly assigned to daily treatment with ezetimibe alone, statin alone, ezetimibe plus statin, or placebo for 12 weeks. Ezetimibe was administered at a dosage of 10 mg once daily, whereas several statin dose levels were evaluated in monotherapy and in coadministration with ezetimibe (atorvastatin and simvastatin: 10 mg, 20 mg, 40 mg, or 80 mg; lovastatin and pravastatin: 10 mg, 20 mg, or 40 mg). In each study, ezetimibe plus statin coadministration was more effective in lowering LDL-C than statin alone (Table 4.6). Notably, the greater efficacy of ezetimibe plus statin coadministration was seen at each statin dose level. Moreover, the coadministration of ezetimibe, 10 mg daily, with the lowest statin dose was as effective as statin monotherapy at the highest dose. For example, calculated LDL-C was equivalently reduced from baseline by ezetimibe, 10 mg, plus simvastatin, 10 mg, and by simvastatin, 80 mg, alone (46% vs. 45%). Similarly, ezetimibe plus atorvastatin, 10 mg, was as effective as atorvastatin, 80 mg, alone (53% vs. 54%); ezetimibe plus lovastatin, 10 mg, was as effective as lovastatin, 40 mg, alone (34% vs. 31%); and ezetimibe plus pravastatin, 10 mg, was as effective at reducing LDL-C as pravastatin, 40 mg, alone (34% vs. 29%, $P <.05$). Coadministration of ezetimibe plus statin (results pooled across doses) was also more effective than statin alone in raising HDL cholesterol (except for ezetimibe plus pravastatin) and reducing TGs and Apo B. Notably, the efficacy of coadministration therapy was not influenced by age, race, gender, or level of CHD risk.

Table 4.6. Percent Changes in Serum Lipids: Ezetimibe Plus Statin Coadministration Therapy versus Statin Monotherapy (Pooled Doses)

	Number of patients	Change in concentration (%)				
		TC	LDL-C	HDL-C	TG	Apo B
Atorvastatin	248	−32	−44	4	−25[b]	−36
+ ezetimibe	255	−41[a]	−56[a]	7[a]	−33[a,b]	−45[a]
Simvastatin	263	−26	−36	7	−17	−30
+ ezetimibe	274	−37[a]	−51[a]	9[a]	−24[a]	−41[a]
Pravastatin	205	−17	−25	7	−8	−20
+ ezetimibe	204	−27[a]	−39[a]	8	−18[a]	−30[a]
Lovastatin	220	−18	−25	4	−11	−21
+ ezetimibe	192	−29[a]	−40[a]	9[a]	−22[a]	−33[a]

Apo B, apolipoprotein B; HDL-C, high-density lipoprotein cholesterol; LDL-C, low-density lipoprotein cholesterol; TC, total cholesterol; TG, triglycerides.
[a]*P <.01 versus statin therapy.*
[b]*Median percent change.*

In a separate study, ezetimibe was added to ongoing statin therapy in primary hypercholesterolemic patients with multiple cardiovascular risk factors or established CHD who did not reach their LDL-C goal with statin monotherapy. These patients had received a stable statin dose for at least 6 weeks and then were randomly assigned to receive concurrent therapy for 8 weeks with ezetimibe, 10 mg, or placebo added to their continuing open-label statin therapy. The addition of ezetimibe was significantly more effective than the addition of placebo in lowering LDL-C (25.1% vs. 3.7%; $P < .001$) and TGs (14.0% vs. 2.9%, $P < .001$) and raising HDL-cholesterol (HDL-C) (2.7% vs. 1.0%, $P < .05$). C-reactive protein (CRP) was also significantly reduced with the coadministration of statin plus ezetimibe compared to statin plus placebo (9.7% vs. 0%, $P < .05$).

Role of Ezetimibe in Dyslipidemic Patients

With the exception of patients with statin intolerance, ezetimibe is most likely to be used in conjunction with statins or other lipid-lowering drugs in a wide variety of patients with dyslipidemia. Statins are generally flat priced above the 10-mg dose, and, thus, there is no cost penalty for titrating the dose of the statin to achieve the NCEP ATP III goals. However, although statins are extremely safe up to doses of 40 mg, the dose titrated from 40 mg to 80 mg is associated with a significant increase in liver function abnormalities and myopathy (.07% to .4% for simvastatin) while only providing an additional 5% to 6% reduction in LDL. As ezetimibe provides an additional 18% to 20% reduction in LDL, with favorable changes in HDL and TGs across the statin dose range safety, the addition of ezetimibe to the 40-mg statin dose appears to provide the best risk-benefit ratio. For patients at high risk for statin side effects, such as the elderly or those taking drugs with pharmacokinetic interactions, adding ezetimibe, 10 mg, to a 10-mg dose of statin would have comparable efficacy to the 80-mg dose of the statin with potentially improved safety.

In addition to the safety and ease of use of combining ezetimibe with a statin, ezetimibe has two unique features as a lipid-altering agent that may provide theoretical benefits. Ezetimibe, by inhibiting intestinal cholesterol and plant sterol absorption, may modify the atherogenicity of the chylomicron remnants, and the reduction in systemic plant sterol levels may reduce cardiovascular risk. Although human plant sterol levels are normally very low, there may be subsets of at-risk populations in which high plant sterol levels significantly increase the risk of CHD. The frequency of modest elevations of plant sterols and the contribution of these particles to atherogenesis is not yet determined, but there are intriguing data indicating that plant sterols contribute to excess CHD risk. As more data become available, these unique benefits may provide a stronger rationale for combining ezetimibe with a statin to further reduce risk in dyslipidemic patients.

NIACIN

Niacin, or nicotinic acid, is a soluble B vitamin that has favorable effects on all major lipid subfractions (Table 4.7) but has not been widely used due to its side-effect profile. Despite the significant lipid-altering effects, pharmaceutical data in the United States have consistently documented that niacin prescriptions are less than 3% of the very large cholesterol drug market. In Europe, the use of niacin is far lower than in the United States. However, the clinical trial data suggest a potentially important role for niacin therapy, and the FDA has approved a modified release (Niacin) that reduces the side-effect profile.

The pharmacokinetics of niacin and its mechanism of action are not well understood, but niacin appears to reduce Apo B secretion, thereby lowering both VLDL and LDL, increasing Apo AI, and lowering lipoprotein(a) [Lp(a)]. On average, niacin lowers LDL by 10% to 20%, TGs by 20% to 40%, and Lp(a) by 10% to 30% and raises HDL by 15% to 30%. Niacin is the only known approved lipid-altering drug (with the exception of estrogen) that lowers Lp(a) and is the most potent drug to raise HDL. Niacin appears to increase HDL by decreasing the hepatic uptake of Apo AI, thereby delaying catabolism. As

Table 4.7. Effects of Niacin

Niacin decreases	Niacin increases
Total cholesterol	HDL-C
Total triglycerides	HDL_2-C
VLDL-C	HDL_3-C (less than HDL_2)
LDL-C	Apo AI, AII
Small dense LDL	LP A-I
Lp(a)	LP A-I + A-II (less than LP A-I)
Apo B	LDL particle size
Total cholesterol/HDL-C	
LDL-C/HDL-C	
Apo B/AI	

Apo, apolipoprotein; HDL-C, high-density lipoprotein cholesterol; LDL-C, low-density lipoprotein cholesterol; Lp(a), lipoprotein(a); VLDL-C, very-low-density lipoprotein cholesterol.
From Kreisberg RA. Am J Med 1994;97:313–316, with permission.

hepatic removal of cholesterol ester is not affected, more efficient reversal cholesterol transport would result because, after unloading the cholesterol ester, the HDL particle containing Apo AI would be able to remove more cholesterol from the peripheral cells.

Niacin can cause significant hepatotoxicity and should be discontinued if liver enzymes (serum glutamic-oxaloacetic transaminase and serum glutamic-pyruvic transaminase) exceed three times the upper limit of normal. Patients who use over-the-counter niacin should worry about the hazard of liver toxicity. Many over-the-counter niacin supplements may not be labeled as sustained release, but, if niacin is combined with a fiber such as oat or rice bran, this can cause a sustained release and adversely affect the liver enzymes. Slo-Niacin is the only over-the-counter sustained-release niacin that has been tested in clinical trials. Patients should generally be advised not to use over-the-counter niacin. Niacin can also increase uric acid levels, aggravating gout. Other side effects of niacin include rash; gastrointestinal problems, including worsening of esophageal reflux and peptic ulcers; and headache. Rarely, skin lesions, usually in the axillary areas or elbows, called *acanthosis nigricans* can develop.

Niacin is often added to a statin in patients with combined hyperlipidemia, especially if the HDL is low or Lp(a) is high. There have been a number of studies that have evaluated the combination of a statin with niacin. The incidence of liver function abnormalities with the combination of a statin plus niacin is generally similar to niacin therapy alone, at least when both drugs in the combination are at the starting doses (i.e., simvastatin, 20 mg; pravastatin, 40 mg; fluvastatin, 40 mg, plus niacin, 1,500 to 2,000 mg per day). Myopathy has been reported with statins plus niacin, but the incidence appears to be less than expected with gemfibrozil. Myopathy has developed with the combination after niacin-induced hepatotoxicity reduces the catabolism of the statin, resulting in markedly elevated statin levels. Therefore, unregulated sustained-release niacins that have a higher incidence of hepatotoxicity should be avoided in combination therapy. The vast majority of combination trials have used either immediate-release niacin or extended-release niacin (Niaspan). In one study, a single tablet containing both extended-release niacin and lovastatin was dose titrated from extended-release niacin, 500 mg, plus lovastatin, 10 mg, to extended-release niacin, 2,000 mg, plus lovastatin, 40 mg, to target levels based on NCEP guidelines over a 16-week period. Once on a stable dose, the patients were followed further for 36 weeks. More than 600 patients were enrolled with LDL levels exceeding the NCEP

ATP II levels for initiating drug therapy. At the 2,000/40 mg dose, LDL was lowered by 47% and TG by 42%, and HDL was increased by 30%. Approximately 7% of patients withdrew as a result of flushing. There were no cases of drug-induced myopathy, and less than 1% had elevated liver enzymes greater than 3 times the upper limit of normal.

Due to the safety data of extended-release niacin in combination with a statin, there has been a resurgence of interest in the use of combination therapy to maximize risk reduction in patients with dyslipidemia. Over the past several years, statins have established a large clinical trial base documenting both safety and outcome benefits. Niacin has also demonstrated CHD outcome benefits either as monotherapy or in combination with other lipid-lowering agents (Table 4.8). The marked reduction in clinical events in the Familial Atherosclerosis Treatment Study and HDL-Atherosclerosis Treatment Study trials (although these were relatively small trials) has provided intriguing data suggesting the importance of combining niacin with other lipid-lowering agents. Statins, in general, have demonstrated a reduction in CHD events of approximately 30%, but, in these small trials combining a statin with niacin, the reduction in CHD events was approximately 75%. This 75% reduction in clinical events by combining a statin with niacin is far more than expected with LDL reduction alone. This marked reduction in CHD events suggests that the other effects of niacin, such as raising HDL and lowering TG and Lp(a), contribute significantly to the benefits. Although the clinical benefits of changing the LDL particle size from small (pattern B) to large (pattern A) are not yet conclusively demonstrated, niacin is one of the most effective agents in modifying LDL particle size, whereas statins are more effective in lowering the total LDL particle numbers.

A subanalysis of the HATS trial demonstrated that statin-niacin therapy significantly increased the large Apo AI–containing α 1 HDL particles. This increase in the larger HDL particles was associated with less progression of coronary stenosis even after adjusting for traditional risk factors (Asztalos B, Batista M, et al. ATVB, 2003). Although statins may also increase larger HDL levels, niacin appears to have the most significant effect on the levels of the large LpA-I particles. These data suggest that niacin was a significant contributor to the benefits of the simvastatin-niacin combination treatment in the regression of atherosclerotic development and CHD event reduction.

The ATP III guidelines, by recommending non-HDL as well as LDL targets if the TGs exceed 200 mg per dL, have also enhanced the need for niacin therapy. Based on a recent evaluation of the safety and pharmacokinetics of statins in combination with fibrates or niacin, an algo-

Table 4.8. Niacin Coronary Heart Disease Endpoint Trials

Study	Population	Results
Coronary Drug Project	8,341 post-MI men Baseline TC, 250 mg/dL—9.9% on trial Baseline TG, 177 mg/dL—26.1% on trial	27% reduction in definite non-fatal MI; 24% reduction in CVA; total mortality decrease, 10.6% at 15 years
Stockholm Ischemia Heart Study	555 consecutive MI survivors <70 yr old; open-label clofibrate/niacin or placebo Baseline TC, 245 mg/dL—13% on trial Baseline TG, 208 mg/dL—19% on trial	36% reduction in CHD deaths
Familial Atherosclerosis Treatment Study	146 men with Apo B ≥125 mg/dL with CHD; conventional therapy vs. niacin/colestipol or lovastatin/colestipol	73% reduction in CHD events in patients who received intensive lipid-lowering therapy
HDL Atherosclerosis Treatment Study (HATS)	160 CHD patients with HDL <35 mg/dL, LDL <145 mg/dL; treated 3 yr with niacin/simvastatin or placebo with or without antioxidants	Reduction of CHD events by 60% (on antioxidants) to 90% (off antioxidants)

CHD, coronary heart disease; CVA, cerebrovascular accident; HDL, high-density lipoprotein; LDL, low-density lipoprotein; MI, myocardial infarction; TC, total cholesterol; TG, triglycerides.

rithm was developed to guide use of appropriate combination treatment if non-HDL goals have not been achieved (Fig. 4.12).

The use of niacin in diabetic patients has, in the past, been considered problematic due to niacin's modest glucose-raising effects. A recent trial and a reevaluation of the Coronary Drug Project (CDP) have provided helpful information on the use of niacin in patients with glucose elevations. A reevaluation of the CDP in the diabetic subpopulation demonstrated a similar reduction in clinical CHD events as in the nondiabetic CHD population. This new information provides support for the use of niacin to treat diabetic dyslipidemia, and, although there may be a modest increase in serum glucose levels, the overall benefit is a marked reduction in cardiovascular events. In the Assessment of Diabetes Control and Evaluation of the Efficacy of Niaspan Trial (ADVENT), 148 patients with type 2 diabetes and dyslipidemia were randomized to

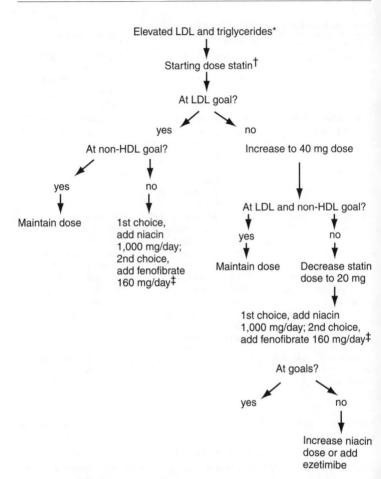

Figure 4.12. Algorithm to maximize safety of lipid-lowering therapy. HDL, high-density lipoprotein; LDL, low-density lipoprotein. *At baseline, check liver function tests, creatine kinase, thyroid profile; document presence of muscle soreness or pain. †U.S. Food and Drug Administration approved starting dose statins: lovastatin, 20, 40 mg; simvastatin, 10, 20, 40 mg; atorvastatin, 10, 20, 40 mg; fluvastatin, 20, 40, 80 mg; pravastatin, 10, 20, 40 mg. ‡Or substitute niacin-ER/lovastatin combination tablet. Alternative options for patients at high risk for statin myopathy include ezetimibe plus niacin or fenofibrate.

extended-release niacin, 1,000 mg per day or 1,500 mg per day, or placebo; 47% of the patients were also taking statins.

In the ADVENT trials, extended-release niacin produced a significant effect on both TG and HDL-C levels. The increase in HDL-C was dose-dependent and was significantly greater at all time points for the niacin-treated groups than for the placebo group. In the 1,000-mg niacin group, HDL-C increased up to 19% at 16 weeks. In the 1,500-mg group, it increased up to 24%. The absolute increases in HDL-C at 16 weeks were 7.6 mg per dL in the 1,000-mg group and 11 mg per dL in the 155-mg group compared with 1.6 mg per dL among placebo-treated patients.

TG reductions were also dose-related. Reductions in the patients receiving lower-dose niacin were not significantly greater than those in placebo-treated patients. TG levels were reduced 28% in the 1,500-mg niacin group at 16 weeks—a significant difference compared with placebo.

Changes in hemoglobin A_{1c} (Hb A_{1c}) levels were small in all treatment groups. Hb A_{1c} values in the 100-mg-per-day treatment group were not significantly different from the placebo group. Changes in Hb A_{1c} levels in the 1,500-mg-per-day group reached marginal significance ($P = .048$) at 16 weeks. Increases in fasting blood glucose occurred between weeks 4 and 8 in the niacin-treated groups; levels returned to baseline by week 16.

ADVENT demonstrated that extended-release niacin, at the doses tested, is effective and well tolerated in patients who have type 2 diabetes and atherogenic dyslipidemia—whether given alone or with a statin. Low doses of extended-release niacin are, therefore, an option for the treatment of dyslipidemia in patients who have type 2 diabetes.

FIBRATES

There are five fibrates currently used in human therapy: clofibrate, gemfibrozil, fenofibrate, bezafibrate, and ciprofibrate. Only gemfibrozil and fenofibrate are available in the United States. Fibrates are peroxisome proliferator–activated receptor-alpha (PPAR-alpha) ligands. PPAR-alpha activated by fibrates form heterodimers with 9-*cis* retinoic acid receptor. The PPAR/9-*cis* retinoic acid receptor heterodimers bind to peroxisome proliferator response elements, upregulating the expression of these genes (Fig. 4.13). PPAR-alpha activation by fibrates leads to the following:

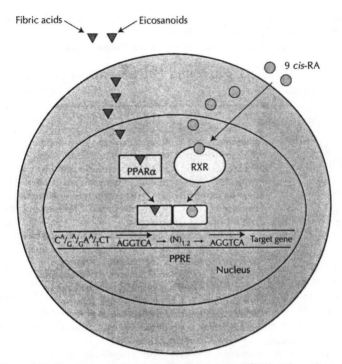

Figure 4.13. Peroxisome proliferator–activated receptor (PPAR)-alpha pathways and their natural (eicosanoids) and synthetic (fibric acids) activators. After activation, PPAR-alpha heterodimerizes with the receptor for 9-*cis* retinoic acid (9 *cis*-RA) (*circles*) and retinoic acid receptor (RXR) and binds to the response elements in the regulatory region of target genes, termed *peroxisome proliferator response elements* (PPRE), which are composed of two degenerate hexanucleotide repeats (*arrows*) arranged in tandem as direct repeats spaced by one or two nucleotides and preceded by an A/T-rich region.

1. Increasing lipoprotein lipase expression and decreasing Apo CIII expression, which results in enhanced catabolism of TG-rich particles.
2. Increased expression of Apo AI and AII. The net result of fibrate therapy is decreased hypertriglyceridemia and an increase in HDL-C. LDL levels may also decrease, most likely due to a reduction of dense LDL, which is more atherogenic than buoyant LDL and has poor affinity for the LDL receptor. However, LDL may also increase in patients with hypertriglyceridemia with

fibrate therapy, but these are usually the less atherogenic buoyant LDL particles. Consequently, fibrates are used almost exclusively for patients with hypertriglyceridemia and low HDL.

There are several outcome trials that have used fibrates. In patients with hypertriglyceridemia or low HDL, or both, these drugs reduce CHD events or the angiographic progression of atherosclerosis. In patients with CHD and low HDL, the Veterans Affairs High Density Lipoprotein Cholesterol Intervention Trial (VA-HIT) study shows that gemfibrozil compares favorably to statin therapy, using a number-needed-to-treat to prevent one event analysis (Fig. 4.14). The Bezafibrate Infarction Prevention (BIP) trial failed to demonstrate a significant overall benefit, but, for patients with TGs greater than 200 mg per dL, there was a 40% CHD risk reduction ($P = .03$). The mean LDL in the VA-HIT study was 111 mg per dL compared to 148 mg per dL in the BIP trial. The lack of benefit for bezafibrate in the BIP trial compared to the significant benefit for gemfibrozil in the VA-HIT study suggests

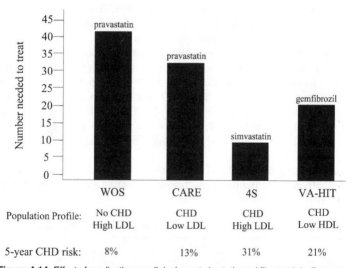

Figure 4.14. Effect of medication on clinical events in statin and fibrate trials. Data are number-needed-to-treat (NNT), which are obtained using the formula: 100/absolute risk reduction. An NNT of 33 or lower is considered as an effective intervention. The 5-year coronary heart disease (CHD) risk presented at the bottom is the actual event rate observed in the placebo group within each study. CARE, Cholesterol and Related Events; HDL, high-density lipoprotein; LDL, low-density lipoprotein; 4S, Scandinavian Simvastatin Survival Study; VA-HIT, Veterans Affairs High Density Lipoprotein Cholesterol Intervention Trial; WOS, West of Scotland Coronary Prevention Study.

that fibrates should be targeted for patients with high TGs or low HDL with a relatively low LDL.

The fibrates are generally well tolerated. The most common side effects are upper gastrointestinal disturbance, headache, myalgia, and loss of libido. Fibrates have absolute contraindications in hepatic or severe renal dysfunction and preexisting gallbladder disease. Fibrates should also not be used in pregnant or nursing mothers.

Gemfibrozil is a potent inhibitor of the CYP2C8 metabolic pathway and the glucuronidation of statins. Cerivastatin is partially cleared by the CYP2C8 pathway and undergoes significant glucuronidation. Gemfibrozil's inhibitory effect on both metabolic pathways for cerivastatin explains the five- to sixfold increase in the AUC for cerivastatin when combined with gemfibrozil, whereas fenofibrate, which does not inhibit the CYP2C8 metabolic pathway or statin glucuronidation, has minimal impact on cerivastatin levels. All statins, including rosuvastatin, require varying degrees of glucuronidation for metabolism, and the AUC for all statins evaluated, except for fluvastatin, are increased when combined with gemfibrozil (Table 4.9). This explains gemfibrozil's greater propensity to increase the risk of rhabdomyolysis when combined with statins compared to fenofibrate.

CYP2C8 is a common metabolic pathway for many of the diabetic treatments such as glimepiride, rosiglitazone, and repaglinide. Gemfibrozil, as an inhibitor of the CYP2C8 metabolic pathway, raises the AUC for all these drugs significantly. Therefore, gemfibrozil should be used with caution in combination with CYP2C8-metabolized drugs (Table 4.10). Alternatively, fenofibrate can be used as a substitute for gemfibrozil without adversely affecting the AUC of CYP2C8-metabolized drugs.

Although gemfibrozil and fenofibrate are both fibrates and activate PPAR-alpha, resulting in similar lipoprotein changes (fenofibrate may

Table 4.9. Statin-Fibrate Combination Therapy: Pharmacokinetic Interactions

	Gemfibrozil	Fenofibrate
Atorvastatin	Not available	Not available
Pravastatin	↑ in C_{max} by twofold	No effect
Fluvastatin		Not available
Simvastatin	↑ in C_{max} by 112%	No effect
Cerivastatin	↑ in C_{max} by two- to threefold	No effect
Rosuvastatin	↑ in C_{max} by twofold	No effect

C_{max}, maximal drug concentration.

Table 4.10. Cytochrome CYP2C8–Metabolized Drugs

CYP2C8 Substrates		CYP2C8 Inhibitors	CYP2C8 Inducers
Amiodarone	Repaglinide	Anastrozole	Carbamazepine
Benzphetamine	Retinoic acid	Gemfibrozil	Phenobarbital
Carbamazepine	Retinal	Nicardipine	Rifabutin
Docetaxel	Rosiglitazone	Quercetin	Rifampicin
Fluvastatin	Tolbutamide	Sulfaphenazole	Rifampin
Isotretinoin	Tretinoin	Sulfinpyrazone	
Paclitaxel	Verapamil	Trimethoprim	
Phenytoin	Warfarin		
Pioglitazone	Zopiclone		

more potently decrease LDL), these drugs have very different pharmacokinetic profiles. Gemfibrozil is a competitive inhibitor of the CYP2C8 metabolic pathway, organic anion transport protein 2, and statin glucuronidation. Fenofibrate is a substrate for the CYP2C9 metabolic pathway but is not an inhibitor and is also a mild inhibitor of Pgp. These metabolic pathways appear to result in little known drug interaction for fenofibrate. The gemfibrozil-statin interaction is most problematic because, frequently, a fibrate must be added to a statin to improve the lipoprotein profile. Both fenofibrate and, perhaps less commonly, gemfibrozil, on rare occasions, may increase serum creatinine by an unknown mechanism. The most likely explanation appears to relate to increases in creatinine production in muscle tissue, but renal filtration changes are also possible. Homocysteine level is increased by both fenofibrate and gemfibrozil (perhaps less so). Although the clinical significance of increased homocysteine level with fibrate therapy is uncertain, based on a correlation between increased homocysteine levels and CHD risk and the demonstrated benefit of folic acid supplementation as a means of decreasing the fenofibrate-associated increase in homocysteine, it appears prudent to consider folic acid supplementation for patients on fibrate therapy. Both fenofibrate and gemfibrozil lower fibrinogen level, but neither fibrate significantly alters Lp(a) level.

Gemfibrozil is usually dosed at 1,200 mg at two divided doses 30 minutes before the morning and evening meals. Micronized fenofibrate, 160 mg, is given with a meal. The pharmacokinetics of micronized fenofibrate are markedly affected by food, and, unless a patient takes the capsule with a meal, the absorption may be suboptimal. A new formulation of micronized fenofibrate is available that does not require intake with food and, therefore, should improve patient compliance. The recommended dose of bezafibrate is 400 g once daily as a sustained-release tablet, and ciprofibrate is given at 100 g daily.

BILE ACID SEQUESTRANTS

Two of the most commonly prescribed bile acid sequestrants, cholestyramine and colestipol, have been in use since the 1980s. Bile acid sequestrants decrease intrahepatic cholesterol by interrupting enterohepatic circulation of bile acids, thereby increasing the synthesis of bile acids from cholesterol in the liver. This upregulates LDL receptor activity and increases clearance of LDL from the blood. Evidence of clinical benefit of bile acid sequestrants has been demonstrated in a number of clinical trials, including the Lipid Research Clinics-Coronary Primary Prevention trial and the Familial Atherosclerosis Treatment study.

Bile acid sequestrants are difficult to use in practice. Adherence to bile acid sequestrants is often an issue with their administration, due in part to the poor palatability of the drug and to the occurrence of adverse gastrointestinal effects, particularly constipation. Compliance with prescribed sequestrant therapy may be as low as 50%. Therefore, colesevelam, a new bile acid sequestrant, has become the preferred drug of this class.

Colesevelam is a polyallylamine cross-linked with epichlorohydrin and alkylated with 1-bromodecane and 6-bromohexyltrimethylammonium bromide. Colesevelam did not inhibit the absorption of lovastatin when administered together.

Colesevelam is a novel, polymeric agent with bile-acid binding activity. The ability of colesevelam to lower serum LDL cholesterol levels has been demonstrated in several clinical trials in which approximately 1,400 patients were evaluated. Compared to historical data with bile acid sequestrants, colesevelam is four to six times more potent. Colesevelam is effective as monotherapy for patients with mild to moderate hypercholesterolemia and when coadministered with an HMG-CoA reductase inhibitor. In terms of its safety and tolerability, colesevelam is well accepted alone and in combination with statin therapy and lacks the constipating effect of typical bile acid sequestrants. There are three types of patients in whom colesevelam may be most appropriate. The first is a patient who has not achieved NCEP ATP III with maximal statin therapy (or maximally tolerated dose). Colesevelam may also be an option for the statin-intolerant patient or the patient who refuses to take a statin because of fear of side effects. In summary, colesevelam is a safe and effective nonsystemic alternative to the currently available lipid-lowering agents. Use of colesevelam has the potential for increasing patient compliance and ultimately contributing to reductions in CHD morbidity and mortality.

COMBINATION DRUGS

Lovastatin/niacin (Advicor), a combination tablet containing 20 mg of lovastatin with 500, 750, or 1,000 mg of extended-release niacin, has been approved by the FDA. This combination tablet at the high dose of 2,000 mg per 40 mg was shown to lower LDL by 45%, TGs by 42%, and Lp(a) by 18%, with a 30% increase in HDL (Fig. 4.15). Flushing was a reason for discontinuation in 9% of patients. No cases of myopathy were reported, and less than 1% (out of 814) of patients had significantly elevated liver enzymes. Random-testing glucose was greater than normal in 33% of participants, but it reached a level of greater than 125 mg per dL in only 3%. Therefore, for patients with combined hyperlipidemia, a combination of niacin/lovastatin may provide an excellent single-tablet option (see Chapter 5, Patient Profile #3: Combined Hyperlipidemia).

Ezetimibe/simvastatin (Vytorin) is a drug that combines a fixed dose of ezetimibe (10 mg) with increasing doses of simvastatin (10, 20, 40, 80 mg). A number of studies demonstrate increased efficacy for LDL-C reduction and HDL-C elevation when ezetimibe is used in com-

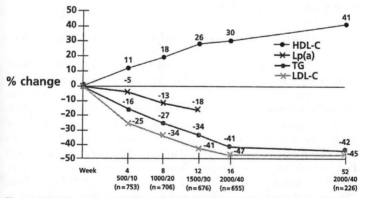

Figure 4.15. Nicostatin long-term study. Niacin dosage: 500 to 2,000 mg; lovastatin dosage: 10 to 40 mg. HDL-C, high-density lipoprotein cholesterol; LDL-C, low-density lipoprotein cholesterol; Lp(a), lipoprotein(a); TG, triglyceride. (Adapted from *J Am Coll Cardiol*; and Kos Pharmaceuticals, Inc.)

bination with simvastatin. In general, with each doubling of a statin's dose, there is an additional 6% reduction in serum LDL-C (the so-called rule of sixes). As the dose of a statin is increased, there is a well-known increase in risk for toxicity. The addition of ezetimibe to a statin can preclude the need for titration in some patients. For example, simvastatin, 10 mg, combined with ezetimibe, 10 mg, reduces LDL-C to an equivalent degree as simvastatin, 80 mg (44%). Moreover, when ezetimibe is combined with simvastatin, the adverse event rate is identical to that observed with simvastatin alone. The addition of ezetimibe to pooled doses of simvastatin (10, 20, 40, or 80 mg) yields an incremental 13.8% decrease in LDL-C, a 2.4% increase in HDL-C, and a 7.5% decrease in TG compared to treatment with simvastatin alone. Atorvastatin is the most commonly used statin for the management of hyperlipidemia. In patients with hypercholesterolemia, atorvastatin, 10 mg, and combinations of ezetimibe with simvastatin at 10/10 and 10/20 mg produced reductions in LDL-C of 37.2, 46.1, and 50.3 mg/dL, respectively, and increases in HDL-C of 5.1, 8.0, and 9.5 mg/dL, respectively. The combination of ezetimibe with simvastatin at 10/80 mg compared to atorvastatin, 80 mg, yields a significantly greater reduction in LDL-C (59.4% vs. 52.5%) and elevation in HDL-C (12.3% vs. 6.5%). Although the ezetimibe component of the ezetimibe/simvastatin combination does not yet have any outcome-based data, the NCEP stresses LDL-C target achievement irrespective of specific drug selection; therefore, this combination therapy may be an especially attractive drug for patients who are committed to attaining their lipid targets with low doses of a statin.

ATORVASTATIN PLUS AMLODIPINE (CADUET)

Sixty-two percent of patients with hypertension (almost two out of every three) also have dyslipidemia, and 44% of patients with dyslipidemia (more than two of every five) also have hypertension. However, although dyslipidemia and hypertension occur frequently together, surveys suggest that only one-third of patients with combined hypertension and dyslipidemia are diagnosed with both conditions, and only 10% of patients with both conditions reach both NCEP ATP III and The Seventh Report of the Joint National Committee on Prevention, Detection, Evaluation, and Treatment of High Blood Pressure goals. The metabolic syndrome, which includes dyslipidemia and hypertension among the characteristic features, increases in prevalence with age; therefore, the prevalence of combined hypertension with dyslipidemia also markedly increases with age. A combination of atorvastatin and amlodipine in a single tablet is available to treat both cardiovascular risk factors simultaneously. Atorvastatin and amlodipine are among the most frequently used therapies for dyslipidemia and hypertension, respectively, and having a combination tablet should improve compliance and reduce costs to the patient. More important, this combination therapy approach helps break down the treatment silos that often occur in CHD risk management. By targeting both dyslipidemia and hypertension simultaneously, global risk reduction and patient outcomes should be improved. The ASCOT trial demonstrated the benefits of reducing CHD events by 36% on atorvastatin in patients with hypertension and supports the role of statin therapy for all patients with a single risk factor such as hypertension. The NCEP ATP III panel based on the ASCOT trial supported an optional target of less than 100 mg per dL for patients with a Framingham global risk score of 10% to 20%, which represents most patients older than age 60 years with hypertension.

SELECTED READING

BIP Study Group. Secondary prevention by raising HDL cholesterol and reducing triglycerides in patients with coronary heart disease. The Bezafibrate Infarction Prevention (BIP) Study. *Circulation* 2000;102:21–27.

Capuzzi DM, Mortan JM, Brusco OA, et al. Niacin dosing: relationship to benefits and adverse effects. *Curr Atheroscler Rep* 2000;2:64–71.

Davidson MH. Does differing metabolism by cytochrome P450 have clinical importance? *Curr Atheroscler Rep* 2000;2:14–19.

Davidson MH. Statin trials in progress: unanswered questions. *Curr Atheroscler Rep* 2000;3:9–13.

Davidson MH. Ezetimibe: a novel option for lowering cholesterol. *Expert Rev Cardiovasc Ther* 2003;1:11–21.

Davidson MH. Emerging therapeutic strategies for the management of dyslipidemia in patients with the metabolic syndrome. *Am J Cardiol* 2004;93:3C–11C.

Davidson MH, Toth PP. Combination therapy in the management of complex dyslipidemias. *Curr Opin Lipidol* 2004;15:423–431.

Davidson MH, Toth PP. Comparative effects of lipid lowering therapies. *Prog Cardiovasc Dis* 2004;47:73–104.

Davignon J, Montigny M, Dufour R. HMG-CoA reductase inhibitors: a look back and a look ahead. *Can J Cardiol* 1992;8:843–864.

Fruchart JC, Brewer HB Jr, Leitersdorf E. Consensus for the use of fibrates in the treatment of dyslipoproteinemia and coronary heart disease. *Am J Cardiol* 1998;81:912–917.

Fruchart J, Staels B, Duriez P. The role of fibric acids in atherosclerosis. *Curr Atheroscler Rep* 2000;3:83–92.

Gotto AM Jr, Whitney E, Stein EA, et al. Relation between baseline and on-treatment lipid parameters and first acute major coronary events in the Air Force/Texas Coronary Atherosclerosis Prevention Study (AFCAPS/TexCAPS). *Circulation* 2000;101:477–484.

Gruer PJK, Vega JM, Mercuri MF, et al. Concomitant use of cytochrome P450 3A4 inhibitors and simvastatin. *Am J Cardiol* 1999;84:811–815.

Grundy SM. Statin trials and goals of cholesterol-lowering therapy. *Circulation* 1998;97:1436–1439.

Heart Protection Study Collaborative Group. MRC/BHF Heart Protection Study of cholesterol-lowering with simvastatin in 5963 people with diabetes: a randomised placebo-controlled trial. *Lancet* 2003;361:2005–2016.

Heinonen TM, Schrott H, McKenney JM, et al. Atorvastatin, a new HMG CoA reductase inhibitor as monotherapy and combined with colestipol. *J Cardiovasc Pharmacol Ther* 1996;1:117–122.

Jones P, Kafonek S, Laurora I, et al., for the CURVES Investigators. Comparative dose efficacy study of atorvastatin versus simvastatin, pravastatin, lovastatin and fluvastatin in patients with hypercholesterolemia (The CURVES study). *Am J Cardiol* 1998;82:582–587.

Linton MF, Fazio S. Re-emergence of fibrates in the management of dyslipidemia and cardiovascular risk. *Curr Atheroscler Rep* 2000;2:29–35.

The Long-Term Intervention with Pravastatin in Ischaemic Disease (LIPID) Study Group. Prevention of cardiovascular events and death with pravastatin in patients with coronary heart disease and a broad range of initial cholesterol levels. *N Engl J Med* 1998;339:1349–1357.

Sacks FM, Pfeffer MA, Moye LA, et al., for the Cholesterol and Recurrent Events Trial Investigators. The effect of pravastatin on coronary events after myocardial infarction in patients with average cholesterol levels. *N Engl J Med* 1996;335:1001–1009.

Scandinavian Simvastatin Survival Study Group. Randomized trial of cholesterol lowering in 4,444 patients with coronary heart disease: the Scandinavian Simvastatin Survival Study (4S). *Lancet* 1994;344:1383–1389.

Sever PS, Dahlof B, Poulter NR, et al., ASCOT investigators. Prevention of coronary and stroke events with atorvastatin in hypertensive patients who have average or lower-than-average cholesterol concentrations, in the Anglo-Scandinavian Cardiac Outcomes Trial—Lipid Lowering Arm (ASCOT-LLA): a multicenter randomized controlled trial. *Lancet* 2003;361(9364):1149–1158.

Shepherd J, Cobbe SM, Ford I, et al., for the West of Scotland Coronary Prevention Study Group. Prevention of coronary heart disease with pravastatin in men with hypercholesterolemia. *N Engl J Med* 1995;333:1301–1307.

Stein EA. New statins and new doses of older statins. *Curr Atheroscler Rep* 2000;3:14–18.

Stein EA, Lane M, Laskarzewski P. Comparison of statins in hypertriglyceridemia. *Am J Cardiol* 1998;81(4A):6B–69B.

Tavintharan S, Kashyap ML. The benefits of niacin in atherosclerosis. *Curr Atheroscler Rep* 2000;3:74–82.

Toth PP, Davidson MH. Simvastatin plus ezetimibe: combination therapy for the management of dyslipidemia. *Expert Opin Pharmacother* 2005;6:131–139.

Vega GL, Grundy SM. Lipoprotein responses to treatment with lovastatin, gemfibrozil, and nicotinic acid in normolipidemic patients with hypoalphalipoproteinemia. *Arch Intern Med* 1994;154:73–82.

Chapter 5

Management of Dyslipidemia by Patient Profiles

PATIENT PROFILE #1: HYPERCHOLESTEROLEMIA

High low-density lipoprotein (LDL), normal triglyceride (TG), and high-density lipoprotein (HDL)	
Patient example: 46-year-old man; nonsmoker; weight (Wt), 180; height (Ht), 5'11"; blood pressure (BP), 130/88	
Family history: Father died of myocardial infarction (MI) at age 74 years	

Lipid profile	
Cholesterol	250 mg/dL
TG	100 mg/dL
HDL	42 mg/dL
LDL cholesterol (LDL-C)	188 mg/dL
Framingham 10-yr risk	10%
Adult Treatment Panel III (ATP III) 10-yr risk	8%
Cardiovascular (CV) age	64 yr
LDL goal	<130
% LDL reduction to achieve goal	31

Treatment Guidelines

Option 1: Starting Dose of Statin and Titrate the Dose to Goal

Table 4.2 depicts the efficacy of various statins throughout the dose range for percent LDL reduction. Many physicians prefer to start with the recommended starting dose of the statin, and, if the patient is not at the appropriate goal after 6 to 12 weeks of treatment, the dose is increased to the next level. After each titration, follow-up lipid profile and liver function tests are recommended at 6- to 12-week intervals.

Once the patient achieves the recommended goal with normal safety laboratory tests, follow-up is usually at 6- to 12-month intervals.

Option 2: Using a Flexible Start Dose

Some physicians prefer a higher start dose based on the percent LDL-C reduction required to achieve the goal. The advantage of this strategy is that a patient is more likely to achieve the recommended goal with fewer titration visits, and having more dramatic results over a shorter period may enhance patient satisfaction. If the patient has an exaggerated response to the higher statin dose, the dose can be down titrated on the follow-up visit. This strategy is probably best advocated for patients at high risk for cardiac events [e.g., patients with coronary heart disease (CHD) or CHD risk equivalent].

Option 3: Starting Dose of Statin Plus Combination Therapy

Bile acid sequestrants (cholestyramine, colestipol, and colesevelam), niacin (Niaspan), and ezetimibe (a cholesterol absorption inhibitor) lower LDL-C, depending on the dose, by 15% to 20%. A 15% to 20% decrease in LDL-C is approximately equivalent to tripling the dose of the statin. For every doubling of the dose of the statin, there is a further decrease in LDL-C of approximately 6%. Therefore, adding one of the aforementioned nonstatin drugs to a starting dose results in LDL-C reductions equivalent to or greater than the highest available dose of the statin. This strategy is being used in patients who are intolerant to a high dose of a statin, in patients who do not achieve the recommended goals despite the use of a high dose of statin, or if more aggressive lipid-modifying therapy is necessary to achieve the desired treatment goals.

Option 4: Nonstatin Therapy for Patients with Mild Low-Density Lipoprotein Elevations

Some patients require an LDL-C reduction of less than 20% to achieve the recommended goals, and for these patients, nonstatin therapy is an option. Although statin therapy may result in LDL-C reduction far below the recommended goals, the proven benefits of statins in clinical trials and the ease of use lead to improved compliance, and, usually, cost issues still make statins the preferred option in most patients with mild LDL-C elevations. Nevertheless, some patients (and physicians) prefer nonsystemic therapies, such as the bile acid sequestrants or ezetimibe, for patients in whom modest LDL-C reduction achieves the recommended goals. For patients with significant cost constraints, over-the-counter immediate-release niacin may be a consideration; however, most pharmaceutical companies provide assistance programs and other options (although not U.S. Food and Drug Administration approved), which include pill cutting or alternate-day dosing of the statin to reduce cost.

PATIENT PROFILE #2: HYPERCHOLESTEROLEMIA WITH LOW HIGH-DENSITY LIPOPROTEIN CHOLESTEROL

High LDL, normal TG, low HDL	
Patient example: 50-year-old man; smoker (two packs/day); Wt, 175 lb; Ht, 5'9"; body mass index (BMI), 25; BP, 130/80 mm Hg	
Family history: Mother died of MI at age 54 years	

Lipid profile	
Cholesterol	248 mg/dL
TG	175 mg/dL
HDL cholesterol (HDL-C)	38 mg/dL
Framingham 10-yr risk	21%
ATP III 10-yr risk	25%
LDL-C	175 mg/dL
CV age	Older than 74 yr
LDL goal	<100 mg/dL
% LDL reduction to achieve goal	43

The treatment options for this patient are similar to those of Patient Profile #1 (high LDL, normal TG and HDL); however, the low HDL and the cigarette smoking confer a much higher global risk for CHD. In addition to achieving the LDL treatment goal, special attention should be paid to attempting to raise the HDL-C. In patients such as this, smoking cessation would usually result in a significant increase in HDL-C. Therefore, smoking cessation should be strongly encouraged. The Mobile Lipid Clinic™ program may help motivate the patient by illustrating the benefits of cigarette-smoking cessation and lipid modification on his CV age. He can reduce his CV age by at least 10 years and reduce his 10-year risk to almost one-third of his baseline risk. Other causes of low HDL-C should also be considered, as in the pneumonic

L—Lack of exercise
O—Obesity
W—Postmenopausal status
H—Hypertriglyceridemia
D—Drugs such as anabolic steroids, testosterone
L—Lack of alcohol
C—Cigarette smoking

Because this patient is overweight, an exercise program should improve weight loss, lower TG values, and raise HDL-C. The Mobile Lipid Clinic™ program also demonstrates the potential benefits of a 5 mg per dL rise in HDL-C.

	Baseline risk	After smoking cessation	Plus lowering LDL ≤100 mg/dL	Plus increasing HDL-C by 5 mg/dL
CV age (yr)	74	74	64	59
Framingham 10-yr risk (%)	21	11	9	7

By raising his HDL by 5 mg per dL to 43 mg per dL, the patient would have a 5-year reduction in his CV age. Physician advice to increase alcohol intake is generally not recommended because of other potentially adverse effects of alcohol. For patients who drink modestly, however, advice regarding the restriction of alcohol intake is not necessary.

Drug Therapy

In patients with high LDL-C and low HDL-C, the drug treatment options are similar to those of patients with isolated high LDL-C, with a potentially greater emphasis on combination drug therapy that may beneficially modify HDL levels. Statins remain the drugs of first choice. Based on the results of the large statin endpoint trials [West of Scotland Coronary Prevention Study, Air Force Coronary Atherosclerosis Prevention Study (AFCAPS)], patients with high LDL and low HDL have significant benefits for statin therapy (Fig. 5.1). The percent reduction of events is even greater in the low HDL-C subjects. The main objective with this patient example is to achieve the LDL goal of less than 100 mg per dL. This requires a 46% reduction in LDL-C; therefore, beginning with a higher starting dose or a more potent statin, or both, is usually advisable. The Canadian guidelines recommend a total cholesterol HDL ratio goal of less than 4.0 for high-risk patients. A ratio goal may be achieved by more aggressive LDL lowering or by potentially increasing HDL. After initiating a statin, the next consideration involves whether to add a second drug (or use a combination of niacin plus lovastatin as a single tablet). Adding niacin to a statin is the most likely combination because niacin has the most significant effects on raising HDL. There have also been a number of trials that have demonstrated the safety of this combination and efficacy in inhibiting the development of atherosclerosis. Adding a fibrate is a less desirable combination for this patient profile because the TGs are not significantly elevated and, in the absence of insulin resistance, fibrates may be of limited clinical value.

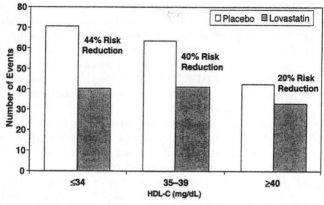

Figure 5.1. Air Force/Texas Coronary Atherosclerosis Prevention Study. Relative risk reduction in primary prevention. HDL-C, high-density lipoprotein cholesterol. (From Downs JR, Clearfield M, Weis S, et al. Primary prevention of acute coronary events with lovastatin in men and women with average cholesterol levels: result of AFCAPS/TexCAPS. Air Force/Texas Coronary Atherosclerosis Prevention Study. *JAMA* 1998;279:1615–1622, with permission.)

PATIENT PROFILE #3: COMBINED HYPERLIPIDEMIA

High LDL (≥130 mg/dL), moderate hypertriglyceridemia (200 to 500 mg/dL), and low HDL (<40 mg/dL)
Patient example: 65-year-old woman; nonsmoker; Wt, 150 lb; Ht, 5'3"; BP, 140/88 mm Hg; BMI, 26
Family history: Father died of MI at age 52 years

Lipid profile	
Cholesterol	260 mg/dL
TG	300 mg/dL
HDL	33 mg/dL
LDL	166 mg/dL
Non-HDL	227 mg/dL
LDL goal	<130 mg/dL
Non-HDL goal	<160 mg/dL
% LDL reduction to achieve goal	22
10-yr risk	9%
CV age	74 yr

Etiology

Familial combined hyperlipidemia is a relatively common genetic disorder associated with the overproduction of apolipoprotein (Apo) B that results in elevations of both LDL and TG. Family members may vary between pure hypercholesterolemia, combined hyperlipidemia, or isolated hypertriglyceridemia. The disorder is dominantly inherited and is also associated with a family history of type 2 diabetes. The ratio of Apo B per LDL is usually greater than or equal to 1.0, dense LDL or pattern B is present, and HDL is often low. On physical examination, premature corneal arcus or xanthelasma is occasionally present, but rarely are there tendon xanthomas.

In patients with mixed dyslipidemia, other potential genetic causes include familial dysbetalipoproteinemia (type 3) or familial hypertriglyceridemia. The treatments are usually similar; however, differentiating the potential genetic causes of hypertriglyceridemia have prognostic implications, and, occasionally, the treatments may vary (see Chapter 2).

In this patient profile, non-HDL becomes the primary target of therapy. Although Apo B may be a more accurate predictor of CHD risk and some physicians advocate direct measurements of LDL, the non-HDL, by incorporating LDL, intermediate-density lipoprotein (IDL), and very-low-density lipoprotein (VLDL), represents a target that contains all of the potentially atherogenic lipoproteins. Apo B, direct LDL, and lipoprotein subparticles are more expensive laboratory tests and not as widely available. If Apo B is measured, a goal of less than 90 mg per dL is the target for high-risk patients. Alternatively, an Apo B/AI ratio of less than 0.7 is an optimal target recommended by the Canadian guidelines.

Treatment Guidelines

Patients with combined hyperlipidemia often respond dramatically to weight loss, exercise, and lower-carbohydrate (lower-calorie) diets. Measurements of weight loss are usually a good guide to ascertain compliance to a prescribed diet and exercise program. Failure to lose weight usually means the patient is noncompliant or unable to adhere to the nonpharmacologic approaches. These are the types of patients in whom a referral to a dietitian or other experienced health professional in nonpharmacologic treatments is cost effective.

Drug Therapy

Drug therapy options are similar to those mentioned in Patient Profile #2. In this example, the patient requires a 22% reduction in LDL-C to achieve the ATP III goal of less than 130 mg per dL and a 30% reduction in non-HDL to achieve the goal of less than 160 mg per dL. These goals should be achieved with statin therapy alone; however, the more potent statins or using a higher dose, or both, usually more effectively lowers TG levels. Combining a statin with niacin or a fibrate (gemfibrozil or fenofibrate) is another possibility that may more effectively lower LDL and TG and raise HDL. Often, the preferred choice is a statin, starting with or titrating to a maximal dose, and if the goals are not achieved with monotherapy, titrate down the dose of the statin and add niacin (or the combination pill of lovastatin plus Niaspan) or a fibrate (fenofibrate preferred). Another option is to add omega-3 fatty acid supplementation, 2 to 6 g per day (marine oil capsules), to a statin that is safe and usually well tolerated. Omega-3 fatty acids do not increase the HDL as much as niacin or a fibrate. After initiation of drug therapy, continued encouragement regarding diet, exercise, and weight loss are vital to the long-term success of the treatment of this patient population (see Chapter 3).

PATIENT PROFILE #4: SEVERE HYPERTRIGLYCERIDEMIA

High cholesterol, TG >500 mg/dL
Patient example: 45-year-old man; nonsmoker; Wt, 250 lb; Ht, 5'11"; BMI, 34
Family history: Father and mother age 67 years, alive and well

Lipid profile	
Cholesterol	300 mg/dL
TG	2,000 mg/dL
Framingham 10-yr risk	16%
ATP 10-yr risk	14%
Glucose	115 mg/dL
LDL	Not able to calculate
HDL	30 mg/dL
Non-HDL	270 mg/dL
Non-HDL goal	<160 mg/dL

Etiology

Severe hypertriglyceridemia is usually due to impairment or deficiency of lipoprotein lipase (LPL), the vascular enzyme that degrades chylomicrons into remnant particles and liberates the TG into free fatty acids for energy use or for fat storage. On occasion, severe forms of familial dysbetalipoproteinemia (type 3) or overproduction of VLDL (familial hypertriglyceridemia) may result in severe hypertriglyceridemia. In these patients, the total cholesterol levels are much higher compared to the TG levels. If the total cholesterol is greater than 300 mg per dL and the TGs are between 500 and 1,000 mg per dL, then perhaps the patient has other genetic causes of dyslipidemia (type 3 or familial hypertriglyceridemia). A simple test to differentiate the various causes of severe hypertriglyceridemia is to place the patient's testing serum in the refrigerator overnight and look for a layer of chylomicrons to separate on the top of the serum. If the serum has a cream-colored layer on top and a clear serum below, the patient has type 1 hyperlipidemia or LPL deficiency. If there is a cream-colored layer on top and a turbid serum below, the patient has type V hyperlipidemia, which means overproduction of VLDL and LPL impairment. If there is no cream-colored layer on top but turbid serum, the patient has elevations of either VLDL (type IV) or IDL (type III). This overnight refrigerator test is usually helpful for both diagnostic and therapeutic purposes. Another important differential feature is the presence on physical examination of eruptive xanthoma. Eruptive xanthomas can appear on the whole body, but most commonly on the back, chest, and buttocks. These skin lesions on biopsy contain chylomicrons, and, often, the diagnosis of LPL deficiency is made by the dermatologist. Tuberoeruptive xanthomas are present with IDL elevations and are most commonly found on the elbows and palms, and distinctive orange streaks can be visualized in the palm creases. If chylomicrons are present in a patient's fasting serum, then low-carbohydrate diets are not advisable. Low-carbohydrate diets often increase fat intake, and because these patients have severe difficulty clearing chylomicrons, adding more fat to the diet can substantially worsen the hypertriglyceridemia and lead to pancreatitis. Pancreatitis, rather than CHD, is the most significant health risk for patients with hyperchylomicronemia. Therefore, patients with this disorder should be placed on a fat-restrictive diet until the hyperchylomicronemia is resolved. In severe cases, or if the patient is experiencing acute pancreatitis, that patient may need to be hospitalized and placed on intravenous fluids for nutrition and, if necessary, undergo plasma exchange.

Treatment Guidelines

Once the patient is stable, it is important to differentiate true LPL deficiency or Apo III deficiency, which is the apoprotein that activates LPL, from LPL impairment. For patients with true LPL deficiency, which is rare, severe fat restriction for the long term is usually effective. Fibrates that upregulate LPL are not helpful because the enzyme is absent and cannot be activated. Much more commonly, however, the LPL enzyme is impaired and not totally absent or inactive. Impaired LPL activity is often an acquired condition due to diabetes, obesity, or hypothyroidism. Therefore, these secondary causes of severe hypertriglyceridemia must be ruled out with appropriate tests. Correction of these secondary causes is effective in decreasing the LPL impairment and improving hypertriglyceridemia.

For patients with impaired LPL activity, both VLDL and chylomicrons are elevated (Fredrickson type V). Once the chylomicrons are reduced by fat restriction, patients may also require simple dietary carbohydrate reduction to further reduce the hypertriglyceridemia by lowering the VLDL. High intake of simple carbohydrates increases VLDL (see Chapter 3).

Therefore, these patients require both dietary fat and simple carbohydrate restriction. Weight control through caloric restriction and exercise is critical for the long-term maintenance of acceptable lipid levels. Omega-3 fatty acid intake either by eating fatty fish, such as salmon, mackerel, or sardines (in the sardine oil), or by supplementing the diet with marine oil capsules may also effectively lower the TG levels.

If dietary therapy fails, the drug therapy options include niacin and fibrates. Fibrates are the drugs of choice in diabetics, but niacin may also be effective with monitoring of the blood glucose. Because most of these patients are diabetic or have impaired fasting glucose, tighter control of the glucose levels may result in substantial improvement in the lipid levels.

PATIENT PROFILE #5: METABOLIC SYNDROME

Normal LDL <130 mg/dL, moderate hypertriglyceridemia (200 to 500 mg/dL), low HDL <40 mg/dL

Patient example: 60-year-old man; nonsmoker; BP, 142/86 mm Hg on 10 mg Norvasc; BMI, 29

Family history: Father died of MI at age 54 years

Lipid profile	
Cholesterol	185 mg/dL
TG	300 mg/dL
Framingham 10-yr risk HDL	19%
ATP 10-yr risk	20%
ATP III LDL goal	118 mg/dL
ATP III non-HDL goal	<130 mg/dL
CV-adjusted age	74 yr
Glucose	<100 mg/dL
LDL	90 mg/dL
HDL	35 mg/dL
Non-HDL	150 mg/dL

Despite a relatively normal LDL, patients with metabolic syndrome are often at high risk for CHD. As in this example, the patient has an LDL of

90 mg per dL but a 20% absolute 10-year probability of CHD. He also has the metabolic syndrome with impaired fasting glucose and hypertension. Because his LDL is already at goal, his secondary treatment goal is a non-HDL of less than 130 mg per dL. Caloric reduction and exercise are critical to reduce body weight in patients with this profile. Usually, weight loss alone effectively achieves the TG lowering necessary to reach the non-HDL goal of less than 130 mg per dL. For patients who are not overweight, a lower-carbohydrate diet significantly improves the lipid profile. Niacin and fibrates are the drugs of first choice but should only be initiated after at least 6 months of dietary therapy.

PATIENT PROFILE #6: ISOLATED LOW HIGH-DENSITY LIPOPROTEIN

TG <200 mg/dL, LDL <130 mg/dL, HDL <40 mg/dL
Patient example: 42-year-old man; nonsmoker; BP, 120/80 mm Hg; BMI, 25
Family history: Father died of MI at age 48 years

Lipid profile	
Cholesterol	190 mg/dL
TG	150 mg/dL
HDL	30 mg/dL
LDL	120 mg/dL
Electron beam computed tomography calcium score	100
Framingham 10-yr risk	6%
ATP 10-yr risk	2%
CV-adjusted age	54 yr
Calcium score–adjusted age	80 yr
Calcium score–adjusted 10-yr probability	13%

Treatment Guidelines

Patients with isolated low HDL associated with a family history of premature CHD have familial hypoalphalipoproteinemia, an autosomal dominant genetic disorder. Nonpharmacologic means to raise HDL should be attempted, but if the HDL level remains markedly depressed, two clinical trials suggest benefits in this patient population. The Veterans Administration High-Density Lipoprotein Intervention Trial (VA-HIT) study evaluated gemfibrozil, 600 mg twice a day, in CHD populations with isolated low HDL, which, despite no change in LDL compared to placebo but a 6% increase in HDL and a 25% decrease in TG, resulted in a 22% reduction in major coronary events. In a post-hoc analysis of the AFCAPS/Texas Atherosclerosis Prevention Study (AFCAPS/Tex-CAPS) trial, patients with an HDL less than or equal to 34 mg per dL had a 45% reduction in clinical events on lovastatin, 40 mg, compared to the placebo group. The mean LDL in the VA-HIT population was 112 mg per dL compared to a mean LDL in the AFCAPS/TexCAPS population of 150 mg per dL. Therefore, both fibrates and statins may be reasonable options in patients with isolated HDL. Niacin appears to have the greatest HDL-raising effect in this population and is another drug treatment option to consider.

Drug Therapy

The main issue regarding the isolated low HDL population is whether to initiate drug treatment. The ATP III states that drug treatment for raising HDL (niacin or fibrates) can be considered; however, treatment for isolated low HDL should mostly be reserved for patients with CHD and CHD risk equivalents. In this patient example, the patient does not have CHD or CHD risk equivalents, but a strong argument can be made to initiate treatment because he has a strong family history of CHD and evidence of significant atherosclerosis by the documentation of a high coronary calcium score on electron beam computed tomography (EBCT). EBCT is most useful in patients with an intermediate CHD risk, in whom the results of the tests would help to decide whether to initiate drug treatment. Measuring lipoprotein(a) [Lp(a)] may also be useful, as a high level would most likely support niacin as the drug treatment of first choice. If the HDL remains low despite niacin or fibrate therapy, a statin may be useful to significantly decrease the LDL. Although statins have not been proven to benefit isolated low-HDL patients, the AFCAPS/TexCAPS data perhaps support more aggressive LDL-lowering in this population. In populations with low HDL but also low LDL (LDL per HDL ratio of less than or equal to 2.0), there is little evidence of significant CHD.

PATIENT PROFILE #7: NORMAL LIPID PROFILE WITH CORONARY HEART DISEASE OR RECURRENT CORONARY HEART DISEASE

LDL ≤100 mg/dL, TG ≤150 mg/dL, HDL ≥40 mg/dL
Patient example: 50-year-old man; post–inferior wall MI (6 months ago); smoked two packs of cigarettes per day for 30 years; quit post-MI; BP, 124/82 mm Hg

Lipid profile	
Cholesterol	170 mg/dL
TG	150 mg/dL
HDL	42 mg/dL
LDL	98 mg/dL

Treatment Guidelines

Approximately 20% of patients with clinical CHD have relatively normal lipid profiles. As in this patient example, there is frequently another major risk factor present, such as cigarette smoking or hypertension. In addition, emerging risk factors, such as Lp(a) or homocysteine, may be present. There is inadequate clinical trial data to support a definitive therapeutic approach. Many experts hold the view that, regardless of the LDL level in a specific patient, if the patient has CHD, the LDL present is too high for that individual and should be lowered. The National Cholesterol Education Program (NCEP) ATP III updates recommend an optional target of an LDL less than 70 mg per dL and a non-HDL less than 100 mg per dL for patients at very high risk, and patients who have an event with an LDL less than 100 mg per dL usually fall into this category. If an obvious major risk factor is present, as in this patient example (cigarette smoking), and this risk factor is corrected, further lipid control is likely to achieve clinical benefits. Ongoing event trials, such as Treating to New Targets, Study of the Effectiveness of Additional Reduction in Cholesterol and Homocysteine, and Incremental Decrease in Endpoints through Aggressive Lipid-Lowering, may show that further LDL reduction in this population could provide additional clinical benefits.

If a relatively young individual has a coronary event with a normal lipid profile and no other major risk factors are present, a more advanced risk factor evaluation is often warranted, such as determination of Lp(a), homocysteine, or lipoprotein particle distribution. Although the widespread evaluation of these emerging risk factors is controversial, most experts would agree that for patients with premature CHD with a normal lipid profile, strong consideration should be given to advanced risk factor evaluation (expanded lipid testing).

PATIENT PROFILE #8: VERY HIGH RISK

The update to NCEP ATP III recommended an optional LDL goal of less than 70 mg per dL and non-HDL less than 100 mg per dL for patients at very high risk. The definition of very high risk included patients with acute coronary syndromes or cardiovascular disease with other significant risk factors, such as diabetes, cigarette smoking, or multiple risk factors of the metabolic syndrome. The Pravastatin or Atorvastatin Evaluation and Infection Therapy trial, which demonstrated the benefits of 80 mg atorvastatin lowering the LDL to 62 mg per dL compared to 40 mg pravastatin lowering the LDL to 95 mg per

Table 5.1. Heart Protection Study Subgroup Analysis: Major Coronary Event Rates[a]

	Simvastatin allocated (%)	Placebo (%)
Overall	8.7	11.8
Diabetes plus elevated creatinine	24.6	27.4
No diabetes plus elevated creatinine	19.9	21.4
CHD plus diabetes	17.4	21
Cerebrovascular with CHD	16.2	19
Diabetes ≥ age 65 yr	13.4	16.9
Peripheral vascular disease with CHD	13.4	16.4
≥ Age 70 yr	12.4	15.2
HDL <35	10.2	14.4
Smoker	8.8	14.2
Diabetes plus HgA$_{1C}$ ≥7.0	10.3	13.7
Hypertensive	10.3	13.4

CHD, coronary heart disease; HDL, high-density lipoprotein; HgA$_{1C}$, hemoglobin A$_{1C}$.
[a]Major coronary events.

dL or cardiovascular outcomes in patients with acute coronary syndrome, was a relatively short 18-month trial.

This very-high-risk group had a cardiovascular event while taking 80 mg atorvastatin of 22% compared to a 26% event rate on 40 mg pravastatin. This study demonstrated the benefits of initiating aggressive LDL lowering to less than 70 mg per dL in patients with acute coronary syndrome as soon as possible in the hospital setting.

Other very-high-risk groups have been identified in the various clinical trials with statins. Table 5.1 lists the patient subgroups in the Heart Protection Study (HPS) that had a very high residual risk even on statin therapy. These data provide a strong rationale to more aggressively treat LDL and non-HDL to therapeutic optional goals of less than 70 mg per dL and non-HDL less than 100 mg per dL in these very-high-risk populations.

PATIENT PROFILE #9: RENAL DISEASE

The incidence of cardiovascular disease is very high in patients with chronic kidney disease (CKD) and in kidney transplant recipients. In HPS, the patients with elevated creatinine were at the greatest risk of any subgroup for coronary events and, although the 40 mg simvastatin group decreased the risk, the residual event rate, even in the statin treatment group, was very elevated. The National Kidney Foundation has issued guidelines for the management of dyslipidemia in patients with CKD and after renal transplant. These guidelines recommend that

Table 5.2. National Kidney Foundation (NKF) Guidelines

	Target population	Recommendations
NKF Task Force on CVD	Women with Cr ≥1.2 mg/dL, men with Cr ≥1.4 mg/dL; patients with proteinuria; patients with ESRD treated with hemodialysis, peritoneal dialysis, or kidney transplantation.	Use NCEP Guidelines but consider patients to be at CVD highest risk.
K/DOQI Guidelines on CKD	At least 3 mo of either structural or functional abnormalities of the kidney, or GFR <60 mL/min/ 1.73 m².	Treat CVD risk factors but consider patients to be at highest risk.
K/DOQI Guidelines on Dyslipidemia	CKD (as defined by the K/DOQI Guidelines on CKD) and kidney transplant recipients with or without CKD.	Specific for stage 1–5 CKD and kidney transplant recipients.

Cr, creatinine; CKD, chronic kidney disease; CVD, cardiovascular disease; ESRD, end-stage renal disease; GFR, glomerular filtration rate; K/DOQI, Kidney Disease Outcomes Quality Initiative; NCEP, National Cholesterol Education Program.

women with creatinine greater than or equal to 1.2 mg per dL, men with creatinine greater than or equal to 1.4 mg per dL, and patients with proteinuria or end-stage renal disease with or without dialysis and after renal transplant should be considered to be in the highest risk category, with an LDL goal of less than 100 mg per dL and non-HDL less than 130 mg per dL (Table 5.2). These guidelines differ from NCEP ATP III in management of dyslipidemia in patients with renal disease (Table 5.3). The rationale for these more aggressive guidelines from the National Kidney Foundation is due to well-recognized increased risk of CVD in this patient population. However, because most lipid-altering drugs are at least partially renally excreted and the vast majority of these patients are taking multiple drugs that may cause interactions, clinicians must be very careful in the management of dyslipidemia in these patients to avoid significant adverse reactions.

Atorvastatin and fluvastatin are the two statins with the least renal clearance and, therefore, require no significant dosage adjustment for declining renal function (Table 5.4). Fluvastatin is least affected by cyclosporine and has been used safely to reduce CV events in patients after renal transplant, and, thus, in this patient population, this statin is probably the drug of choice. Fluvastatin is also not affected by gemfibrozil, although other statins have significantly increased area under

Table 5.3. Key Features of the National Kidney Foundation-Kidney Disease Outcomes Quality Initiative (NKF-K/DOQI) Guidelines That Differ from Those of the National Cholesterol Program Adult Treatment Panel III and the Expert Panel on Children

NKF-K/DOQI Guidelines	Adult Treatment Panel III Guidelines	Expert Panel on Children
CKD and kidney transplant patients should be considered to be in the highest risk category.	CKD and kidney transplant patients are not managed differently from other patients.	Adolescents with CKD are not managed differently from other patients.
Evaluation of dyslipidemias should occur at presentation, after a change in status, and annually.	Evaluation of dyslipidemias should occur every 5 yr.	If LDL >130 mg/dL, start TLC Step I AHA diet, followed in 3 mo by Step II AHA diet if LDL >130 mg/dL.
Drug therapy should be used for LDL 100–129 mg/dL after 3 mo of TLC.	Drug therapy is considered optional for LDL 100–129 mg/dL.	If LDL ≥160 mg/dL and family history of CHD or two or more CVD risk factors, start drug therapy.
Initial drug therapy for high LDL should be with a statin	Initial drug therapy for high LDL should be with a statin, bile acid sequestrant, or nicotinic acid.	
Recommendations are made for patients age <20 yr.	No recommendations are made for patients age <20 yr.	
Fibrates may be used in stage 5 CKD for patients with triglycerides ≥500 mg/dL and for patients with triglycerides ≥200 mg/dL and non-HDL cholesterol ≥130 mg/dL who do not tolerate statins.	Fibrates are contraindicated in stage 5 CKD.	
Gemfibrozil may be the fibrate of choice for treatment of high triglycerides in patients with CKD and kidney transplant patients.	No preferences are indicated for which fibrate should be used to treat hypertriglyceridemia.	
Adolescents with CKD or kidney transplants should be considered to be in the highest risk category.		

continued

Table 5.3. *Continued*

NKF-K/DOQI Guidelines	Adult Treatment Panel III Guidelines	Expert Panel on Children
Evaluation of dyslipidemias in adolescents with kidney transplants should occur at presentation, after a change in kidney status, and annually. If LDL ≥160 mg/dL, start TLC plus a statin.		

AHA, American Heart Association; CHD, coronary heart disease; CKD, chronic kidney disease; CVD, cardiovascular disease; HDL, high-density lipoprotein; LDL, low-density lipoprotein; TLC, therapeutic lifestyle changes.
Note: To convert mg/dL to mmol/L, multiply triglycerides by 0.01129 and cholesterol by 0.02586.
Note: Currently atorvastatin is the only statin approved by the U.S. Food and Drug Administration for use in children.
From Kasiske B. Am J Transplant 2004;4(Suppl 7):13–53, with permission.

Table 5.4. Recommended Daily Statin Dose Ranges

	Level of glomerular filtration rate (mL/min/1.73 m^2)		
Statin	≥30[a]	>30 or dialysis	With cyclosporine
Atorvastatin	10–80 mg	10–80 mg	10–80 mg
Fluvastatin	20–80 mg	10–80 mg	10–80 mg
Lovastatin	20–80 mg	10–40 mg	10–40 mg
Pravastatin	20–40 mg	20–40 mg	20–40 mg
Simvastatin	20–80 mg	10–40 mg	10–40 mg

[a]Adult Treatment Panel III recommendations for GFR≥30 mL/min/1.732. Most manufacturers recommend once daily dosing, but consider giving 50% of the maximum dose twice daily.
From Kasiske B. Am J Transplant 2004;4(Suppl 7):13–53, with permission.

Table 5.5. Recommended Daily Fibrate Dose Ranges

	Dose [mg by level of glomerular filtration rate (mL/min/1.73 m^2)]			
Fibrate	>90	60–90	15–59	<15
Bezafibrate	200 t.i.d.	200 b.i.d.	200 q.d.	Avoid
Clofibrate	1,000 b.i.d.	1,000 q.d.	500 q.d.	Avoid
Ciprofibrate	200 q.d.	?	?	?
Fenofibrate	201 q.d.	134 q.d.	67 q.d.	Avoid
Gemfibrozil	600 b.i.d.	600 b.i.d.	600 b.i.d.	600 b.i.d.

From Kasiske B. Am J Transplant 2004;4(Suppl 7):13–53, with permission.

the curve in combination with this fibrate. This is of clinical importance because fenofibrate requires dosage adjustments in patients with renal impairment but gemfibrozil does not (Table 5.5). Therefore, for renal patients with combined dyslipidemia, a combination of fluvastatin and gemfibrozil is a good option. Alternatively, other statins should be used in dosages not to exceed 5 to 10 mg in combination with gemfibrozil or low dose of fenofibrate (54 mg). Colesevelam, a bile acid sequestrant, is a nonsystemic drug and, therefore, is appropriate to use in combination with any lipid-lowering therapy. Ezetimibe may be affected by fibrates and cyclosporine and, thus, should be used with caution in combination with these drugs; ezetimibe can, however, be safely be used in conjunction with statins without adversely affecting blood levels. In addition, as many patients with kidney disease or posttransplant receive antifungal drugs, macrolide antibiotics, or calcium channel blockers, caution is necessary if statins, which are metabolized by the cytochrome P450 3A4 pathway, are initiated. In general, only low doses of statins, such as 5 mg of simvastatin or rosuvastatin, 10 mg of atorvastatin, or 80 mg of fluvastatin XL, should be used if the creatinine is greater than 2.0 mg per dL. For further LDL lowering, colesevelam or ezetimibe can be added, if necessary, to achieve the LDL goal of less than 100 mg per dL. If additional triglyceride lowering is necessary, fish oil capsules (1 g of omega-3 fatty acids) are a good option. Gemfibrozil, or a low dose of fenofibrate (54 mg), is the fibrate of choice. Niacin, up to 1,000 to 1,500 mg, is an option to manage low HDL. Niacin is also renally excreted to some degree, so caution is still necessary.

Outcome data for patients with CKD receiving lipid-lowering therapy are not yet available, but the Study of Heart and Renal Protection trial is evaluating the benefits of simvastatin plus ezetimibe in comparison to placebo in a high-risk population with elevated creatinine. The benefits of lipid management for the high-risk population with CKD are likely, but due to safety issues, caution is required.

PATIENT PROFILE #10: HUMAN IMMUNODEFICIENCY VIRUS–ASSOCIATED DYSLIPIDEMIC LIPODYSTROPHY

Since the development of highly active antiretroviral therapy for the treatment of patients with human immunodeficiency virus (HIV) infection, a drug-induced metabolic syndrome has developed characterized by anthropometric changes and severe dyslipidemia. The mechanism underlying the development of HIV-associated dyslipidemia lipodystrophy is not well understood but most likely involves a defect in fatty acid metabolism in peripheral adipocytes. These patients frequently have markedly elevated TGs, low HDL, and increased glucose levels with dorsocervical fat accumulation ("buffalo hump") and loss of fat in the face and gluteus.

Statins may be helpful in improving the lipid abnormalities, but the protease inhibitors also markedly impair metabolism by the cytochrome P450 3A4 pathway. Therefore, pravastatin, rosuvastatin, and fluvastatin are the statins of choice. Agents that inhibit adipocyte lipolysis, such as niacin, or the fibrates that increase fatty-acid oxidation by effectively targeting the underlying biochemical defects may significantly improve the dyslipidemia. Low-carbohydrate diets (50 g per day) are generally useful in improving the glucose levels and the dyslipidemia. Therefore, the general approach for patients with HIV-associated dyslipidemia lipodystrophy is to institute a low-carbohydrate diet (see Appendix A), and, if LDL remains elevated, use a statin that does not require cytochrome P450 3A4 metabolism (or do not exceed 10 mg of cytochrome P450 3A4–metabolized statins). For triglyceride elevation, a fibrate should be initiated, and, if the glucose is well controlled, niacin therapy is an option. In most cases, combination therapy with a statin and a fibrate is required.

SPECIAL POPULATIONS

Women

To the surprise of most women, CHD is the leading cause of death in women by a wide margin over cancer (the majority of women believe cancer is their leading cause of death). Although there have been many reports on the differences between men and women regarding CHD risk, in reality, men and women have basically the same risk factors. On average, the onset of CHD is delayed by 10 to 15 years in women compared to men. Women have lower LDL and higher HDL than men, and their hormonal status appears to account for these differences. Until puberty, boys and girls have similar HDL levels. At puberty, with the concurrent rise in testosterone, the HDL levels in young men decline to lower adult levels. Therefore, the HDL differences between men and women may be an androgen effect, not an estrogen effect. The 20% difference in HDL probably accounts for a decrease in CHD over a lifetime of at least 20%, which may entirely explain the gender difference in CHD risk.

Women more often present with angina as the first symptom whereas men more often present with acute MI or sudden death. How ever, once women have an acute MI, they have a higher mortality than men, with a 12-month mortality of 45% compared to 20% for men, based on the Framingham Heart Study. The higher mortality in women is probably due to their older age and prevalence of other risk factors such as diabetes, hypertension, and hyperlipidemia.

In both men and women, the lipoprotein levels predict a CHD event, but these are modest differences regarding the magnitude of risk associated with each lipid level. The data do not support the concept that the relative impact of LDL may be smaller and that of HDL greater in women than in men. Based on a large pooled univariate analysis for women younger than 65 years, a total cholesterol of 240 mg per dL or higher compared to less than 200 mg per dL was associated with a 144% excess risk of CHD, whereas for men, the excess was 73%. For LDL and HDL (LDL greater than 160 mg per dL vs. less than 130 mg per dL and HDL less than 50 mg per dL vs. greater than 60 mg per dL), the excess risk for women was 227% and 113%, respectively, and 92% and 131% for men. The most striking difference appears to be for TG greater than 130 mg per dL versus less than 100 mg per dL; the excess risk for women increased to 98% compared to 16% for men. In men and women older than 65 years, the excess risk for each lipid parameter is less pronounced, but for women, HDL and TGs remain the most powerful predictors of excess risk. Therefore, as judged from univariate analysis, the lipid risk factors are similar for men and women, with the possible exception of TGs, which appear to be a more powerful predictive factor for CHD in women.

In the major statin trials that included women (Scandinavian Simvastatin Survival Study, Cholesterol and Recurrent Events, Long-term Intervention with Pravastatin in Ischemic Disease, and HPS) (Table 5.6), there appear to be no greater differences regarding the benefits of therapy. Therefore, based on these post-hoc analyses, women should receive the same lipid-lowering therapy as men.

Selective estrogen receptor modulators (SERMs) also have potentially beneficial effects on serum lipids. A SERM (raloxifene) is approved for the prevention and treatment of osteoporosis. SERMs do not reduce vasomotor symptoms, and raloxifene may actually increase the incidence of hot flashes in women. Raloxifene has been compared to conjugated estrogen plus medroxyprogesterone acetate on CHD risk factors (Fig. 5.2). Raloxifene lowers LDL to a similar degree as hormone replacement therapy (HRT) but does not increase TG, and, therefore, Apo B decreases significantly more with raloxifene compared to HRT. Raloxifene also lowers

Table 5.6. Coronary Events in Women in Major Cardiovascular Trials of Statins or Hormone Replacement Therapy (HRT)

Study	No. of women	Statin	Coronary events/treatment group, n (%)	
			Placebo	Risk reduction (%)
Statin trials				
Primary prevention				
AFCAPS/Tex-CAPS	997	7/499 (1.4)[a]	13/498 (2.6)	37 (NR)
Secondary prevention				
4S	827	59/407 (14.5)[b]	91/420 (21.6)	35 (53, 9)
CARE	576	39/290 (13.4)[c]	23/286 (8.0)	46 (22, 62)
LIPID	1,516	90/756 (12.0)[c]	104/760 (13.7)	11 (−18, 33)
Pooled CARE/LIPID	2,092	129/1,046 (12.3)	127/1,046 (12.1)	20 (38, −2)
HRT trials		HRT	Placebo	
HERS	2,763	172/1,380 (12.5)[c]	176/1,383 (12.7)	1 (−20, 22)

4S, Scandinavian Simvastatin Survival Study; AFCAPS/TexCAPS, Air Force/Texas Coronary Atherosclerosis Prevention Study; CARE, Cholesterol and Recurrent Events; CI, confidence interval; HERS, Heart and Estrogen/Progestin Replacement Study; LIPID, Longterm Intervention with Pravastatin in Ischemic Disease; NR, not reported.
[a]*Fatal or nonfatal myocardial infarction (MI), unstable angina, or sudden cardiac death.*
[b]*Coronary death, nonfatal MI, silent MI, resuscitated cardiac arrest.*
[c]*Coronary heart disease death and nonfatal MI.*

C-reactive protein (CRP) compared to HRT that increases CRP levels. Raloxifene, however, does not raise HDL or Apo AI and, therefore, the CHD risk modifying effects are uncertain. In animal experiments, raloxifene was less effective than conjugated estrogen in reducing atherosclerosis in oophorectomized monkeys (Fig. 5.3). The ongoing Raloxifene Use for The Heart (RUTH) trial will hopefully answer many of the questions regarding the cardiovascular effects of SERMs.

In conclusion, the treatment of dyslipidemia for women is similar to men. Hypertriglyceridemia may be a more important risk factor in postmenopausal women compared to men, and, in this group of women, the use of oral HRT (conjugated estrogen plus medroxyprogesterone acetate) must be used with caution. Parenteral estrogen (patch, nasal or lingual spray) may also provide an alternative for women with hypertriglyceridemia and, due to their lack of first-pass hepatic metabolism, may mimic more closely the effects of endogenous estrogen. Statins plus HRT may be an excellent option in general for women, but there is no evidence that this combination provides

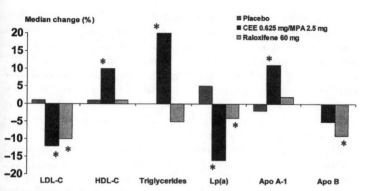

Figure 5.2. Conjugated equine estrogen (CEE)/medroxyprogesterone (MPA) versus raloxifene. Apo A-1, apolipoprotein A-1; HDL-C, high-density lipoprotein-cholesterol; LDL-C, low-density lipoprotein-cholesterol; Lp(a), lipoprotein(a). *significantly ($P <.05$) different from placebo. (From Walsh BW, Kuller LH, Wild RA, et al. Effects of raloxifene on serum lipids and coagulation factors in healthy postmenopausal women. *JAMA* 1998;279:1445–1451, with permission.)

greater benefit than statins alone. The prevailing wisdom regarding HRT is to individualize the treatment according to the patient's history. For women in whom HRT may be a good option, a lifetime strategy should be considered. This lifetime strategy involves low-dose oral contraceptives in the perimenopausal period and standard HRT doses

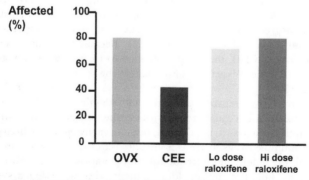

Figure 5.3. Atherosclerosis: raloxifene. Prevalence of atherosclerosis measured as the percentage of animals affected. CEE, conjugated equine estrogen; OVX, ovariectomized. (From Clarkson TB, Anthony MS, Jermone CP, et al. *J Clin Endocrinol Metab* 1998;83:721–726, with permission.)

for the first 5 years after menopause to reduce vasomotor symptoms, prevent bone loss, and maintain an improved lipid profile. After 5 years of menopause, perhaps a lower dose of HRT is sufficient to maintain bone density, and after 10 years postmenopause, switch to a SERM to continue to provide protection against osteoporosis while reducing LDL levels and, perhaps, reducing the risk of breast cancer. This lifetime strategy has become increasing popular and may provide the best long-term approach regarding the use of hormone therapy to maximize the quality of life for women.

The American Heart Association recently issued evidence-based guidelines for cardiovascular disease prevention in women. In light of the Heart and Estrogen/Progestin Replacement Study and Women's Health Initiative trials in postmenopausal women, which demonstrated no cardiovascular benefits for hormone therapy, including estrogen therapy alone, these guidelines recommend that hormones not be initiated for either primary or secondary prevention of cardiovascular disease. Table 5.7 lists the clinical recommendations.

Elderly

Age is the most powerful risk factor for CHD. Every decade of life approximately doubles the risk. The Framingham risk score gives the greatest number of points to age and, therefore, an older patient is more likely to receive a more aggressive goal for LDL than a younger patient (Table 5.8). In addition, the elderly represent the population with the greatest burden of disease (Fig. 5.4). Therefore, the misconception that an older person is perhaps immune from CHD is not based on the data. The elderly also appear to benefit to an equal or greater degree than younger individuals from statin therapy in the endpoint trials (Table 5.9 and Fig. 5.5). Because the elderly are at greater risk of CHD, the number needed to treat to avoid one CHD event in the elderly is actually lower than in the younger patient cohort (Table 5.10).

The main issue regarding treating dyslipidemia in the elderly is the cost of treatment because the elderly bear the burden of out-of-pocket prescription purchases. In addition, because many elderly patients are taking multiple drugs, there is a greater risk of drug interactions. In general, the elderly more frequently have comorbid disease that may complicate lipid therapy. All elderly patients with dyslipidemia should be screened with a thyroid-stimulating hormone level to rule out hypothyroidism and a urinalysis to evaluate proteinuria. Impaired liver function is more common in the elderly, and although statin therapy is

Table 5.7. Guide to Cardiovascular Disease (CVD) Prevention in Women: Clinical Recommendations

Lifestyle interventions
    Cigarette smoking
        Consistently encourage women not to smoke and to avoid environmental tobacco. (Class I, Level B)$_{GI=1}$
    Physical activity
        Consistently encourage women to accumulate a minimum of 30 min of moderate-intensity physical activity (e.g., brisk walking) on most, and preferably all, days of the week. (Class I, Level B)$_{GI=1}$
    Cardiac rehabilitation
        Women with a recent acute coronary syndrome or coronary intervention, new-onset or chronic angina should participate in a comprehensive risk-reduction regimen, such as cardiac rehabilitation or a physician-guided home- or community-based program. (Class I, Level B)$_{GI=2}$
    Heart-healthy diet
        Consistently encourage an overall healthy eating pattern that includes intake of a variety of fruits, vegetables, grains, low-fat or nonfat dairy products, fish, legumes, and sources of protein low in saturated fat (e.g., poultry, lean meats, plant sources). Limit saturated fat intake to <10% of calories, limit cholesterol intake to <300 mg/d, and limit intake of transfatty acids. (Class I, Level B)$_{GI=1}$
    Weight maintenance/reduction
        Consistently encourage weight maintenance/reduction through an appropriate balance of physical activity, caloric intake, and formal behavioral programs when indicated to maintain/achieve a BMI between 18.5 and 24.9 kg/m^2 and a waist circumference <35 in. (Class I, Level B)$_{GI=1}$
    Psychosocial factors
        Women with CVD should be evaluated for depression and referred/treated when indicated. (Class IIa, Level B)$_{GI=2}$
    Omega-3 fatty acids
        As an adjunct to diet, omega-3 fatty acid supplementation may be considered in high risk[a] women. (Class IIb, Level B)$_{GI=2}$
    Folic acid
        As an adjunct to diet, folic acid supplementation may be considered in high-risk[a] women (except after revascularization procedure) if a higher-than-normal level of homocysteine has been detected. (Class IIb, Level B)$_{GI=2}$
Major risk factor interventions
    Blood pressure—lifestyle
        Encourage an optimal blood pressure of <120/80 mm Hg through lifestyle approaches. (Class I, Level B)$_{GI=1}$
    Blood pressure—drugs
        Pharmacotherapy is indicated when blood pressure is ≥140/90 mm Hg or an even lower blood pressure in the setting of blood pressure–related target-organ damage or diabetes. Thiazide diuretics should be part of the drug regimen for most patients unless contraindicated. (Class I, Level A)$_{GI=1}$

continued

Table 5.7. *Continued*

Lipid, lipoproteins
> Optimal levels of lipids and lipoproteins in women are LDL-C <100 mg/dL, HDL-C >50 mg/dL, triglycerides <150 mg/dL, and non-HDL-C (total cholesterol minus HDL-C) <130 mg/dL and should be encouraged through lifestyle approaches. (Class I, Level B)$_{GI=1}$

Lipids—diet therapy
> In high-risk women or when LDL-C is elevated, saturated fat intake should be reduced to <7% of calories, cholesterol to <200 mg/d, and transfatty acid intake should be reduced. (Class I, Level B)$_{GI=1}$

Lipids—pharmacotherapy—high risk[a]
> Initiate LDL-C-lowering therapy (preferably a statin) simultaneously with lifestyle therapy in high-risk women with LDL-C ≥100 mg/dL (Class I, Level A)$_{GI=1}$, and initiate statin therapy in high-risk women with an LDL-C <100 mg/dL unless contraindicated (Class I, Level B)$_{GI=1}$.
> Initiate niacin[b] or fibrate therapy when HDL-C is low, or non-HDL-C elevated in high-risk women. (Class I, Level B)$_{GI=1}$

Lipids—pharmacotherapy—intermediate risk[c]
> Initiate LDL-C-lowering therapy (preferably a statin) if LDL-C level is ≥130 mg/dL on lifestyle therapy (Class I, Level AB)$_{GI=1}$, or niacin[b] or fibrate therapy when HDL-C is low or non-HDL-C elevated after LDL-C goal is reached. (Class I, Level B)$_{GI=1}$

Lipids—pharmacotherapy—lower risk[d]
> Consider LDL-C–lowering therapy in low-risk women with 0 or 1 risk factor when LDL-C level is ≥190 mg/dL or if multiple risk factors are present when LDL-C is ≥160 mg/dL (Class IIa, Level B) or niacin[b] or fibrate therapy when HDL-C is low or non-HDL-C elevated after LDL-C goal is reached. (Class IIa, Level B)$_{GI=1}$

Diabetes
> Lifestyle and pharmacotherapy should be used to achieve near normal HgA$_{1c}$ (<7%) in women with diabetes. (Class I, Level B)$_{GI=1}$

CVD prevention strategies for clinical practice
> Assess and stratify women into high, intermediate, lower, or optimal risk categories.
> Lifestyle approaches (smoking cessation, regular exercise, weight management, and heart-healthy diet) to prevent CVD are Class I recommendations for all women and a top priority in clinical practice.
> Other CVD risk-reducing interventions should be prioritized on the basis of strength of recommendation (Class I > Class IIa > Class IIb) and within each class of recommendation on the basis of the level of evidence, with the exception of lifestyle, which is a top priority for all women (A > B > C).
> Highest priority for risk intervention in clinical practice is based on risk stratification: (high risk > intermediate risk > lower risk > optimal risk).
> Avoid interventions designated as Class III.

continued

Table 5.7. *Continued*

Priorities for prevention in practice based on risk classification
  Women at high risk (>20% risk)
    Class I recommendations
      Smoking cessation/environmental smoke avoidance
      Physical activity/cardiac rehabilitation
      Diet therapy
      Weight maintenance/reduction
      Blood pressure control
      Lipid control/statin therapy
      Aspirin therapy (75–162 mg)
      Beta-blocker therapy unless contraindicated
      ACE inhibitor therapy (ARBs if contraindicated)
      Glycemic control in diabetics
    Class IIa recommendation
      Evaluation/referral for depression
    Class IIb recommendations
      Omega-3 fatty-acid supplementation
      Folic acid supplementation
  Women at intermediate risk (10% to 20% risk)
    Class I recommendations
      Smoking cessation/environmental smoke avoidance
      Physical activity
      Heart-healthy diet or lipid-lowering diet
      Weight maintenance/reduction
      Blood pressure control
      Lipid control
    Class IIa recommendation:
      Aspirin therapy (75–162 mg)
  Women at lower risk (<10% risk)
    Class I recommendations:
      Smoking cessation/environmental smoke avoidance
      Physical activity
      Heart-healthy diet or lipid-lowering diet
      Weight maintenance/reduction
      Treat individual CVD risk factors as indicated
  Stroke prevention among women with atrial fibrillation
    Class I recommendations:
      High-intermediate risk of stroke
        Warfarin therapy
      Low risk of stroke (<1%/year) or contraindication to warfarin
        Aspirin therapy (325 mg)
    Class III (not recommended for CVD prevention):
      Hormone therapy in postmenopausal women
      Antioxidant supplements
      Aspirin therapy in low-risk women

continued

Table 5.7. *Continued*

	Classification and levels of evidence
	Strength of recommendation
Classification	
Class I	Intervention is useful and effective
Class IIa	Weight of evidence/opinion is in favor of usefulness/efficacy
Class IIb	Usefulness/efficacy is well established by evidence/opinion
Class III	Intervention is not useful/effective and may be harmful
Level of evidence	
A	Sufficient evidence from multiple randomized trials
B	Limited evidence from single randomized trial or other non-randomized studies
C	Based on expert opinion, case studies, or standard of care
GI	
1	Very likely that results generalize to women
2	Somewhat likely that results generalize to women
3	Unlikely that results generalize to women
0	Unable to project whether results generalize to women

ACE, angiotensin-converting enzyme; ARB, angiotensin receptor blocker; BMI, body mass index; GI, generalizability index; HDL-C, high-density lipoprotein cholesterol; LDL-C, low-density lipoprotein cholesterol.
[a]High-risk is defined as coronary heart disease (CHD) or risk equivalent, or 10-year absolute CHD risk >20%.
[b]Dietary supplement niacin must not be used as a substitute for prescription niacin, and over-the-counter niacin should only be used if approved and monitored by a physician.
[c]Intermediate risk is defined as 10-year absolute CHD risk of 10% to 20%.
[d]Lower risk is defined as 10-year absolute CHD risk <10%.
From Mosca L. J Am Coll Cardiol 2004;43:900–921, with permission.

contraindicated in patients with active liver disease, patients with non-alcoholic fatty liver disease can usually receive statin therapy without adverse outcomes. Most drugs that are used by the elderly are metabolized hepatically by the cytochrome P450 3A4 pathway. Lovastatin, sim-

Table 5.8. Effect of Age on Global Risk

68-yr-old man		40-yr-old man	
Blood pressure	138/85	Blood pressure	138/85
Total cholesterol	198	Total cholesterol	198
Triglycerides	90	Triglycerides	90
High-density lipoprotein cholesterol	42	High-density lipoprotein cholesterol	42
Low-density lipoprotein cholesterol	138	Low-density lipoprotein cholesterol	138
Estimate of 10-yr risk for coronary heart disease	20%	Estimate of 10-yr risk for coronary heart disease	2%

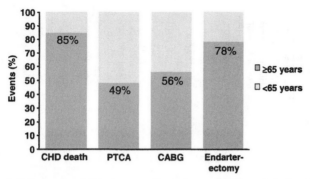

Figure 5.4. Proportion of clinical coronary heart disease (CHD) events in the elderly. CABG, coronary artery bypass graft; PTCA, percutaneous transluminal coronary angioplasty. (From American Heart Association. 1999 Heart and Stroke Statistical Update. AHA;1998, with permission.)

vastatin, and atorvastatin are also metabolized as substrates through this pathway, whereas fluvastatin is metabolized by P450 2C9 and pravastatin and rosuvastatin do not require P450 metabolism. Potent P450 3A4 inhibitors, which include cyclosporine, ketoconazole, nefazodone, and erythromycin, should be avoided, if possible, in combination with these P450 3A4 metabolized statins. In general, because the elderly may have decreased hepatic and renal function and are frequently on polypharmacy, caution should be used in initiating statin therapy, especially at higher doses. This is especially true for elderly women who have a smaller BMI and appear to be more prone to drug interactions. The best strategy with the elderly is to start with lower doses and titrate the dose gradually as needed to achieve the NCEP ATP III goals.

Children, Adolescents, and Young Adults

The earliest atherosclerotic lesion, the fatty streak, often begins in childhood, and autopsy data have correlated the extent of fatty streaks in children with serum cholesterol. By adolescence, fibrous coronary arterial plaques may be ubiquitous and also appear to depend on the number of risk factors present. The preponderance of evidence supports a lifelong pathology for atherosclerotic disease. However, considerable controversy exists about the treatment of lipid disorders in children, adolescents, and even young adults. There are two categories of children that require special attention: the obese child and the child with a strong family history of premature CHD. According to the Bogalusa Heart Study, the obese child is far

Table 5.9. Clinical Trials with a Significant Number of Elderly Subjects

Study	Age range, yr	Subjects, n	Entry criteria	Intervention	Net mean change in lipids	Follow-up, yr	Selected outcomes[a]
HPS	40–80 (28% >70)	20,536	Primary and secondary prevention	Simvastatin, 40 mg, vs. placebo	TC: ↓ 20% LDL: ↓ 29% HDL: ↑ 3% TG: ↓ 14%	5	All-cause mortality: OR (0.87) CHD: 18% RRR of CHD death Stroke: 30% RRR of ischemic stroke
ASCOT-LLA	40–79 (64% >60)	10,305	Primary prevention	Atorvastatin, 10 mg, vs. placebo	TC: ↓ 18% LDL: ↓ 28% HDL: No change TG: ↓ 12%	3.3 (planned for 5)	All-cause mortality: Not significant CHD: 30% RRR in total coronary events Stroke: 29% in fatal and nonfatal stroke
PROSPER	70–82	5,804	Primary and secondary prevention	Pravastatin, 40 mg, vs. placebo	TC: no data LDL: ↓ 32% HDL: ↑ 5% TG: ↓ 12%	3.2	All-cause mortality: Not significant CHD: 17% RRR in CHD death or nonfatal MI Stroke: No difference

Trial	Age	N	Prevention	Drug	Lipid effects	Years	Outcomes
ALLHAT-LLT	>55	10,355	Primary and secondary prevention	Pravastatin, 40 mg, vs. placebo	TC: ↓ 14% LDL: ↓ 16% HDL: No change TG: ↓ 3.5%	4.8	All-cause mortality: Not significant CHD: Not significant Stroke: Not significant
PROVE-IT	>18	4,162	Secondary prevention after acute coronary syndrome	Pravastatin, 40 mg, vs. atorvastatin, 80 mg	TC: No data LDL: ↓ 10% HDL: ↑ 8.1% TG: No data TC: No data LDL: ↓ 42% HDL: ↑ 6.5% TG: No data	2	All-cause mortality: Not significant CHD: 12% RRR in MI, revascularization, or CHD death Stroke: Not significant

ALLHAT-LLT, Antihypertensive and Lipid-Lowering Treatment to Prevent Heart Attack Trial—Lipid-Lowering Trial; ASCOT-LLA, Anglo-Scandinavian Cardiac Outcomes Trial—Lipid Lowering Arm; CHD, coronary heart disease; HDL, high-density lipoprotein; HPS, Heart Protection Study; LDL, low-density lipoprotein; MI, myocardial infarction; OR, odds ratio; PROSPER, Prospective Study of Pravastatin in the Elderly at Risk; PROVE-IT, Pravastatin or Atorvastatin Evaluation and Infection Therapy trial; RRR, relative risk ratio; TC, total cholesterol; TG, triglyceride.
[a]All reach statistical significance unless otherwise indicated.

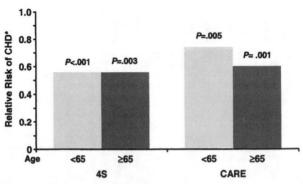

Figure 5.5. Statins in secondary prevention of cardiovascular disease in the elderly. CARE, Cholesterol and Recurrent Events; CHD, coronary heart disease; 4S, Scandinavian Simvastatin Survival Study. *CHD death only. [Adapted from Miettinen TA, Pyorala K, Olsson AG, et al. Cholesterol-lowering therapy in women and elderly patients with myocardial infarction of angina pectoris: findings from the Scandinavian Simvastatin Survival Study (4S).*Circulation* 1997:96:4211–4218; and Lewis SI, Moge LA, Sacks FM, et al. Effect of pravastatin on cardiovascular events in older patients with myocardial infarction and cholesterol levels in the average range. Results of the Cholesterol and Recurrent Events (CARE) trial. *Ann Intern Med* 1998;129:681–689.]

more likely to have dyslipidemia, and obese children usually become obese adults with metabolic syndrome. Obesity in children has become an epidemic in the United States, with adolescents between the ages of 10 and 20 years the fastest growing population with type 2 diabetes. A child with a body weight greater than the ninety-fifth percentile for his or her age is cause for concern requiring dietary counseling. The Dietary Intervention in School Children trial demonstrated that comprehensive dietary counsel-

Table 5.10. Number-Needed-to-Treat (NNT) to Avoid One Coronary Heart Disease Event, Death, or Myocardial Infarction in Secondary Prevention Trials

Trial	NNT by patient age (yr)[a]	
	Older	Younger
4S	11	12
CARE	15	67
LIPID	20	34

4S, Scandinavian Simvastatin Survival Study; CARE, Cholesterol and Recurrent Events; LIPID, Long-term Intervention with Pravastatin in Ischemic Disease.
Note: Although secondary prevention in elderly patients appears to be very cost effective, the cost effectiveness of primary prevention in the elderly remains an open question.
[a] ≥65 versus <65 in 4S and CARE; 65–69 versus 55–64 in LIPID.

Table 5.11. Major Lipid Cutpoints in Children and Adolescents

Category	Level (mg/dL)
Blood cholesterol	
High	200 or higher
Borderline high	170–199
Desirable	Below 170
Low-density lipoprotein	
High	130 or higher
Borderline high	110–129
Desirable	Below 110
High-density lipoprotein	
Low	Below 35
Borderline low	35–45
Desirable	Above 45

ing in children effectively lowered saturated fat intake and LDL cholesterol without adversely affecting growth and development. Along with caloric restriction, increasing physical activity is critical for the long-term success of weight management. The American Heart Association (AHA) and the American Academy of Pediatrics both endorse the Step I diet in children 2 years of age or older; however, total fat intake should not be less than 30% of calories in the pediatric population.

The NCEP expert panel on blood cholesterol levels in children and adolescents issued detailed guidelines for the recognition and treatment of hypercholesterolemia in young people (between the ages of 2 and 19 years) in 1992. This panel discouraged mass screening but recommended evaluating lipid profiles after the second year in children with certain risk factors. Lipid profiles should be determined in children whose parents or grandparents have premature CHD or hypercholesterolemia (serum cholesterol greater than or equal to 240 mg per dL). Physicians may also choose to measure cholesterol levels for children and adolescents whose parental or grandparental history is unobtainable, particularly those children with other risk factors such as obesity or cigarette smoking. Although not specifically stated in the guidelines, all children above the ninetieth percentile of body weight to age should also have a screening lipid profile. The cardiologist is probably the physician most responsible for recommending that the children or grandchildren of high-risk adults be screened for hyperlipidemia. Table 5.11 lists the major lipid cutpoints in children and adolescents (between the ages of 2 and 19 years).

The treatment of hyperlipidemia in children should be dietary therapy only before age 10 years, except for the rare child with homozygous or severe heterozygous familial hypercholesterolemia. Familial hypercholesterolemia is detectable at birth, with homozygous familial hypercholesterolemia occurring in only 1 in 1 million people. In children with homozygous fit, cutaneous xanthomas develop in the first few months of life, and the treatment is LDL apheresis.

If the child is older than 10 years of age and a Step I diet is unsuccessful, including the addition of viscous soluble fibers, plant sterols, and soy protein to lower the LDL cholesterol below 160 mg per dL, then pharmacologic therapy may be considered. Drug therapy should not be considered in children without other risk factors or a family history of premature CHD unless the LDL cholesterol exceeds 190 mg per dL. The minimum goal to achieve is an LDL less than 130 mg per dL. The NCEP expert panel only recommended bile acid sequestrants because these drugs are nonsystemic and data on statin safety were not available in 1992. However, the Lovastatin Adolescent Male Study demonstrated the efficacy and safety of 1 year of lovastatin, 40 mg, in boys between the ages 10 and 14 years in their rapid growth phase. Lovastatin-treated males had the same growth and development as the placebo-treated population. Because bile acid sequestrants, with the exception of colesevelam, are unpalatable to most children, statins should be considered if the child is noncompliant with resin therapy. Although the Lovastatin Adolescent Male Study trial demonstrated excellent safety, statins should ideally be initiated after boys develop some facial hair and girls begin menstruating. For elevated plasma TG in pediatric patients, dietary caloric restriction (especially simple carbohydrates) and exercise should be recommended. Drug therapy should be reserved for only extreme elevations.

After age 21 years, the NCEP ATP III guidelines should be enacted. The Cardiac Assessment Risk in Adolescents study has provided useful information regarding the prevalence of CHD risk factors in young adults between the ages of 18 and 30 years. Table 5.12 shows selected percentiles for men and women for total cholesterol in young adults. Special lifestyle attention should be directed to men and women who are above the fiftieth percentile for total cholesterol. Studies have demonstrated that these are the individuals who develop premature CHD, and early dietary counseling and management of other risk factors are likely to significantly benefit this population in later years.

Diabetic Patients

The diabetic patient is one of the most common but also one of the most difficult patients in which to achieve all the recommended goals. Due to the high risk for CHD, the NCEP ATP III, the American Diabetes Associa-

Table 5.12. Coronary Artery Risk Development in Young Adults Study: Total Cholesterol (Selected Percentiles)

Percentile	White men		White women		Black men		Black women	
	18–24 (n = 424)	25–30 (n = 698)	18–24 (n = 472)	25–30 (n = 806)	18–24 (n = 576)	25–30 (n = 495)	18–24 (n = 706)	25–30 (n = 705)
Total cholesterol (mg/dL)								
95	228	243	227	230	225	249	238	240
90	204	226	214	220	211	231	222	228
75	186	202	192	197	187	203	197	204
50	166	177	170	174	166	183	173	178
25	147	158	152	156	145	160	152	157
10	132	140	139	141	128	140	136	138
5	122	132	130	131	120	130	128	129
Mean (SD)	168.1 (31.6)	181.0 (33.9)	173.5 (29.7)	177.8 (31.1)	167.8 (31.5)	183.7 (36.1)	176.3 (34.3)	181.1 (33.1)

tion, and the Seventh Report of the Joint National Convention on Prevention, Detection, Evaluation, and Treatment of High Blood Pressure have recommended more aggressive goals for the diabetic patient. Combining the recommendation of all three panels, the goals are as follows: LDL less than 100 mg per dL, non-HDL less than 130 mg per dL, TG less than 150 mg per dL, HDL greater than 40 mg per dL, BP less than or equal to 130/80 mm Hg, and hemoglobin A_{1c} less than 7.0%.

The statin and fibrate trials have demonstrated that diabetic patients benefit from either drug class for reducing cardiovascular events (Table 5.13). Therefore, in most respects, the diabetic, similar to the nondiabetic, should be treated according to their dyslipidemia profile (American Diabetes Association guidelines, Table 5.14). However, because the diabetic patient usually has more aggressive goals than the nondiabetic patient and is often taking other drugs to modify other cardiovascular risk factors, the potential risk of drug side effects is significantly greater in this population. Therapeutic lifestyle changes can be effective in patients with diabetes and should be the first line of treatment. Intensive diet and exercise therapy should be initiated and continued even if drug therapy is used. Hopefully, lifestyle changes will ameliorate the need to use multiple drug therapies.

Nevertheless, it is common for a diabetic patient to be taking multiple drugs for each risk factor present. In regard to dyslipidemia, bile acid resins are rarely used, as they tend to raise TG levels. Niacin can worsen glucose control and, therefore, is usually avoided. However, more recent data have demonstrated that niacin may be used successfully in patients with diabetes and should be considered in diabetic patients with a low HDL or high Lp(a).

The most commonly used drugs in the diabetic patient are statins or fibrates. In a diabetic patient with impaired renal function, fenofibrate must be used with caution, and a statin dose must be adjusted accordingly (see Patient Profile #9: Renal Disease). For patients with hypertriglyceridemia and renal failure, marine oil capsules are an option instead of a fibrate, and niacin may be used cautiously. If patients have normal renal function (creatinine greater than 2.0 mg per dL), statins are the first option if the LDL is greater than or equal to 130 mg per dL and TGs are less than 400 mg per dL. If TGs are greater than 400 mg per dL, a fibrate should be used first. If combination therapy with a statin is anticipated (e.g., non-HDL greater than 160 mg per dL), fenofibrate or, if available, bezafibrate or ciprofibrate should be considered, as the myopathy rate appears to be lower when these fibrates are combined with statins. Fenofibrate in the Diabetes

Table 5.13. Summary of Secondary Prevention Trials in Subgroups of Patients with Diabetes

Study	Drug/dose	No. patients with MCE/ total no. of patients (%)		% Reduction in RR (95% CI)	P value
		Placebo	Active treatment		
Scandinavian Simvastatin Survival Study	Simvastatin, 20–40 mg/d				
Diabetic		44/97 (45%)	24/105 (23%)	55 (24–74)	.002
Nondiabetic		578/2,126 (27%)	407/2,116 (19%)	32 (23–40)	<.00001
Cholesterol and Recurrent Events	Pravastatin, 40 mg/d				
Diabetic		112/304 (37%)	81/282 (29%)	25 (0–43)	.05
Nondiabetic		437/1,774 (25%)	349/1,799 (19%)	23 (11–33)	<.001
Long-term Intervention with Pravastatin in Ischemic Disease	Pravastatin, 40 mg/d				
Diabetic		88/386 (23%)	76/396 (19%)	19 (−10 to 41)	
Nondiabetic		627/4,116 (15%)	481/4,116 (12%)	25 (15–33)	
Veterans Administration High-Density Lipoprotein Intervention Trial	Gemfibrozil, 1,200 mg/d				
Diabetic		116/318 (36%)	88/309 (28%)	24 (−0.1 to 43.0)	.05
Nondiabetic		214/949 (23%)	170/955 (18%)	24 (6–30)	.009

CI, confidence interval; MCE, major coronary events; RR, relative risk.

Table 5.14. Order of Priorities for Treatment of Diabetic Dyslipidemia in Adults[a]

Low-density lipoprotein cholesterol lowering[a]
  First choice
    Hepatic 3-methylglutaryl coenzyme A reductase inhibitor (statin)
  Second choice
    Bile acid binding resin (resin)
High-density lipoprotein cholesterol raising
  Behavioral interventions, such as weight loss, increased physical activity, and
    smoking cessation, may be useful
  Difficult except with nicotinic acid, which is relatively contraindicated
Triglyceride lowering
  Glycemic control first priority
  Fibric acid derivative (gemfibrozil)
  Statins are moderately effective at high dose in hypertriglyceridemic subjects
    who also have high low-density lipoprotein cholesterol
Combined hyperlipidemia
  First choice
    Improved glycemic control plus high-dose statin
  Second choice
    Improved glycemic control plus statin[b] plus gemfibrozil[b]
  Third choice
    Improved glycemic control plus resin plus gemfibrozil
    Improved glycemic control plus statin[b] plus nicotinic acid[b] (glycemic control
      must be monitored carefully)

[a]Decision for treatment of high low-density lipoprotein before elevated triglyceride is based on clinical trial data indicating safety as well as efficacy of the available agents.
[b]The combination of statins with nicotinic acid and especially with gemfibrozil may carry an increased risk of myositis.

Atherosclerosis Intervention Study showed a 40% reduction in the progression of coronary atherosclerosis compared to a placebo angiographically. In the fenofibrate group, there was a decrease of 23% in the combined events, which was not significant because the sample size of only 418 type 2 diabetic patients was probably too small. When the LDL is between 100 and 130 mg per dL, only gemfibrozil has been shown to benefit patients with a low HDL level in the VA-HIT trial. However, if TGs are not elevated (less than 500 mg per dL), many experts would still consider a statin the first option, even though the clinical outcome data only support gemfibrozil at this time.

Often in diabetic patients, monotherapy is insufficient to achieve the combined goals of LDL less than 100 mg per dL, non-HDL less than 130 mg per dL, TG less than 150 mg per dL, and HDL greater than 40 mg per dL, and, thus, combination therapy is required. A statin-fibrate combination is logical, but close follow-up is necessary.

Other options include statin-niacin, especially if HDL is low or Lp(a) is high, but increasing the glucose control may be necessary. A third option is to add marine oil capsules containing 3 to 6 g of omega-3 fatty acids (three to nine capsules, depending on omega-3 concentration). This option adds fat calories and also may require tighter glucose control. Triple drug therapy is sometimes required, but extreme caution should be used because the potential for drug interaction is significant.

Statin Intolerant

Approximately 5% of hyperlipidemic patients do not tolerate statins, usually due to myalgias or, occasionally, gastrointestinal disturbance. Less than 1% discontinue statin use because of liver function abnormalities or myopathy (creatine phosphokinase greater than ten times the upper limits of normal with symptoms). Patients with liver function abnormalities or myopathy usually tolerate a lower dose of the statin, but patients with myalgias (muscle aches without creatine phosphokinase elevations) or gastrointestinal complaints may continue to have symptoms on lower doses or different statins. The cause of myalgias is uncertain, and in controlled trials, the incidence is far less than in clinical practice and similar to the placebo rate. Switching from one statin to another sometimes results in a statin the patient can tolerate. Although only anecdotal, some physicians have found success in preventing statin-induced myalgia by coadministering 50 mg of coenzyme Q10 (ubiquinone). Statins may decrease ubiquinone levels in skeletal muscles. Nonstatin therapy, such as the bile acid–binding polymer colesevelam, the cholesterol absorption inhibitor ezetimibe, niacin, or fibrates, may also be used if statin intolerance is unavoidable. Many patients may tolerate an every-other-drug dosing of a low-dose statin alternating with an every-other-drug dosing of ezetimibe.

Cardiac Transplant

The heart transplant patient is relatively rare, but also one of the most difficult patients to manage with dyslipidemia. Lipid abnormalities are common after heart transplantation, with up to 80% of recipients developing total cholesterol levels greater than 220 mg per dL. In addition, allograft coronary vasculopathy (ACV), an accelerated form of atherosclerotic disease, is considered to be due to chronic rejection and increases progressively to 20% to 45% by 3 years. Because hyperlipidemia is a significant factor for ACV (Table 5.15), the aggressive

Table 5.15. Fasting Serum Lipid and Lipoprotein Values

Variable	No ACV (n = 97)	ACV (n = 33)	P value[a]
Total cholesterol (mmol/L)	6.3 (1.7)	7.1 (2)	.02
Low-density lipoprotein cholesterol (mmol/L)	4.4 (1.0)	4.9 (1.6)	.03
Triglycerides (mmol/L)	2.0 (1.0)	2.3 (1.3)	.54
High-density lipoprotein cholesterol (mmol/L)	1.15 (0.3)	1.4 (0.9)	.68
Lipoprotein(a) (mg/dL)	22 (1–170)	71 (3–193)	.0006

ACV, allograft coronary vasculopathy.
Note: Results as mean (standard deviation) except for Lipoprotein(a), which is given as median (range).
[a]P value calculated using Mann-Whitney test.
From Barbir, et al., with permission.

management of lipid levels in cardiac transplant is of paramount importance to improve long-term organ survival.

The reasons for the high prevalence of dyslipidemia in cardiac transplant patients is multifunctional. First, many patients who undergo cardiac transplants have ischemic heart disease with concomitant hyperlipidemia. In one study, patients with a pretransplant diagnosis of ischemic cardiomyopathy had significantly higher posttransplant total cholesterol levels of 282 mg per dL compared with 224 mg per dL in those with a diagnosis of dilatated cardiomyopathy. In addition, the immunosuppressive regime with cyclosporin A, azathioprine, and oral prednisolone used to prevent allograft rejection adversely affects lipoprotein levels.

The treatment of dyslipidemia in cardiac transplant patients may prevent ACV and improve survival. In a nonblind trial, 97 transplant patients received pravastatin or placebo. After a 1-year follow-up, the patients treated with pravastatin showed a significant reduction in mortality rate, as well as a significantly lower incidence of ACV. In a larger, uncontrolled series of 244 heart transplant recipients with hyperlipidemia, those who responded well to statin therapies, simvastatin, pravastatin, or fluvastatin and were followed for a mean of 10 years tended to survive longer. Statins, in addition to improving elevated lipoproteins, may have other effects that improve allograft survival. Statins have been shown to decrease antibody-dependent cellular cytotoxicity and natural killer-cell function. Simvastatin has been shown to reduce ACV without significant changes in lipoprotein concentrations in a rat model of heart transplantation of FK506 immunosuppressive therapy.

Statins would appear to be ideal drugs to use in cardiac transplant patients, except for the major issue that cyclosporine has significant pharmacokinetic interactions with statins, and numerous cases of rhabdomyolysis have been reported with concomitant use. Cyclosporine is a potent inhibitor of the cytochrome P450 3A4 pathway that provides the major hepatic catabolism of lovastatin, simvastatin, atorvastatin, and cerivastatin. These cytochrome P450 3A4–metabolized statins have a higher incidence of reported rhabdomyolysis when combined with cyclosporine than pravastatin and fluvastatin. Pharmacokinetic studies have demonstrated that cyclosporine markedly increases the area under the curve for lovastatin compared to a far smaller increase for pravastatin. However, pravastatin has also been reported to induce rhabdomyolysis in posttransplant patients treated with cyclosporine, so other pharmacokinetic interactions, in addition to cytochrome P450 inhibition, may also be involved. Fluvastatin is metabolized by P450 CY9 and appears to have a significantly lower incidence of rhabdomyolysis in transplant patients. In the Assessment of Lescol in Renal Transplantation trial, approximately 1,000 post–renal transplant patients taking cyclosporine and fluvastatin have had no reported cases of rhabdomyolysis. Simvastatin, at lower doses (up to 20 mg), has also been shown to be relatively safe. It is advisable that patients on statin therapy be informed about the potential side effects of muscular ache and weakness, and their creatinine kinase levels should be measured on a regular basis.

Many cardiac transplant centers are performing annual intravascular ultrasounds to evaluate the progression of ACV. If ACV develops, more aggressive lipid lowering with statin or combination therapies may be beneficial, and many experts lower their target LDL cholesterol to less than 75 mg per dL in these patients. Lp(a) appears to be a potent risk factor for ACV (Fig. 5.6). In patients with high Lp(a) and ACV, consideration should be given to combining niacin with a statin (with the usual precautions), but if the ACV is severe and especially if the patient is statin intolerant, LDL apheresis, which also lowers Lp(a), should be strongly considered. Table 5.16 summarizes the potential therapies for treating ACV.

TREATMENT OF EMERGING RISK FACTORS

Lipoprotein(a)

Lp(a) is an LDL particle with an Apo(a) attached. Apo(a) is linked to LDL by a disulfide bond with a repeating kringle structure (named for a looped Scandinavian pastry) (Fig. 5.7). This structure has significant homology to plasminogen, and the enhanced CHD risk associated with Lp(a) is reportedly due to the inhibiting effects of this lipoprotein particle on plasminogen activation, leading to enhanced thrombosis.

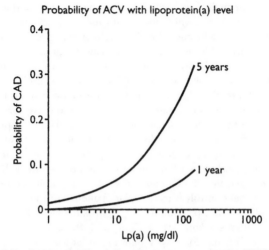

Figure 5.6. Predicted probability of allograft coronary vasculopathy (ACV) versus lipoprotein(a) [Lp(a)] level for men without hypertension 1 and 5 years after transplant. CAD, coronary artery disease. (From Barbir, et al., with permission.)

Lp(a) may also increase the atherogenicity of LDL. The majority of observational trials (10 of 15) support the association of Lp(a) with enhanced cardiovascular risk. Every 30 mg per dL increase in Lp(a) approximately doubles the risk of CHD. The distribution of Lp(a) levels in the population is different from the bell-shaped curve for serum cholesterol, but the majority of Americans have low levels (less than 10 mg per dL), with a small percentage having greater than 30 mg per dL. Elevated Lp(a) is more common in the Asian Indian and Turkish population.

Therapeutically modifying Lp(a) is controversial, and only two pharmacologic treatments, niacin and estrogen, modestly lower Lp(a). Both niacin and estrogen lower Lp(a) by approximately 20%. A post-hoc analysis of the Heart and Estrogen/Progestin Replacement Study demonstrated that for women with CHD with the highest quartile of Lp(a), HRT resulted in a significant reduction in subsequent coronary events. In the Familial Atherosclerosis Treatment Study, the lowering of Lp(a) with niacin appeared to beneficially modify atherosclerotic progression as determined by quantitative angiography. These trials are supportive, but not conclusive, that lowering Lp(a) with either

Table 5.16. Treating Allograft Arteriopathy

Antiproliferative agents
  Angiopeptin
  Low-molecular-weight heparin (Enoxiparin)
Newer immunosuppressive agents
  Mycophenolate mofetil
  Rapamycin
  Anticytokine/TAC monoclonal antibodies as induction
Older immunosuppressive strategies
    (added to conventional agents)
  Methotrexate
  Cyclophosphamide
  Induction lymphocytolytic strategies
    (monoclonal/polyclonal antibodies)
Antihypertensive agents
  Calcium channel blockers
    Diltiazem
  Angiotensin-converting enzyme inhibitors
Lipid-lowering agents
  Hepatic 3-methylglutaryl coenzyme A reductase inhibitors
Antioxidants/vitamins
  Fish oil
  Omega-3 fatty acids
  Vitamin E
  Vitamin B_6
  Folic acid
Prophylactic antimicrobial therapy
  Ganciclovir infusions
  Chronic prophylactic antimicrobial administration
Photophoresis
Lipoprotein aphoresis (HELP therapy)
Coronary revascularization
  Percutaneous transluminal angioplasty/stent placement
  Percutaneous rotablator/atherectomy
  Coronary artery bypass
Transmyocardial laser revascularization
Aspirin

HELP, heparin-induced extracorporeal low-density lipoprotein precipitation.

estrogen or niacin may be beneficial. Another approach for the patient with elevated Lp(a) is to significantly lower LDL. Transgenic mice expressing human Apo(a) developed vascular lesions only when fed a lipid-rich diet, not when fed normal chow. In addition, the odds ratio for having significant angiographic CHD in patients with high (greater

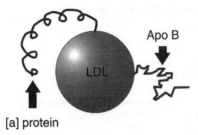

[a] protein

Figure 5.7. See text for explanation. Apo B, apolipoprotein B; LDL, low-density lipoprotein.

than 30 mg per dL) versus low (less than or equal to 5 mg per dL) Lp(a) levels increased from 1.67 to 6.0, as concomitant LDL concentrations increased. Therefore, Lp(a) may be a significantly less important risk factor if LDL is less than 100 mg per dL. If Lp(a) is elevated and treatment is deemed necessary in the judgment of the physician, the decision to use niacin or estrogen for women is enhanced, but the primary focus of therapy should be to aggressively lower LDL or non-HDL to the appropriate goals.

Homocysteine

Homocysteine is an amino acid that, if elevated, results in an increased risk of CHD. The strength of this association is debatable, but, clearly, patients with an inherited defect in homocysteine catabolism resulting in hyperhomocysteinuria have a marked increased risk of premature atherosclerosis and thrombosis. These rare genetic deficiencies of either methylenetetrahydrofolate reductase or of cobalamin metabolism result in homocysteinuria in which 30% of untreated patients have thrombotic events by age 20 years. These genetic enzyme deficiencies are rare, but many other factors may affect homocysteine levels (Table 5.17). The most important acquired causes of increased homocysteine levels are nutritional deficiency of either folate, vitamin B_{12}, or vitamin B_6. Because homocysteine levels can be effectively lowered with vitamin supplementation, this risk factor is an intriguing target for therapeutic intervention.

A metaanalysis of both retrospective and prospective trials demonstrates a moderate but relatively consistent association between homocysteine and increased CHD and cerebrovascular events (Fig. 5.8). Because factors that raise homocysteine such as a folate-deficient diet

Table 5.17. Determinants of Plasma Homocysteine (Hcy) Level

Personal characteristics	
Increasing age	↑
Male gender	↑
Menopause	↑
Genetic	
Enzyme defects	
Homozygous/heterozygous defects in cystathionine β-synthase	↑↑↑
Homozygous/heterozygous defects in methylenetetrahydrofolate reductase	↑↑↑
Thermolabile methylenetetrahydrofolate reductase	↑↑
Methionine synthase	↑
Cobalamin transport and metabolism	↑↑↑
Acquired	
Nutritional deficiency of	
Folate	↑↑
Vitamin B_{12}	↑↑
Vitamin B_6	↑
Disease states	
Renal impairment	↑↑
Hypothyroidism	↑
Liver disease	↑
Diabetic retinopathy	↑
Psoriasis	↑
Acute lymphoblastic leukemia	↑
Convalescent period after myocardial infarction	↑
Convalescent period after stroke	↑
Drugs	
Nitrous oxide	↑↑
Anticonvulsants—phenytoin, carbamazepine	↑
Theophylline	↑
Methotrexate	↑
Tamoxifen	↓
Azarabine	↑
Nicotinic acid	↑
Oral contraceptive	↓
Fish oil	↓
Penicillamine	↓
Lifestyle characteristics	
Tobacco smoking	↑
Sedentary lifestyle	↑
Caffeinated coffee	↑
Alcohol	↑↓

↓, reduced plasma + tHcy level; ↑, mildly increased plasma Hcy level (<15 μmol/L); ↑↑, moderate hyperhomocysteinemia (15–30 μmol/L); ↑↑↑, severe hyperhomocysteinemia (>30 μmol/L).

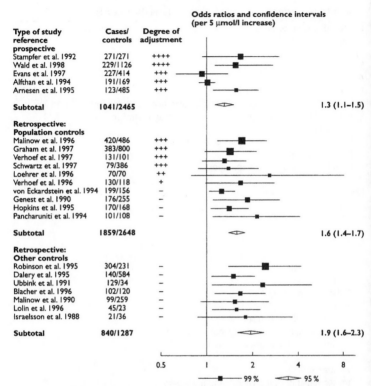

Figure 5.8. Metaanalysis of case control and prospective epidemiologic studies up to 1998. Odds ratios in epidemiologic studies of plasma total homocysteine and coronary heart disease. Odds ratios compare a 5 μmol per L increase in baseline concentration of plasma total homocysteine in the different studies. Black squares indicate the odds ratio in each study plotted on a doubling scale, with the square size proportional to the number of cases and the horizontal lines representing the 99% confidence intervals. The combined odds ratio in each subtotal and its 95% confidency interval are indicated by unshaded diamonds. Degree of adjustment for confounders denoted as: – for no adjustment at all, + for age and sex only, ++ for age and sex plus smoking, +++ for these plus some other standard vascular risk factors, ++++ for these plus markers of social class. (Adapted from Danesh J. *J Cardiovasc Risk* 1998;5:229–232.)

(low in green vegetables), hypothyroidism, and renal failure may be independently associated with increased CHD risk, the value of measuring and treating high homocysteine levels is uncertain. Furthermore, after the fortification of the U.S. food supply with folate to reduce the incidence of neural tube birth defects, the number of patients with moderate hyperhomocysteinemia is likely to be small. Therefore, neither the American College of Cardiology nor the AHA advocates population-based screening for homocysteine. In addition, due to the high cost of measuring homocysteine and the relatively low cost of folate (the cost of one homocysteine blood test is approximately equivalent to at least 2 years of folate therapy), many experts advocate folate, B_{12}, and B_6 supplementation but not routine homocysteine measurements for patients with or at high risk for CHD. There is also a lack of proven clinical trial evidence that lowering homocysteine levels with folate and other B vitamin supplementation results in reduced ischemic events. There are several ongoing vitamin trials that are prospectively evaluating the benefits of homocysteine reduction on CHD risk.

Although there is no clear consensus on whom to test or treat for elevated homocysteine, in patients with premature or a strong family history for CHD or recurrent CHD with a relatively benign lipid profile, measuring homocysteine may provide useful guidance in a comprehensive risk management strategy. A normal homocysteine level is less than 10 µmol per L, and, similar to serum cholesterol, the risk for CHD increases in a relatively linear manner for homocysteine levels between 10 and 15 µmol per L. If homocysteine is elevated, often a multivitamin with 400 mg of folate is sufficient to lower the level to normal, but certain patients require higher doses of folate or other factors that enhance homocysteine catabolism to satisfactorily lower the level to below 10 µmol per L.

C-Reactive Protein

CRP is a marker of general inflammation reflecting the formation of foam cells formed from macrophages engulfing oxidized LDL particles. Foam cells secrete interleukin-6 that induces the liver to secrete CRP. CRP is the best studied of a series of inflammatory markers that appear to predict CHD risk (Table 5.18). The concentration of CRP associated with atherosclerosis is substantially below those of most routine CRP assays (3 mg per L), and, thus, a more sensitive assay termed *high-sensitivity CRP* (hs-CRP) has been developed. Several studies suggest that measurement of CRP may provide a useful method of assessing the risk of CHD in apparently healthy people, particularly when

Table 5.18. Potential Inflammatory Biochemical Surrogates

General
   C-reactive protein
   Serum amyloid A
   Fibrinogen
Cytokines
   Interleukin-6
   Tissue necrosis factor-α
Endothelium adhesion molecules
   Vascular cellular adhesion molecules
   Intervascular cellular adhesion molecules
   E-selectin
Lesion lytic enzymes
   MMP-1, MMP-2, MMP-3, MMP-9
   Enzyme activated by oxidized low-density lipoprotein, lipoprotein-associated
      phospholipase A_2

MMP, matrix metalloproteinase.

LDL is low. In addition, the endpoint trials (AFCAPS and Cholesterol and Recurrent Events) have demonstrated that statins lower CRP and that this reduction of CRP is associated with a reduction in endpoints, but this effect of statin may be independent of its effect on cholesterol. All statins appear to lower CRP. In a crossover study, with equal lowering of LDL, atorvastatin, simvastatin, and pravastatin lowered CRP equally. There appears to be a greater difference in that in apparently healthy women, CRP levels greater than 1.5 mg per L predict three to seven times the risk for MI or stroke, but for men, a CRP level greater than 2.11 mg per L predicts three times the risk for MI and two times the risk for ischemic stroke. There also appears to be a lag time between the detection of elevated CRP and when an atherosclerotic event occurs. The test is most predictive for risk of an event 4 to 6 years later. CRP as a risk predictor alone is comparable to the total cholesterol to HDL ratio and is additive to the ratio when used in combination (Fig. 5.9).

The more criteria for the metabolic syndrome the patient has, the more likely CRP will be elevated (Fig. 5.10B). However, even for those patients with the metabolic syndrome, the presence of an elevated CRP is associated with an increased risk of CHD (Fig. 5.10C). In the AFCAPS/TexCAPS trial, a post-hoc analysis demonstrated that patients with an LDL below the median but a CRP above the median has the same relative risk reduction on statin therapy as those with high LDL (Fig. 5.10A). The hypothesis that patients with elevated CRP levels but

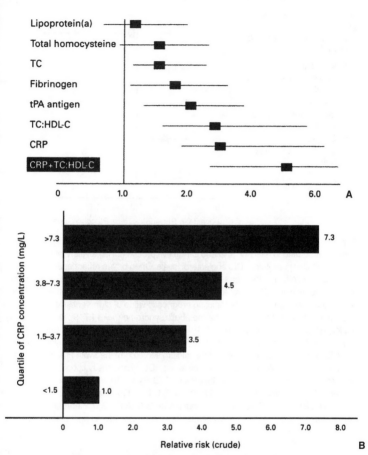

Figure 5.9. A: C-reactive protein (CRP) and total cholesterol (TC) to high-density lipoprotein cholesterol (HDL-C) ratio together are a stronger predictor of myocardial infarction (MI). **B:** Relative risk of future MI or stroke. tPA, tissue plasminogen activator. (Adapted from Ridker.)

LDL levels that are below the NCEP ATP III drug treatment initiation thresholds will benefit from lipid-lowering therapy is being tested in the ongoing Justification for Use of statins in Primary prevention: an Intervention Trial Evaluating Rosuvastatin. Justification for Use of statins in Primary prevention: an Intervention Trial Evaluating Rosuvastatin is a randomized trial of 15,000 patients with a CRP level

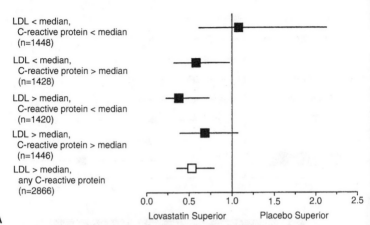

A

Figure 5.10. A: Relative risks (and 95% confidence intervals) associated with lovastatin therapy, according to baseline lipid and C-reactive protein (CRP) levels. Data are shown for low-density lipoprotein (LDL) cholesterol levels. Open boxes reflect analyses for all participants with LDL cholesterol levels higher than the median. **B:** Graph depicting the relationship between CRP level and Adult Treatment Panel III (ATP III) definition of the metabolic syndrome. **C:** Graph depicting prognostic value of high-sensitivity CRP in relation to the ATP III definition of the metabolic syndrome (n = 14,719). **D:** Graph depicting how the prognostic value of CRP adds to the Framingham Risk Score and LDL cholesterol (LDL-C). **E:** Hazard ratio for coronary death or nonfatal myocardial infarction (MI) based on coronary artery calcium score combined with Framingham risk score (n = 1,029). CVD, cardiovascular disease; HDL, high-density lipoprotein; TG, triglyceride. *P <.05; †P <.001; ‡P <.03; §P <.006; □ P <.01; ¶P <.005; #P <.002. (**B** from Ridker PM, et al. *Circulation* 2003;107:391–397; **C** from Greenland et al. *JAMA* 2003;291:210; **D** from Ridker, et al. *N Engl J Med* 2002;347:1557. Reproduced with permission. Copyright © 2002 Massachusetts Medical Society. All rights reserved.)

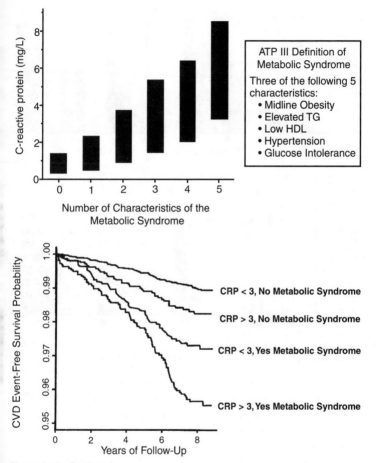

ATP III Definition of
Metabolic Syndrome

Three of the following 5
characteristics:
- Midline Obesity
- Elevated TG
- Low HDL
- Hypertension
- Glucose Intolerance

Figure 5.10. *Continued*

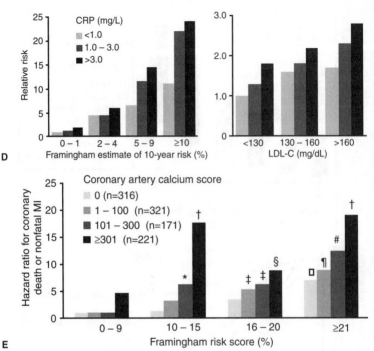

Figure 5.10. *Continued*

greater than 2.0 mg per dL but an LDL level less than 130 mg per dL treated with rosuvastatin, 20 mg, or with placebo. Besides statins, other lipid-lowering agents, such as niacin, fibrates, and ezetimibe, have been shown to lower CRP levels. According to the AHA/Centers for Disease Control Scientific Statement on Markers of Intervention and Cardiovascular Disease, the patient with an intermediate Framingham ATP III 10-year risk score of 10% to 20% with an LDL level below the cutpoint for initiation of drug therapy is the most appropriate patient in whom to measure CRP level (Fig. 5.10D). The basis for this recommendation is that in this intermediate risk group, an elevated CRP level would provide a rationale to initiate lipid-lowering therapy. In patients already known to be at high risk, such as those with diabetes, CHD or a greater than 20% Framingham 10-year risk score, measuring CRP level would not be necessary because the initiation of lipid-lowering therapy is clearly indicated.

Table 5.19. American Heart Association/Centers for Disease Control Panel: Recommendations for High-Sensitivity C-Reactive Protein (hs-CRP) Laboratory Testing

Measurements of hs-CRP
   Should be performed twice (2 wk apart)
   Results averaged, expressed as mg/L
   Fasting or nonfasting, in metabolically stable patients
   If level >10 mg/L, test should be repeated, patient examined for sources of infection or inflammation
Relative risk categories for hs-CRP levels
   Low: <1 mg/L
   Average: 1.0–3.0 mg/L
   High: >3.0 mg/L

Data from Pearson, et al., Circulation 2003;107:499.

The AHA/Centers for Disease Control panel considered recommending more widespread testing of CRP level, such as in those patients with a family history of CHD or the metabolic syndrome, but considered the evidence inadequate at this time (Table 5.19). For patients with CHD, more aggressive treatment of LDL in those with an elevated CRP has not yet been demonstrated to be beneficial in clinical trials. As more evidence accumulates regarding the benefits of CRP testing, the recommendation as to which patients are likely to benefit from testing is likely to broaden.

Lipoprotein-Associated Phospholipase A$_2$

Lipoprotein-associated phospholipase A$_2$ (Lp-PLA$_2$) is a subtype of the phospholipase A$_2$ superfamily, a family of enzymes that hydrolyze phospholipids. Lp-PLA$_2$, also known as *platelet-activating factor acetylhydrolase*, is a 50-kD, Ca^{2+}-independent phospholipase that is distinct from another macrophage product, secretary PLA$_2$, a 14-kD, Ca-dependent enzyme. Increasing evidence suggests that Lp-PLA$_2$ plays a critical role in the vascular inflammatory process that leads to the development of atherosclerosis and its clinical sequelae. Lp-PLA$_2$ activity is upregulated in atherosclerotic plaques and, when released into circulation, binds specifically to LDL.

The key role of Lp-PLA$_2$ in atherogenesis is its hydrolysis of oxidized LDL, which is generated when LDL becomes oxidized in the milieu of the artery wall. The hydrolysis of oxidized LDL by Lp-PLA$_2$ produces the proinflammatory, atherogenic byproducts lysophosphatidylcholine and oxidized fatty acids. Lysophosphatidylcholine plays a critical role in atherogenesis. It acts as a chemoattractant for monocytes, impairs endothelial function, causes cell death by disrupting

Table 5.20. Lipoprotein-Associated Phospholipase A$_2$ (Lp-PLA$_2$) and C-Reactive Protein (CRP): Independent and Distinct Inflammatory Markers

CRP	Lp-PLA$_2$
Marker of systemic inflammation	Marker of vascular inflammation
Produced by liver in response to inflammatory reactions—acute phase reactant	An enzyme produced by macrophages
Specific role in cardiovascular disease unclear	Appears to be involved in the initiation of the early stage of the vascular inflammatory process
Not usable in all patients due to existing inflammatory conditions	Minimal biovariability
Not a specific target for therapeutic intervention	Not affected by other inflammatory conditions
	A specific target for pharmacologic intervention for the treatment of coronary heart disease

plasma membranes, and induces apoptosis in smooth muscle cells and macrophages.

Based on clinical data obtained from a number of recent epidemiologic studies, it appears that the determination of Lp-PLA$_2$ levels may aid in the identification of individuals at high risk for CHD and stroke. Elevated levels of Lp-PLA$_2$ have been shown to indicate a greater risk of plaque formation and rupture independent of traditional risk factors and CRP (Table 5.20). The PLAC™ test is an enzyme immunoassay developed for the quantitative determination of Lp-PLA$_2$ in human plasma to be used in conjunction with clinical evaluation and patient risk assessment in predicting risk for CHD. Results are reliable and reproducible when the assay procedure is carried out with adherence to good laboratory practice.

Lipoprotein Subfractions

Many lipid specialists use advanced laboratory testing to determine subfractions of LDL, HDL, and VLDL. The three most popular technologies that have been developed by commercial laboratories are ultracentrifugation (Berkeley Heart Labs, Berkeley, CA), vertical autoprofile (Atherotec, Birmingham, AL), and nuclear magnetic resonance (NMR) (LipoMed, Raleigh, NC). The price for the lipoprotein subfraction tests ranges from $75 to $300. The main purpose of these tests is to identify patients at higher risk for CHD due to small, dense LDL or pattern B. These tests also determine VLDL and HDL subfractions. Generally, patients with high TG and low HDL have dense LDL, but between

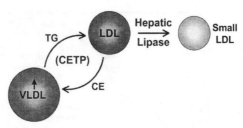

Figure 5.11. See text for explanation. CE, cholesterol ester; CETP, cholesterol ester transfer protein; LDL, low-density lipoprotein; TG, triglycerides, VLDL, very-low-density lipoprotein.

TG levels of 100 and 200 mg per dL, the likelihood of pattern B varies significantly. In the presence of hypertriglyceridemia, LDL particles are TG enriched and relatively cholesterol poor and are catalyzed by cholesterol ester transfer protein. The TG-enriched LDL particles are further degraded by hepatic lipase to form a small, dense, more atherogenic LDL particle (Fig. 5.11). Therefore, the total LDL level may be normal, but the number of LDL particles is significantly increased. The Quebec Cardiovascular Study followed 2,000 men over a 5-year period. This study demonstrated that the denser the LDL particle, the greater the increased risk for CHD, and the risk was extremely high (odds ratio of 6.2) if both the LDL particles were small and the particle concentration was high (LDL greater than 120 mg per dL).

Subfactoration of VLDL and HDL have also demonstrated differences in CHD risk. Increased large VLDL particles in testing plasma correlate with impaired rates of chylomicron clearance, which independently predict CHD risk. For HDL, the larger subclasses appear to confer most of the protection from CHD, compared to the smaller HDL particles. The NMR LipoProfile determines all the various lipoprotein subclasses (Fig. 5.12). Figure 5.13 provides an example of an NMR LipoProfile with an annotated explanation of the various lipoprotein subclasses.

The basic question regarding advanced lipoprotein testing is whether these tests should be used routinely. Because non-HDL incorporates all of the potentially atherogenic lipoproteins, perhaps simply targeting non-HDL as recommended by ATP III in patients with TG greater than 200 mg per dL sufficiently reduces CHD risk. The superiority of lipoprotein subclass testing over non-HDL to further reduce CHD risk requires further investigation. However, the tests have become more economical ($75 per test) and provide a relatively accurate standard lipid profile as well. Therefore, these tests may provide clinically useful information

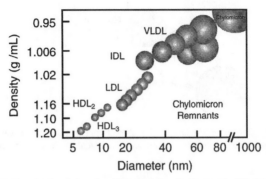

Figure 5.12. See text for explanation. HDL, high-density lipoprotein; IDL, intermediate-density lipoprotein; LDL, low-density lipoprotein; VLDL, very-low-density lipoprotein.

without significantly adding cost. In patients with premature CHD or a strong family history of CHD with a relatively benign lipid profile, these tests may provide the greatest value. The most promising advanced lipoprotein test is the LDL particle concentration, which determines the total number of LDL particles (nmol per L) in the blood determined by direct measurement of four LDL subclasses, including IDL. LDL particle concentration may be more strongly linked with CHD risk than LDL cholesterol and, therefore, may be a better target of therapy. Fibrates or niacin may more likely convert a patient from pattern B (dense LDL) to pattern A (large LDL) by lowering TG more than a statin, but statins are more effective at lowering LDL particle concentrations. The results of advanced lipid testing often lead to the use of combination therapy or higher dose statins to achieve the optimal targets for all the lipoprotein subclasses. Proponents of these tests believe that ultimately CHD risk assessment will be better defined and targeted treatment will more successfully prevent atherosclerosis progression. This hypothesis requires further clinical evaluation.

Noninvasive Tests for Preclinical Disease

The ability of traditional risk factors to predict the development of clinical atherosclerosis is, at best, 80% accurate. Advocates of noninvasive tests to evaluate the severity of preclinical atherosclerotic plaque maintain that these tests indicate the actual presence of disease rather than risk factors to disease and are, therefore, better predictors of CHD events. In addition, improvement in these surrogate markers of

Produced under patent licenses to U.S. Patent Nos. 4,933,844 and 5,343,389

© LipoMed, Inc. 2001

NMR LipoProfile®

LipoMed, Inc.
3009 New Bern Avenue
Raleigh, NC 27610
877-547-6837
www.lipoprofile.com

Page 1 of 2

Patient Name	Sex	Age
	M	63

Patient ID	Birth Date	Accession Number
	7-29-36	18820

Clinician Name & Address

Clinician — Client #/Route #
Client Name
Address 1
Address 2
Phone:
Fax:

Date Collected	Date Received	Report Date and Time	Requisition Number	Comment
08/24/2001	08/25/2001	08/26/2001 6:15 pm (R)	LM314906	see page 3

LIPOPROTEIN PANEL

Coronary Heart Disease (CHD) Risk Categories

		Optimal*	Near optimal	Borderline-high	High	Very high
LDL Particle Number	nmol/L 1654	under 1100	1100 - 1399	1400 - 1799	1800 - 2100	over 2100

* *Goal for patients with CHD or CHD risk equivalents*

		Pattern A (large LDL)	Pattern B (small LDL)
LDL Particle Size	nm 19.1	22.0 - 20.6	20.5 - 19.0
		Lower-Risk	Higher-Risk

		Negative Risk Factor	Intermediate	Positive Risk Factor
Large HDL (cholesterol)	mg/dL 10	greater than 30	30 - 11	less than 11

		Lower-Risk	Intermediate	Higher-Risk
Large VLDL (triglyceride)	mg/dL 35	less than 7	7 - 27	greater than 27

LDL particle number risk categories correspond to NCEP risk categories for LDL cholesterol (20th, 50th, 80th, & 95th percentile cutpoints).

LDL particle sizes are referenced to those measured by electron microscopy and are 5 nm smaller than gradient gel electrophoresis estimates. Pattern A and B definitions correspond to those of Austin et al. (JAMA 1988;260:1917).

Large HDL is the protective component of HDL; levels < 11mg/dL (30th percentile) indicate higher risk and > 30 mg/dL (75th percentile) lower risk.

Large VLDL levels are correlated with plasma triglyceride levels and delayed chylomicron clearance; values > 27 mg/dL (75th percentile) indicate higher risk and < 7 mg/dL (25th percentile) lower risk.

RISK ASSESSMENT PANEL

Elevated LDL particle number and the lipoprotein traits of the metabolic syndrome affect CHD risk interactively. Risk is highest when both are present.

Elevated LDL Particle Number — >1400 nmol/L ✓

Lipoprotein Traits of the Metabolic Syndrome* — ≥2 traits ✓

Lipoprotein Traits of the Metabolic Syndrome*

Small LDL Pattern B (≤ 20.5 nm)	Reduced Large HDL (<11 mg/dL)	Elevated Large VLDL (>27 mg/dL)
✓	✓	✓

* *Other identifiers of the metabolic syndrome include abdominal obesity, elevated blood pressure, and fasting glucose ≥110 mg/dL.*

Figure 5.13. Understanding the nuclear magnetic resonance (NMR) LipoProfile. NMR LipoProfile testing helps to better evaluate a patient's need for therapy and measures treatment response in a consistent, quantifiable manner. Follow-up NMR analysis is essential to determining effectiveness of a prescribed course of treatment. HDL, high-density lipoprotein; IDL, intermediate-density lipoprotein; LDL, low-density lipoprotein; VLDL, very-low-density lipoprotein.

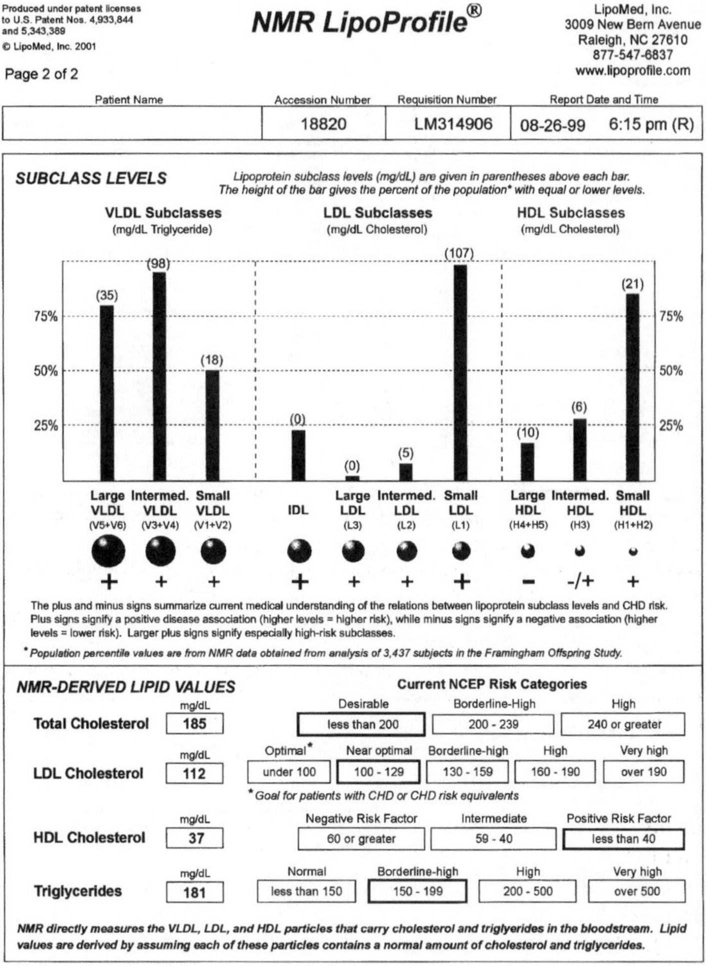

Produced under patent licenses to U.S. Patent Nos. 4,933,844 and 5,343,389

© LipoMed, Inc. 2001

Page 2 of 2

NMR LipoProfile®

LipoMed, Inc.
3009 New Bern Avenue
Raleigh, NC 27610
877-547-6837
www.lipoprofile.com

Patient Name	Accession Number	Requisition Number	Report Date and Time
	18820	LM314906	08-26-99 6:15 pm (R)

SUBCLASS LEVELS

Lipoprotein subclass levels (mg/dL) are given in parentheses above each bar. The height of the bar gives the percent of the population with equal or lower levels.*

The plus and minus signs summarize current medical understanding of the relations between lipoprotein subclass levels and CHD risk. Plus signs signify a positive disease association (higher levels = higher risk), while minus signs signify a negative association (higher levels = lower risk). Larger plus signs signify especially high-risk subclasses.

** Population percentile values are from NMR data obtained from analysis of 3,437 subjects in the Framingham Offspring Study.*

NMR-DERIVED LIPID VALUES

Current NCEP Risk Categories

	mg/dL					
Total Cholesterol	185	Desirable: less than 200	Borderline-High: 200 - 239	High: 240 or greater		
LDL Cholesterol	112	Optimal*: under 100	Near optimal: 100 - 129	Borderline-high: 130 - 159	High: 160 - 190	Very high: over 190
HDL Cholesterol	37	Negative Risk Factor: 60 or greater	Intermediate: 59 - 40	Positive Risk Factor: less than 40		
Triglycerides	181	Normal: less than 150	Borderline-high: 150 - 199	High: 200 - 500	Very high: over 500	

** Goal for patients with CHD or CHD risk equivalents*

NMR directly measures the VLDL, LDL, and HDL particles that carry cholesterol and triglyerides in the bloodstream. Lipid values are derived by assuming each of these particles contains a normal amount of cholesterol and triglycerides.

Figure 5.13. *Continued*

atherosclerosis may better indicate the benefits of therapy, or a lack of a beneficial change in these markers may mean more aggressive therapeutic interventions are necessary. The National Institutes of Health has initiated the Multi-Ethnic Study of Atherosclerosis to determine if the noninvasive assessment of preclinical disease improves risk predict-

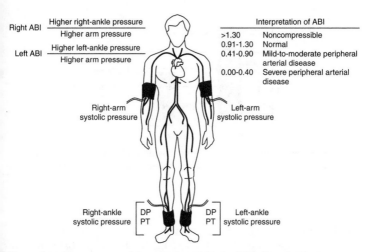

Figure 5.14. Measurement of the ankle-brachial index (ABI). Systolic blood pressure is measured by Doppler ultrasonography in each arm and in the dorsalis pedis (DP) and posterior tibial (PT) arteries in each ankle. The higher of the two arm pressures is selected, as is the higher of the two pressures in each ankle. The right and left ABI values are determined by dividing the higher ankle pressure in each leg by the higher arm pressure. The ranges of the ABI values are shown, with a ratio greater than 1.30 suggesting a noncompressible, calcified vessel. In this condition, the true pressure at that location cannot be obtained, and additional tests are required to diagnose peripheral arterial disease. Patients with claudication typically have ABI values ranging from 0.41 to 0.90, and those with critical leg ischemia have values of 0.40 or less.

ability and provides clinical value beyond the traditional risk assessment scores.

One of the easiest to perform and least costly noninvasive measures of preclinical atherosclerosis is the ankle-brachial index (ABI) (Fig. 5.14). This test shows goal reproducibility, with 95% confidence variability of a single measurement being approximately 16%. An ABI of less than 0.90 is commonly used as a cutpoint to define peripheral vascular disease. The NCEP ATP III also defines peripheral vascular disease as an ABI of less than 0.90, and, therefore, the LDL goal for these patients is less than 100 mg per dL. The severity of the ABI abnormality predicts cardiovascular disease mortality, and for each risk factor, the coexistence of an ABI less than 0.90 significantly increases the CHD mortality (Fig. 5.15). Although ABI abnormalities increase sharply with age, for adults between the ages of 40 and 59 years, only 2% to 3% have

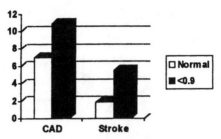

Figure 5.15. Percentage of elderly men with coronary artery disease (CAD) and stroke by presence or absence of abnormal ankle-brachial index. (Adapted from *Arterioscler Thromb Vasc Biol.*)

an abnormal ABI. Therefore, the ABI is a helpful screening tool to identify high-risk individuals for CHD. ABI should probably be conducted routinely on smokers older than age 40 years, because although their NCEP ATP III Framingham risk score may not be 20% or greater, an ABI of less than 0.90 would automatically place the patient in the CHD risk-equivalent category with an LDL goal of less than 100 mg per dL. In addition, these patients should be on aspirin or other antiplatelet therapy and, based on the Heart Outcomes Prevention Evaluation trial, may benefit from ACE inhibitors, such as ramipril, used in this trial. The Mobile Lipid Clinic™ program calculates the ABI, and if the ABI is less than 0.90, establishes an LDL goal of less than 100 mg per dL for the patient.

Carotid ultrasound has been extensively evaluated as a tool to assess CHD risk and as a surrogate to demonstrate the benefits of therapeutic interventions. B-mode ultrasounds to measure the intima media thickness (IMT) of the common carotid (near and far wall) and the internal carotid have been fairly well standardized (Fig. 5.16). Although the far wall of the common carotid is the easiest and most standardized of the measurements, most epidemiologic studies have found that a combined score of the near and far wall of the common carotid plus the internal carotid is the best predictor of CHD risk. The Cardiovascular Health Study showed that IMT at the adjustment for other risk factors was significantly associated with risk of MI and stroke (Fig. 5.17). One study showed that each 0.1-mm increase in common carotid IMT is associated with a 1.91 total risk of CHD. In patients with documented CHD, the Cholesterol-Lowering Atherosclerosis Study showed that each 0.03-mm increase per year in carotid IMT conferred a relative risk

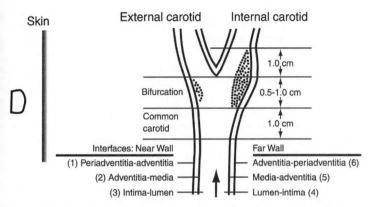

Figure 5.16. B-mode ultrasound: measurements technique. Schematic diagram of high-resolution B-mode ultrasound showing measures of maximal intima-media thicknesses of the common carotid and internal carotid artery in the near and far walls. [Adapted from the MIDAS Research Group. Design features. *Am J Med* 1989;86(Suppl 4A):37–39.]

of 2.2 for nonfatal MI or coronary deaths and 3.1 for any cardiovascular event. Therefore, carotid IMT screening may be useful to predict increased risk in patients without documented CHD and may also be a helpful guide to intensity treatment if the IMT continues to progress. The small changes in carotid IMT (0.03-mm increase per year) that

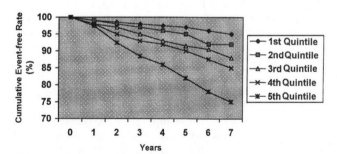

Figure 5.17. Unadjusted cumulative event-free rates for the combined endpoint of myocardial infarction or stroke, according to quintile of combined intima-medial thickness. (Adapted from *N Engl J Med.*)

predict increased risk for events may be difficult to visualize unless the ultrasonography is well standardized. Feinstein and Macioch have demonstrated that bubble contrast can greatly assist the measurements of the near and far wall and, therefore, perhaps better identify the patients in whom the atherosclerotic progression continues despite adequate LDL reduction (Fig. 5.18). In the patients who continue to have progression of carotid IMT thickness, more aggressive LDL treatment or evaluation of other risk factors may be necessary. The Atorvastatin Simvastatin Atherosclerosis Project trial comparing simvastatin, 40 mg, to atorvastatin, 80 mg, in patients with familial hypercholesterolemia has demonstrated that in the simvastatin-treated patients, the carotid IMT continued to progress, but in the more aggressive LDL-treated group with atorvastatin, there was slight regression. This study highlights the potential ability of carotid IMT measurements as a useful tool to adequately treat patients with preclinical atherosclerosis.

One of the most popular, but also perhaps the most controversial, noninvasive measures of preclinical atherosclerosis is the EBCT measurement of coronary calcification. Coronary calcification can be detected by means of traditional spiral CT scans, but these scanners use technology that is too slow to obtain clear and motionless pictures of the heart. EBCT provides image acquisition rapidly (50 to 100 milliseconds per slice) to accurately detect the coronary calcium density and volume. Coronary calcium accumulates at a relatively late stage in the atherosclerotic plaque development.

Coronary calcification is quantitated via a score calculated according to the Agatston method. The area of a calcified plaque is multiplied by a coefficient estimated on the basis of the peak density of the calcified lesion. For a density of 130 to 200 Hounsfield units, the density coefficient is 1, for 201 to 300 it is 2, for 301 to 400 it is 3, and for greater than or equal to 401 the density coefficient is 4. A calcium score greater than 300 or 400 generally indicates the need for a cardiac stress test to rule out significant ischemia.

Nomograms of calcium scores obtained by submitting symptomatic individuals to EBCT screening indicate the expected distribution of coronary calcification in the general population. In one study, Raggi et al. published tables of calcium score percentiles derived from scoring 9,728 individuals asymptomatic for coronary artery disease (Table 5.21). Men demonstrate a rapid increase in prevalence and extent of coronary calcification after age 40 years. In women, on the contrary, calcium scores increase slowly compared to men, and a significant growth is not seen until approximately 10 years later. Fur-

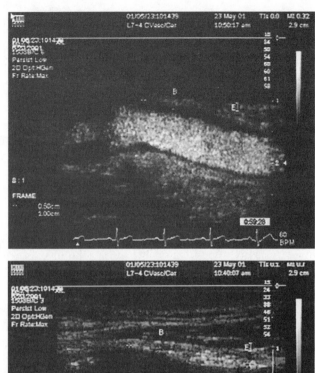

Figure 5.18. See text for explanation.

thermore, the calcium score values in women never reach the same extent as in men.

The main controversy regarding the use of EBCT scanning is whether the presence of coronary calcium can be a better predictor of

Table 5.21. Normal Distribution of Calcium Scores in 9,728 Asymptomatic Patients

					Age in yr			
Men (n = 5,433)	35–39 (n = 479)	40–44 (n = 859)	45–49 (n = 1,066)	50–54 (n = 1,085)	55–59 (n = 853)	60–64 (n = 613)	65–70 (n = 478)	
25th percentile	0	0	0	0	3	14	28	
50th percentile	0	0	3	16	41	118	151	
75th percentile	2	11	44	101	187	434	569	
90th percentile	21	64	176	320	502	804	1,178	
Women (n = 4,297)	35–39 (n = 288)	40–44 (n = 589)	45–49 (n = 822)	50–54 (n = 903)	55–59 (n = 693)	60–64 (n = 515)	65–70 (n = 485)	
25th percentile	0	0	0	0	0	0	0	
50th percentile	0	0	0	0	0	4	24	
75th percentile	0	0	0	10	33	87	123	
90th percentile	4	9	23	66	140	310	362	

events than the Framingham risk score. A study was conducted in a group of 491 patients with chest pain symptoms who were submitted to sequential cardiac catheterization and EBCT imaging. After a follow-up time of 30 ± 13 months, 13 deaths and eight nonfatal MIs were recorded, and patients with a score above the median (median = 75.3) showed a risk sixfold greater than those below the median. In logistic regression analyses that included age, gender, the number of angiographically diseased vessels, and log calcium score, the latter was the only independent predictor of an event. However, another trial evaluating younger patients demonstrated an independent effect of a high calcium score (>300) in combination with the Framingham score (Fig. 5.10E).

In a second study performed by the same investigators in a group of 1,196 high-risk, older, and asymptomatic individuals, the predictive ability of coronary calcium scores was no greater than that of conventional risk factors. However, the use of a suboptimal imaging protocol, which could cause the loss of significant imaging information in a group of patients already at high risk of events because of the presence of multiple risk factors, weakened the conclusions of this study.

In a study by Raggi et al., the authors followed 632 asymptomatic patients screened by EBCT for an average of 3 years. At the end of the follow-up period, 19 MIs and eight deaths were recorded. Events were clustered in patients demonstrating a calcium score in the upper quartile for age and gender. Furthermore, the event in the upper quartile of calcium score percentile was approximately 20 times higher than in the lowest quartile, whereas the event rate in the upper quartile of risk factors was six times higher than in the lowest group. Therefore, the hazard ratio was much larger for relative calcium score differences than for cardiovascular risk factor groups.

EBCT screening is probably best used in asymptomatic individuals at intermediate to high risk of coronary artery disease to assess the presence and extent of atherosclerotic disease and to follow up the progression of disease. Screening is best suited for particular age groups. Specifically, men should probably undergo screening between the ages of 30 and 35 years and 55 to 60 years. However, for women, screening could be useful in almost any patient older than age 40 years (Fig. 5.19).

Because the Framingham risk score is a proven equation to predict CHD events and the coronary calcium score percentile for age also appears to independently predict CHD event, perhaps combining the two scores improves the risk predictability of each score used independently. Grundy has proposed adjusting the Framingham age score based on the coronary calcium percentile for age (Table 5.22). If the total calcium

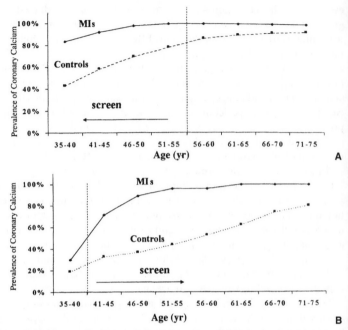

Figure 5.19. These paired curves indicate the age at which electron beam tomography screening is most appropriate in men **(A)** and women **(B)** to identify patients at risk of having a hard coronary event. MI, myocardial infarction.

score is entered into the Mobile Lipid Clinic™ program, the patient's Framingham risk score and the cardiovascular risk equivalent age is adjusted either higher or lower, depending on percentile ranking of the calcium score. The rationale for this adjustment is that the coronary cal-

Table 5.22. Adjustment of the Weight Assigned to Age in the Framingham Index Score by Using the Calcium Score Percentiles

Percentile	Point adjustment
0–24th	−2
25–49th	−1
50–74th	+1
75–90th	+2
>90th	+3

Adapted from Am J Cardiol.

cium score may more effectively predict CHD events than the biologic age. As more data accumulate regarding the CHD predictive value of EBCT, hopefully the combination of the Framingham with the calcium score will provide a clinically useful enhancement of risk predictability.

In addition to ABI, carotid IMT, and coronary calcium by EBCT, there are other emerging measures of preclinical disease that may provide clinical value. Perhaps the most promising is brachial artery endothelial reactivity. This noninvasive method involves the use of high-resolution ultrasound to measure changes in brachial artery diameter in response to increased flow induced by reactive hyperemia after 5 minutes of cuff occlusion of the brachial artery. In normal arteries lined by healthy endothelium, the increased flow causes dilatation of the brachial artery comparable to a sublingual nitroglycerin control. If endothelial dysfunction is present, however, the brachial artery does not dilate normally, and this impairment can be measured by the ultrasound. This technique requires some skill, and the variability and interpretation have not been well standardized. Although some data have linked brachial artery reactivity to the presence of CHD, data are lacking as to whether an abnormal test predicts CHD events or an improvement in the vasodilatation correlates with a reduction in CHD rates.

As the data regarding the use of noninvasive measures of preclinical atherosclerosis continue to evolve, these tests should help determine which patients may most benefit from risk factor modification. The National Institutes of Health has launched the Multi-Ethnic Study of Atherosclerosis to help determine the most cost-effective measures or the best combination of measures to efficiently identify patients at the highest risk of clinical disease outcomes.

SELECTED READING

Angelin B. Therapy for lowering lipoprotein(a) levels. *Curr Opin Lipidol* 1997;8:337–341.

Arad Y, Spadaro LA, Goodman K, et al. Prediction of coronary events with electron beam computed tomography. *J Am Coll Cardiol* 2000;36:1253–1260.

Austin MA, King MC, Vranizan KM, et al. Atherogenic lipoprotein phenotype. A proposed genetic marker for coronary heart disease risk. *Circulation* 1990;82:495–506.

Berenson GS, Srinivasan SR, Bao W, et al. Association between multiple cardiovascular risk factors and atherosclerosis in children and young adults. *N Engl J Med* 1998;338:1650–1656.

Berenson GS, Wattigney WA, Tracy RE, et al. Atherosclerosis of the aorta and coronary arteries and cardiovascular risk factors in persons aged 6 to 30 years and studies at necropsy (the Bogalusa Heart Study). *Am J Cardiol* 1992;70:851–858.

Black DM. Statins in children: What do we know and what do we need to do? *Curr Atheroscler Rep* 2000;3:29–34.

Bowen PH, Guyton JR. Nonpharmacologic and pharmacologic treatment of patients with low levels of high-density lipoprotein cholesterol. *Curr Atheroscler Rep* 2000;2:58–63.

Boushey CJ, Beresford SA, Omenn GS, et al. A quantitative assessment of plasma homocysteine as a risk factor for vascular disease. *JAMA* 1995;274:1049–1057.

Budde T, Fechtrup C, Bosenberg E, et al. Plasma Lp(a) levels correlate with number, severity, and length-extension of coronary lesions in male patients undergoing coronary arteriography for clinically suspected coronary atherosclerosis. *Arterioscler Thromb* 1994;14:1730–1736.

Chambless LE, Heiss G, Folsom AR, et al. Association of coronary heart disease incidence with carotid arterial wall thickness and major risk factors: the Atherosclerosis Risk in Communities (ARIC) Study. *Am J Epidemiol* 1997;146:483–494.

Criqui MH, Coughlin SS, Fronek A. Noninvasively diagnosed peripheral arterial disease as a predictor of mortality: results from a prospective study. *Circulation* 1985;72:768–773.

Farnier M, Picard S. Diabetes: statins, fibrates, or both? *Curr Atheroscler Rep* 2000;3:19–28.

Gardner CD, Fortmann SP, Krauss RM. Association of small low-density lipoprotein particles with the incidence of coronary artery disease in men and women. *JAMA* 1996;276:875–881.

Giles WH, Crost JB, Greenlund KJ, et al. Association between total homocyst(e)ine and the likelihood for a history of acute myocardial infarction by race and ethnicity: Results from the Third National Health and Nutrition Examination Survey. *Am Heart J* 2000;139: 446–453.

Greenland P, Abrams J, Aurigemma GP, et al. Prevention Conference V: Beyond secondary prevention: identifying the high-risk patient for primary prevention: noninvasive tests of atherosclerotic burden: Writing Group III. *Circulation* 2000;101:E16–22.

Grundy SM, Bazzarre T, Cleeman J, et al. Prevention Conference V: Beyond secondary prevention: identifying the high-risk patient for primary prevention: medical office assessment: Whiting Group I. *Circulation* 2000;101:E3–E11.

Herrington DM, Klein KP. Statins, hormones, and women: benefits and drawbacks for atherosclerosis and osteoporosis. *Curr Atheroscler Rep* 2000;3:35–42.

Herrington DM, Reboussin DM, Brosnihan KB, et al. Effects of estrogen replacement on the progression of coronary-artery atherosclerosis. *N Engl J Med* 2000;343:522–529.

Hulley S, Grady D, Bush T, et al. Randomized trial of estrogen plus progestin for secondary prevention of coronary heart disease in postmenopausal women. *JAMA* 1998;20:605–613.

Kannel WB, Hjortland MC, McNamara PM, et al. Menopause and risk of cardiovascular disease: the Framingham Study. *Ann Intern Med* 1976;85:447–452.

Klag MJ, Ford DE, Mead LA, et al. Serum cholesterol in young men and subsequent cardiovascular disease. *N Engl J Med* 1993;328:313–318.

Kobashigawa J. What is the optimal prophylaxis for treatment of cardiac allograft vasculopathy? *Curr Atheroscler Rep* 2000;1:166–171.

Koenig W, Sund M, Frohlich M, et al. C-reactive protein, a sensitive marker of inflammation, predicts future risk of coronary heart disease in initially healthy middle-aged men: results from the MONICA (Monitoring Trends and Determinants in Cardiovascular Disease) Augsburg Cohort Study, 1984–1992. *Circulation* 1999;99:237–242.

Leng GC, Fowkes FG, Lee AJ, et al. Use of ankle brachial pressure index to predict cardiovascular events and death: a cohort study. *BMJ* 1996;313:1440–1444.

Marcovina SM, Hegele RA, Koschinsky ML. Lipoprotein(a) and coronary heart disease risk. *Curr Cardiol Rep* 1999;1:105–111.

Marcovina SM, Koschinsky ML. Lipoprotein(a) as a risk factor for coronary artery disease. *Am J Cardiol* 1998;82:57U–66U; discussion 86U.

McKenna M, Wolfson S, Kuller L. The ratio of ankle and arm arterial pressure as an independent predictor of mortality. *Atherosclerosis* 1991;87:119–128.

Meigs JB, Mittleman MA, Nathan DM, et al. Hyperinsulinemia, hyperglycemia, and impaired hemostasis: the Framingham Offspring Study. *JAMA* 2000;283:221–228.

Mendall MA, Strachan DP, Butland BK, et al. C-reactive protein: relation to total mortality, cardiovascular mortality and cardiovascular risk factors in men. *Eur Heart J* 2000;21:1584–1590.

Morrisett JD. The role of lipoprotein(a) in atherosclerosis. *Curr Atheroscler Rep* 2000;2:243–250.

Mosca L. Hormone replacement therapy in the prevention and treatment of atherosclerosis. *Curr Atheroscler Rep* 2000;2:297–302.

Mosca L, Appel LJ, Benjamin EJ, et al. Evidence-based guidelines for cardiovascular disease prevention in women. *J Am Coll Cardiol* 2004;43:900–921.

O'Rourke RA, Brundage BH, Froelicher VF, et al. American College of Cardiology/American Heart Association Expert Consensus document on electron-beam computed tomography for the diagnosis and prognosis of coronary artery disease. *Circulation* 2000;102:126–140.

Raggi P. Electron beam tomography as an endpoint for clinical trials of antiatherosclerotic therapy. *Curr Atheroscler Rep* 2000;2:284–289.

Raggi P, Callister TQ, Cooil B, et al. Identification of patients at increased risk of first unheralded acute myocardial infarction by electron-beam computed tomography. *Circulation* 2000;101:850–855.

Ridker PM, Buring JE, Shih J, et al. Prospective study of C-reactive protein and the risk of future cardiovascular events among apparently healthy women. *Circulation* 1998b;98:731–733.

Ridker PM, Glynn RJ, Hennekens CH. C-reactive protein adds to the predictive value of total and HDL cholesterol in determining risk of first myocardial infarction. *Circulation* 1998a;97:2007–2011.

Ridker PM, Hennekens CH, Buring JE, et al. C-reactive protein and other markers of inflammation in the prediction of cardiovascular disease in women. *N Engl J Med* 2000;342:836–843.

Ridker PM, Rifai N, Pfeffer MA, et al. Long-term effects of pravastatin on plasma concentration of C-reactive protein. The Cholesterol and Recurrent Events (CARE) Investigators. *Circulation* 1999;100:230–235.

Rossouw JE. Debate: the potential role of estrogen in the prevention of heart disease in women after menopause. *Curr Atheroscler Rep* 2000;1: 135–138.

Seman LJ, DeLuca C, Jenner JL, et al. Lipoprotein(a)-cholesterol and coronary heart disease in the Framingham Heart Study. *Clin Chem* 1999;45:1039–046.

Smith SC Jr, Amsterdam E, Balady GJ, et al. Prevention Conference V: Beyond secondary prevention: identifying the high-risk patient for primary prevention: tests for silent and inducible ischemia: Writing Group II. *Circulation* 2000;101:E12–16.

Smith SC Jr, Greenland P, Grundy SM. AHA Conference Proceedings. Prevention Conference V: Beyond secondary prevention: identifying the high-risk patient for primary prevention: executive summary. American Heart Association. *Circulation* 2000;101:111–116.

Stehouwer CD, Weijenberg MP, van den Berg M, et al. Serum homocysteine and risk of coronary heart disease and cerebrovascular disease in elderly men: a 10-year follow-up. *Arterioscler Thromb Vasc Biol* 1998;18:1895–1901

Stubbs P, Seed M, Lane D, et al. Lipoprotein(a) as a risk predictor for cardiac mortality in patients with acute coronary syndromes. *Eur Heart J* 1998;19:1355–1364.

Superko HR. Small, dense, low-density lipoprotein and atherosclerosis. *Curr Atheroscler Rep* 2000;2:226–231.

Walsh BW, Kuller LH, Wild RA, et al. Effects of raloxifene on serum lipids and coagulation factors in healthy postmenopausal women. *JAMA* 1998;279:1445–1451.

Young JB. Perspectives on cardiac allograft vasculopathy. *Curr Atheroscler Rep* 2000;2:259–271.

Chapter 6

Management of Other Risk Factors: Hypertension, Diabetes, Obesity, and Cigarette Smoking

HYPERTENSION

The Seventh Report of the Joint National Committee on Prevention, Evaluation, and Treatment of High Blood Pressure (JNC 7) established guidelines for the management of hypertension (Fig. 6.1). Nonpharmacologic therapies should be the front line of treatment for mild to moderate hypertension. A low-sodium, high-potassium, high-calcium, low-fat, and high-fiber diet (e.g., Dietary Approaches to Stop Hypertension) may obviate the need for antihypertensive therapy (Table 6.1). Other nonpharmacologic approaches include weight loss, exercise, and biofeedback. JNC 7 differs from the previous blood pressure guidelines (JNC 6) in several ways. First, a new blood pressure (BP) classification system was developed by adding the category "prehypertension," which includes people with BP in the range of 120/80 to 139/89 mm Hg (Table 6.1). The JNC 7 panel decided to create the prehypertension category to underscore that cardiovascular risk begins to increase in a linear fashion starting at a BP of 115/75 mm Hg based on data from the Framingham Heart Study. The risk doubles with each 20/10 mm Hg incremental increase in BP. In addition, whereas JNC 6 called for goal BP of less than 130/85 mm Hg for patients with diabetes or kidney disease, JNC 7 lowered the goal to less than 130/80 mm Hg.

Based on the results of the Antihypertensive and Lipid-Lowering Treatment to Prevent Heart Attack Trial–Lipid-Lowering Trial, which showed that coronary event rates were similar in patients receiving a thiazide-like diuretic, an angiotensin converting enzyme (ACE) inhibitor, or a calcium channel blocker, JNC 7 endorsed the concept of using diuretics as first-

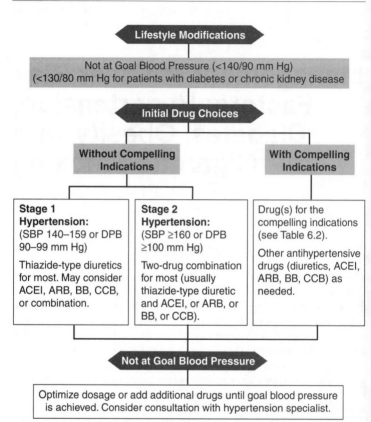

Lifestyle Modifications

Not at Goal Blood Pressure (<140/90 mm Hg)
(<130/80 mm Hg for patients with diabetes or chronic kidney disease

Initial Drug Choices

Without Compelling Indications

With Compelling Indications

Stage 1 Hypertension:
(SBP 140–159 or DPB 90–99 mm Hg)

Thiazide-type diuretics for most. May consider ACEI, ARB, BB, CCB, or combination.

Stage 2 Hypertension:
(SBP ≥160 or DPB ≥100 mm Hg)

Two-drug combination for most (usually thiazide-type diuretic and ACEI, or ARB, or BB, or CCB).

Drug(s) for the compelling indications (see Table 6.2).

Other antihypertensive drugs (diuretics, ACEI, ARB, BB, CCB) as needed.

Not at Goal Blood Pressure

Optimize dosage or add additional drugs until goal blood pressure is achieved. Consider consultation with hypertension specialist.

Figure 6.1. Algorithm for treatment of hypertension. ACEI, angiotensin-converting enzyme inhibitor; ARB, angiotensin receptor blocker; BB, beta blocker; CCB, calcium channel blocker; DBP, diastolic blood pressure; SBP, systolic blood pressure.

line therapy for most patients with hypertension due to the lower cost. However, JNC 7 emphasized the importance of using more than one antihypertensive agent when necessary to control BP. Low-dose combination therapy has gained wide support in recent years because of its efficacy and reduction in side effects associated with high-dose monotherapy. JNC 7 recommended that diuretics are part of any combination therapy. As with JNC 6, JNC 7 also recognized that there may be compelling reasons to use specific antihypertensive therapies. These compelling reasons are listed in Table 6.2. The treatment algorithm for BP control is shown in Figure 6.1.

Table 6.1. Classification and Management of Blood Pressure (BP) for Adults[a]

BP classification	SBP (mm Hg)[a]	DBP (mm Hg)[a]	Lifestyle modification	Initial drug therapy	
				Without compelling indication	With compelling indication (see Table 6.2)
Normal	<120	and <80	Encourage	—	—
Prehypertension	120–139	or 80–89	Yes	No antihypertensive drug indicated.	Drug(s) for compelling indications.[c]
Stage 1 hypertension	140–159	or 90–99	Yes	Thiazide-type diuretics for most. May consider ACEI, ARB, BB, CCB, or combination.	Drug(s) for the compelling indications.[c] Other antihypertensive drugs (diuretics, ACEI, ARB, BB, CCB) as needed.
Stage 2 hypertension	≥160	or ≥100	Yes	Two-drug combination for most[b] (usually thiazide-type diuretic and ACEI, ARB, BB, or CCB)	

ACEI, angiotensin-converting enzyme inhibitor; ARB, angiotensin receptor blocker; BB, beta blocker; CCB, calcium channel blocker; DBP, diastolic blood pressure; SBP, systolic blood pressure.

[a]Treatment determined by highest BP category.

[b]Initial combined therapy should be used cautiously in those at risk for orthostatic hypotension.

[c]Treat patients with chronic kidney disease or diabetes to BP goal of <130/80 mm Hg.

Table 6.2. Clinical Trial and Guideline Basis for Compelling Indications for Individual Drug Classes

Compelling indications[a]	Recommended drugs						Clinical trial basis[b]
	Diuretic	BB	ACEI	ARB	CCB	Aldo ANT	
Heart failure	•	•	•	•		•	ACC/AHA Heart Failure Guideline, MERIT-HF, COPERNICUS, CIBIS, SOLVD, AIRE, TRACE, ValHeFT, RALES
Postmyocardial infarction		•	•			•	ACC/AHA Post-MI Guideline, BHAT, SAVE, CAPRICORN, EPHESUS
High coronary disease risk	•	•	•		•		ALLHAT, HOPE, ANBP2, LIFE, CONVINCE, ALLHAT
Diabetes	•	•	•	•	•		NKF-ADA Guideline, UKPDS, ALLHAT
Chronic kidney disease			•	•			NKF Guideline, Captopril Trial, RENAAL, IDNT, REIN, AASK
Recurrent stroke prevention	•		•				PROGRESS

AASK, The African American Study of Kidney Disease and Hypertension; ACC, American College of Cardiology; ACEI, angiotensin-converting enzyme inhibitor; ADA, American Diabetes Association; AHA, American Heart Association; AIRE, Acute Infarction Ramipril Efficacy; ARB, angiotensin receptor blocker; Aldo ANT, aldosterone antagonist; ALLHAT, Antihypertensive and Lipid-Lowering Treatment to Prevent Heart Attack Trial; ANBP2, Second Australian National Blood Pressure Study; BB, beta blocker; BHAT, Beta-blocker Heart Attack Trial; CAPRICORN, Carvedilol Post-Infarct Survival Control in LV Dysfunction; CCB, calcium channel blocker; CIBIS, Cardiac Insufficiency Bisoprolol Study; COPERNICUS, Carvedilol Prospective Randomized Cumulative Survival Study; EPHESUS, Eplerenone Post-Acute Myocardial Infarction Heart Failure Efficacy and Survival Study; HOPE, Heart Outcomes Prevention Evaluation; IDNT, Irbesartan Diabetic Nephropathy Trial; MERIT-HF, Metoprolol CR/XL Randomized Intervention Trial in Heart Failure; MI, myocardial infarction; NKF, National Kidney Foundation; PROGRESS, Perindopril Protection Against Recurrent Stroke Study; RALES, Randomized Aldactone Evaluation Study; REIN, Ramipril Efficacy In Nephropathy; RENALL, Reduction of Endpoints in Non-Insulin-Dependent Diabetes Mellitus with the Angiotensin II Antagonist Losartan; SAVE, Survival and Ventricular Enlargement; SOLVD, Studies of Left Ventricular Dysfunction; TRACE, Trandolapril Cardiac Evaluation; UKPDS, UK Prospective Diabetes Study; ValHeFT, Valsartan Heart Failure Trial.

[a]Compelling indications for antihypertensive drugs are based on benefits from outcome studies or existing clinical guidelines; the compelling indication is managed in parallel with the blood pressure.

[b]Conditions for which clinical trials demonstrate benefit of specific classes of antihypertensive drugs.

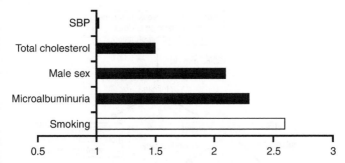

Figure 6.2. Relative risk of developing ischemic heart disease. Multivariate analysis shows that microalbuminuria is associated with a 2.3-fold increased risk of ischemic heart disease (P = .002), which is of the same magnitude as that for men (2.1, P = .01) and current smoking (2.6, P = .0004). n = 2,085. 10-year follow-up. SBP, systolic blood pressure.

Microalbuminuria was initially demonstrated to be associated with cardiovascular risk in patients with diabetes; however, this risk has recently also been demonstrated in the general population. Microalbuminuria is associated with a 2.3-fold increase in the risk of coronary heart disease (CHD), which is similar in magnitude to that for male sex and cigarette smoking (Fig. 6.2). The Microalbuminuria, Cardiovascular, and Renal Outcomes–Heart Outcomes Prevention Evaluation (HOPE) trial, a substudy of HOPE that included 3,577 patients with diabetes, showed that long-term ACE inhibition with ramipril was associated with a significant reduction in both the albumin to creatinine ratio and in development of overt nephropathy. Also in the HOPE trial, the risk reduction in total mortality with ACE inhibitors was 43% in patients with renal insufficiency (creatinine, 71.4 mg per dL) and 10% in patients without renal insufficiency. The JNC 7 has recommended ACE inhibitors as the antihypertensive treatment of choice in patients with diabetes, especially in the presence of nephropathy (Fig. 6.3). The HOPE results have, therefore, expanded the potential benefits of ACE inhibition beyond patients with diabetes, patients with left ventricular (LV) dysfunction, and post–myocardial infarction patients to include patients with microalbuminuria and also support the use in other high-risk groups to reduce cardiovascular events, such as those with a history of peripheral vascular disease and stroke.

LV hypertrophy (LVH) is another important predictor of CHD risk in patients with hypertension. LV mass predicts cardiovascular mortal-

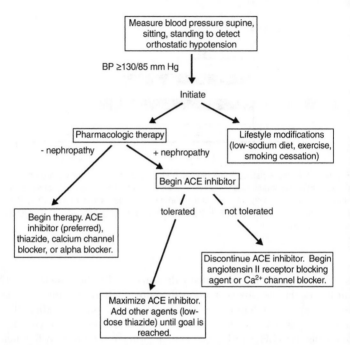

Figure 6.3. Joint National Committee VI recommendations for the treatment of hypertension in diabetics. ACE, angiotensin-converting enzyme; BP, blood pressure. (Adapted from JNC VI. The sixth report of the Joint National Committee on Prevention, Detection, Evaluation, and Treatment of High Blood Pressure. *Arch Intern Med* 1997;157:2413–2446.)

ity (Fig. 6.4), and in the Framingham equation, the presence of LVH adds at least six points to the risk of stroke or CHD (similar to adding 20 years of age). The electrocardiogram is a useful screening test for LVH, but an echocardiogram is far more sensitive. In patients with hypertension of uncertain duration or severity, an echocardiogram to evaluate LV mass may help decide the aggressiveness of treatment.

Due to the results of a large number of clinical trials, the role of specific classes of antihypertensive agents in various hypertensive groups is fairly well defined. Ongoing clinical trials should clarify more definitively the optimal use of antihypertensives for additional endpoints beyond stroke reduction and identify more appropriate goals for patients at higher risk of events.

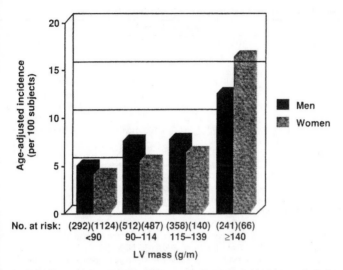

Figure 6.4. Effect of left ventricular (LV) mass on age-adjusted incidence of cardiovascular disease over a 4-year period in the Framingham Heart Study. (Adapted from Levy D, Garrison KJ, Savage DD, et al. *N Engl J Med* 19990;322:1561–1566.)

GLUCOSE CONTROL IN DIABETES

Table 6.3 compares the various guidelines for lipid control, and Table 6.4 lists the risk factor goals for patients with diabetes. In both type 1 and type 2 diabetes, glucose control has been proven to reduce the development of microvascular disease; however, the benefits of glucose reduction on cardiovascular events have not been conclusively demonstrated. Glycosylated hemoglobin (HbA_{1C}) is a powerful predictor of CHD mortality and events (Fig. 6.5), and the United Kingdom Prospective Diabetes Study (UKPDS) showed a statistically nonsignificant ($P = .052$) 21% reduction in myocardial infarction rates (Table 6.5). Although the reduction in CHD rates in UKPDS was not so statistically significant, this study, which evaluated tight control with glyburide, chlorpropamide, and insulin versus usual care, demonstrated a significant reduction in any diabetes-related endpoints and microvascular disease. In UKPDS, low-density lipoprotein and high-density lipoprotein ranked above HbA_{1C} as predictors of CHD events (Table 6.6). These data support the concept that glucose control is very important in reducing diabetes-related complications, but the benefits of lipid modification are more powerful in reducing CHD mortality.

Table 6.3. Guidelines at a Glance

Parameter	ATP III + Update[a]	Women[b]	ADA position[c]
Optimal LDL-C	<100 mg/dL	<100 mg/dL	<100 mg/dL
Very high risk (2004 update)[d]	<70 mg/dL	—	—
Optimal TG	<150 mg/dL	<150 mg/dL	<150 mg/dL
Optimal HDL-C	>40 mg/dL	>50 mg/dL	>40 mg/dL (men) >50 mg/dL (women)
LDL-C goal for CHD or equivalents	<100 mg/dL	<100 mg/dL	<100 mg/dL
Non-HDL goal	<130 mg/dL	<130 mg/dL	—

ADA, American Diabetes Association; ATP III, Adult Treatment Panel III; HDL-C, high-density lipoprotein cholesterol; LDL-C, low-density lipoprotein cholesterol; TG, triglycerides.
[a]Expert Panel on Detection Evaluation and Treatment of High Blood Cholesterol in Adults. Executive Summary of The Third Report of The National Cholesterol Education Program (NCEP) Expert Panel on Detection, Evaluation, and Treatment of High Blood Cholesterol in Adults (Adult Treatment Panel III). JAMA 2001;285:2486–2497.
[b]Mosca L, Appel LJ, Benjamin EJ, et al. Evidence-based guidelines for cardiovascular disease prevention in women. Circulation 2004;109:672–693.
[c]Hafner SM; American Diabetes Association. Dyslipidemia management in adults with diabetes. Diabetes Care 2004;27[Suppl 1]:S68–S71.
[d]Grundy SM, Cleeman JI, Merz CN, et al. Implications of recent clinical trials for the National Cholesterol Education Program Adult Treatment Panel III guidelines. Circulation 2004;110:227–239.

The American Diabetes Association has established treatment goals for glycemic control (Table 6.3). The initial treatment aimed at glycemic control in type 2 diabetes is a diet and exercise program. If, after 3 months, the patient has not achieved the HbA_{1C} goal of less than 8%, then pharmacologic therapy is recommended. Drug therapy should be

Table 6.4. Risk Factor Goals for Patients with Diabetes

ABCs	ADA goal
A_{1C}	<7%
Blood pressure	<130/80 mm Hg
Cholesterol	
Total	Below 200 mg/dL
LDL	Below 100 mg/dL
HDL	Above 45 mg/dL (men)
	Above 55 mg/dL (women)
Triglycerides	Below 150 mg/dL

ADA, American Diabetes Association; A_{1C}, glycosylated hemoglobin; HDL, high-density lipoprotein; LDL, low-density lipoprotein.

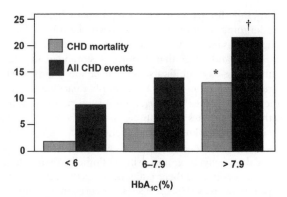

Figure 6.5. Glycosylated hemoglobin (HbA$_{1C}$) as a predictor of coronary heart disease (CHD) mortality and events. *P <.01 compared with HbA$_{1C}$ <6%; †P <.05 compared with HbA$_{1C}$ <6%. (From Kuusisto J, Mykkanen L, Pyorala K, et al. NIDDM and its metabolic control predict coronary heart disease in elderly subjects. *Diabetes* 1994;43:960–964, with permission.)

**Table 6.5. United Kingdom Prospective Diabetes Study:
Glucose Control Study Results**

	Intensive blood glucose control[a]	
	Change in absolute risk (%)	P value
Any diabetes-related endpoint	↓ 12	.029
Diabetes-related deaths	↓ 10	NS
Myocardial infarction (fatal/nonfatal)	↓ 16	.052
Stroke (fatal/nonfatal)	↑ 11	NS
Microvascular disease	↓ 25	.0099

NS, non-significant; ↑, increased; ↓, decreased.
[a]With glyburide, chlorpropamide, or insulin.
From United Kingdom Prospective Diabetes Study Group. Lancet *1998;352:837–853, with permission.*

Table 6.6. United Kingdom Prospective Diabetes Study

Priorities for coronary heart disease risk reduction
    Low-density lipoprotein cholesterol
    High-density lipoprotein cholesterol
    Glycosylated hemoglobin
    Systolic blood pressure
    Smoking

From Turner RC, Millns H, Neil HA, et al. Risk factors for coronary artery disease in non-insulin dependent diabetes mellitus: United Kingdom Prospective Diabetes Study. BMJ *1998;316:823–828, with permission.*

the initial therapy for patients with symptoms of hyperglycemia, for patients undergoing surgery, and for those with ketosis.

The drug options include the sulfonylureas, metformin, thiazolidinediones (glitazones), and drugs that improve postprandial hyperglycemia, such as alpha-glucosidase inhibitors and nateglinide (Starlix). The sulfonylureas are often recommended as initial pharmacologic intervention because these drugs increase endogenous insulin production and most patients with type 2 diabetes are relatively insulin deficient. The biguanide metformin improves insulin sensitivity, slightly improves lipid levels, and promotes weight loss. The glitazones are more potent insulin sensitizers and may have direct effects on improving endothelial dysfunction, which is a prominent disorder in diabetic patients. Drugs that affect postprandial glucose appear to decrease HbA_{1C} to a lesser degree than sulfonylureas or metformin. Usually, the basic approach to the pharmacologic treatment of diabetes is to start with a single agent, usually a sulfonylurea or metformin, and readily add a second drug rather than titrating the dose of the oral agent to the maximal dose. As the effectiveness of oral agents decreases, insulin therapy is usually required to maintain control. The recent availability of glargine insulin (a long-acting insulin) may markedly improve the treatment of both type 1 and type 2 diabetes. Using insulin in the early treatment of type 2 diabetes, which was once discouraged, has become a more prominent treatment due to data demonstrating that early insulin use may spare beta cells from deterioration.

Diabetes is increasing to epidemic proportions throughout the world. Clearly, the high obesity rates are driving the increasing prevalence of type 2 diabetes. The prevention of diabetes, therefore, requires a more aggressive approach to lifestyle changes in patients with the metabolic syndrome or a body mass index (BMI) greater than 25 kg per m². This is especially true in school-age children because young adults between the ages of 15 and 20 years are the fastest growing population developing type 2 diabetes. The term "adult-onset diabetes" is becoming a misnomer.

OBESITY MANAGEMENT:
A PHARMACOLOGIC APPROACH

The National Institutes of Health has developed a classification system for overweight and obese. BMI, in conjunction with waist circumference (measured at the umbilicus), predicts the severity of comorbid conditions associated with obesity. In patients with a BMI greater than or equal to 27 kg per m², 65% exhibit the comorbidities of hypertension, dyslipidemia, or type 2 diabetes. Two large-scale studies, the Nurses'

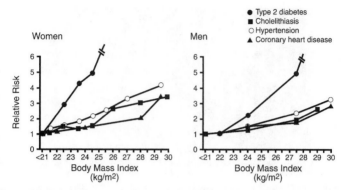

Figure 6.6. Relation between body mass index (BMI) and comorbidities. Two large-scale studies, the Nurses' Health Study and the Health Professionals Follow-Up Study, followed large groups of subjects for several years. Among these subjects, the risk of various diseases was closely related to BMI. Cholelithiasis, hypertension, and coronary heart disease all increased at comparable rates—a person with a BMI of 30 had approximately three to four times the risk of a person with a BMI of 21. The risk of type 2 diabetes, however, increased much more sharply. (From Willet WC, Dietz WH, Colditz GA. Guidelines for healthy weight. *N Engl J Med* 1999;341:427–434, with permission.)

Health Study and the Health Professionals Follow-Up Study, followed large groups of subjects for several years to evaluate the risk of various diseases associated with BMI (Fig. 6.6). The Mobile Lipid Clinic™ program automatically calculates the BMI and provides a relative risk of developing type 2 diabetes compared to a BMI of 21 kg per m². BMI also correlates a total mortality risk, with the lowest mortality in patients with a BMI between 20 and 25 kg per m². BMI less than 20 kg per m² may be associated with wasting diseases, poor nutrition, or generalized illness that may cause increased mortality, but there is no evidence that losing weight to a BMI less than 20 kg per m² is harmful (Fig. 6.7).

Weight loss improves the comorbidities associated with obesity (Fig. 6.8), and, in a 12-year follow-up of more than 15,000 middle-aged, overweight women (BMI greater than or equal to 27 kg per m²) with obesity-related health conditions at baseline, intentional weight loss was associated with dramatic reductions in mortality from various causes (Fig. 6.9).

The National Institutes of Health guidelines for the treatment of obesity recommend physician intervention with a BMI greater than or equal to 30 kg per m², or a BMI between 25 and 29 kg per m², or a high waist circumference with two or more risk factors. The recommended

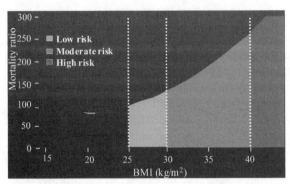

Figure 6.7. Relationship between body mass index (BMI) and mortality ratio. (Adapted from Bray GA. *Ann Intern Med* 1985;103:1052–1062.)

initial goal of weight loss is approximately 10% of body weight in the first 6 months. This initial loss, if successful, can be followed by further weight reduction, but, perhaps more important, are the measures to be taken to ensure that the weight loss is sustained.

The initial treatment for obesity should be diet and exercise (see Chapter 3); however, a conjunctive pharmacotherapy may be necessary if, after 6 months, the patient has lost less than 5% of his or her body weight. There are three approved drugs to treat obesity. These include the appetite suppressants phentermine and sibutramine, as well as

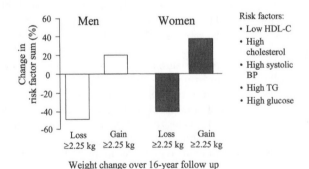

Figure 6.8. Change in weight and coronary heart disease risk-factor clustering: Framingham offspring study. BP, blood pressure; HDL-C, high-density lipoprotein cholesterol; TG, triglyceride. (Adapted from Wilson PW, et al. *Arch Intern Med* 1999;159: 1104–1109.)

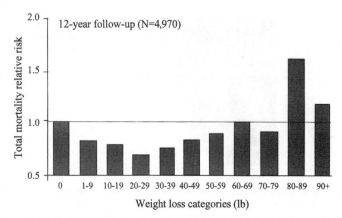

Figure 6.9. Intentional weight loss reduces mortality in overweight patients with type 2 diabetes. Weight loss reduces not only risk factors, but also mortality. In a 12-year follow-up of more than 15,000 middle-aged, overweight women (body mass of 27 or greater) with obesity-related health conditions at baseline, intentional weight loss was associated with dramatic reductions in mortality from various causes. Even modest weight loss (1 to 19 lb) had notable results. The most marked mortality reductions were from cancer and diabetes. (From Williamson DF, et al. *Diabetes Care* 2000;23:1499–1504, with permission.)

orlistat, which inhibits fat absorption (Table 6.7). Phentermine stimulates norepinephrine and dopamine release, and sibutramine inhibits the reuptake of norepinephrine, serotonin, and dopamine. Sibutramine is the better studied of the two appetite suppressants, and in these trials,

Table 6.7. Obesity Pharmacotherapy

System	Mechanism	Examples
Systemically acting		
CNS	Noradrenergic	Phentermine
	Stimulate norepinephrine and dopamine release	
CNS	Noradrenergic and serotonergic	Sibutramine
	Block norepinephrine, serotonin, and dopamine reuptake	
Nonsystemically acting		
Digestive	Inhibition of lipase	Orlistat

CNS, central nervous system.
Note: There have been no comparative safety and efficacy trials between orlistat and sibutramine or phentermine.

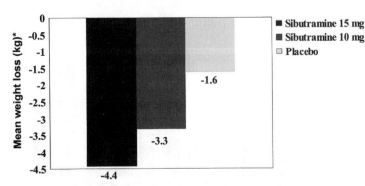

Figure 6.10. Effect of sibutramine on body weight at 1 year. Sibutramine was studied in three phase III trials of 6 months or longer. In these studies, weight loss was greater with sibutramine, 10 or 15 mg, than with placebo. The chart shows weight loss in excess of that of placebo. $P <.01$ sibutramine versus placebo. *Mean weight loss (kg) in intent-to-treat population, n = 485. (From Jones SP, et al. *Int J Obes Relat Metab Disord* 1995;19:41, with permission.)

sibutramine reduced body weight approximately 8 to 12 lb beyond the placebo effect (Fig. 6.10). The main side effects of sibutramine are headaches, dry mouth, constipation, and insomnia. Sibutramine is contraindicated in patients receiving monamine oxidase inhibitors and should be avoided in patients with a history of severe hypertension, CHD, chronic heart failure, arrhythmia, or stroke. These contraindications make the use of sibutramine difficult in patients with combined conditions because they have a high prevalence of these conditions.

Orlistat is a nonsystemic inhibitor of pancreatic lipase. Orlistat inhibits the absorption of approximately one-third of the daily fat intake, approximately equivalent to a 200- to 300-calorie weight loss per day. A 300-calorie deficit per day equates to a weight loss of approximately 2 lb per month (3,500 calories per lb). Orlistat has been well studied in at least seven large multicenter trials. The weight loss, as predicted by the mechanism of action of the drug, is modest, with approximately 60% of patients losing more than 5% of their body weight and 33% losing more than 10% of their weight compared with 41% and 17%, respectively, for patients taking placebo but also undergoing an extensive dietary program (Fig. 6.11). After 2 years, more than one-half of orlistat-treated patients had maintained more than a 5% weight loss and 27% had main-

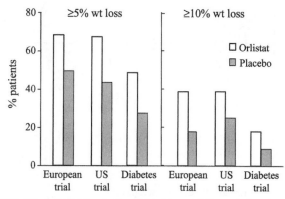

Figure 6.11. Effect of orlistat on body weight at 1 year. At the end of 1 year, 58.9% of patients taking orlistat had lost more than 5% of their weight, and 32.5% had lost more than 10%, compared with 40.8% and 16.5%, respectively, of patients taking placebo. After 2 years, more than one-half of orlistat-treated patients had maintained more than 5% weight loss and 27.3% had maintained more than 10% weight loss. (Adapted from Sjostrom L, Rissanen A, Anderson T, et al. Randomized placebo-controlled trial of orlistat for weight loss and prevention of weight regain in obese patients. *Lancet* 1998;352:167–173; Davidson MH, Hauptman J, DiGirolamo M, et al. *JAMA* 1999; 281:235–242; and Hollander PA, Elbein SC, Hirsch IB, et al. Role of orlistat in the treatment of obese patients with type 2 diabetes. A 1-year randomized double-blind study. *Diabetes Care* 1998;21:1288–1294.)

tained a weight loss of more than 10%. Patients who lost more than 3% of their body weight in the first 12 weeks (responders) had an average weight loss of almost 19 lb at 52 weeks compared to those who lost less than 3% during the first 12 weeks (nonresponders) who lost only 3.5 lb on average. Therefore, the first 12 weeks of therapy for orlistat appears to be critical for long-term success. Orlistat has also been shown to reduce low-density lipoprotein (–8% in placebo), improve blood pressure, and lower HbA_{1C} in diabetic patients (Figs. 6.12 and 6.13). The combined benefits of modifying all three risk factors from a global-risk perspective are substantial.

The main difficulty with orlistat therapy is the side-effect profile. In the first year, approximately one-third of patients experience oily spotting, flatus with discharge, or fecal urgency. These side effects are usually transient and may be improved by increasing the fiber content in the diet. The side-effect profile may also increase if the patient binges on high-fat food. However, if the diet is too fat restrictive, orlistat is not as

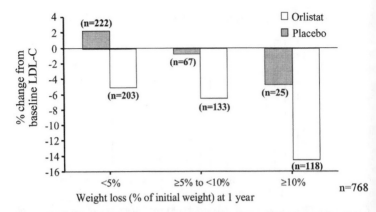

Figure 6.12. Effect of weight loss on cholesterol at year 1: pooled data from five trials. At 1 year, patients receiving orlistat had experienced a 2% reduction in total cholesterol, compared to a 5% increase for patients receiving placebo (P <.001). Low-density lipo-protein cholesterol (LDL-C) levels decreased by 4% in orlistat-treated patients, whereas they increased by 5% in patients receiving placebo (P <.001). The LDL/high-density lipoprotein ratio decreased more in orlistat-treated patients than in placebo-rated patients. These data represent results from the treated population as a whole. The long-term effects of orlistat on morbidity and mortality have not been established.

effective because the drug needs to inhibit fat absorption to induce weight loss. Orlistat, 120 mg, should be taken with meals containing fat. The diet should contain approximately 30% of calories from fat to avoid significant side effects but have enough fat in the diet to promote weight loss via inhibition of fat absorption. Orlistat in conjunction with higher-fat, high-protein diets has not been carefully evaluated, but, anecdotally, in some patients on these diets, orlistat improves the weight loss without intolerable side effects. Ideally, the fat should be distributed across three daily meals to minimize the side effects. Orlistat also may inhibit some fat-soluble vitamin absorption, and, therefore, a daily multivitamin is advised.

Long-term compliance is the most difficult challenge in the treat-ment of obesity. Physicians and other health professionals, therefore, should consider obesity a chronic disease that requires long-term man-agement. Physicians feel more comfortable with the pharmacologic treatment of the comorbid effects of obesity, such as dyslipidemia, hypertension, and diabetes, than with treating the underlying abnor-mality (obesity) with drug therapy. As drug therapies for obesity con-

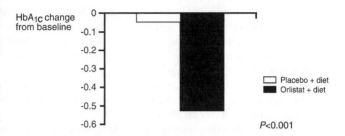

- ≥5% weight loss with orlistat + diet was associated with a decrease of 1.22% in HbA$_{1C}$ ($P \le 0.05$)

Figure 6.13. Improvement in glycosylated hemoglobin (HbA$_{1C}$) from randomization in obese patients with type 2 diabetes (HbA$_{1C}$ >8%). In a 1-year study of obese patients with diabetes (n = 321), orlistat treatment was associated with a 0.53% reduction in HbA$_{1C}$ from baseline in high-risk patients (patients with HbA$_{1C}$ >8% at baseline) compared with a 0.05% reduction for placebo. In all patients in the study, the numbers were –0.18% for orlistat and +0.28% for placebo. Orlistat-treated patients who lost 5% or more of body weight and had HbA$_{1C}$ of greater than 8% at baseline had a mean decrease in HbA$_{1C}$ of 1.22%. The long-term effects of orlistat on morbidity and mortality have not been established. (From Hollander PA, Elbein SC, Hirsch IB, et al. Role of orlistat in the treatment of obese patients with type 2 diabetes. A 1-year randomized double-blind study. *Diabetes Care* 1998;21:1288–1294, with permission.)

tinue to improve, the stigma of considering obesity a medical condition rather than purely a cosmetic problem diminishes.

SMOKING CESSATION

Cigarette smoking is ranked as one of the most potent risk factors for CHD, but often the physician spends little time advising the patient on smoking-cessation programs. The American Lung Association and the Agency for Health Care Policy and Research have provided excellent guides to assist the physician in helping his or her patients quit smoking (see Appendix B).

SELECTED READING

American Diabetes Association. Clinical practice recommendations 1998: screening for type 2 diabetes. *Diabetes Care* 1998;21[Suppl 1]:1–98.
Diabetes Control and Complications Trial Research Group. The effect of intensive treatment of diabetes on the development and progres-

sion of long-term complications in insulin-dependent diabetes mellitus. *N Engl J Med* 1993;329:977–986.

JNC 7. The seventh report of the Joint National Committee on Prevention, Detection, Evaluation, and Treatment of High Blood Pressure. Hypertension. 2003;42(6):1206–1252.

Kottke TE, Solberg LI, Brekke ML, et al. A controlled trial to integrate smoking cessation advice into primary care practice. Doctors Helping Smokers, Round III. *J Fam Pract* 1992;34:701–708.

McBride PE. The health consequences of smoking. Cardiovascular diseases. *Med Clin North Am* 1992;76:333–353.

UK Prospective Diabetes Study (UKPDS) Group. Intensive blood-glucose control with sulfonylureas or insulin compared with conventional treatment and risk of complications in patients with type 2 diabetes (UKPDS 33). *Lancet* 1998a;352:837–853.

Chapter 7

Hospital-Based Intervention Programs: Improving National Cholesterol Education Program Guideline Adherence and Patient Compliance

A major concern regarding the new National Cholesterol Education Program Adult Treatment Panel (NCEP ATP) III guidelines is that the complexities of the recommendations confuse physicians and reduce guideline adherence. Numerous surveys have demonstrated that the NCEP ATP II guidelines, which are less complex and require drug treatment for significantly fewer patients (20 million Americans for ATP II versus 39 million Americans for ATP III require drug therapy), were not followed in the majority of patients with coronary heart disease (CHD). Only approximately 18% to 25% of patients with CHD were at the recommended goal of low-density lipoprotein (LDL) less than or equal to 100 mg per dL based on chart reviews and physician surveys. The failure of most patients with CHD to achieve ATP II goals was not due to a lack of knowledge of the guidelines (because most physicians surveyed were aware of the LDL goal of less than or equal to 100 mg per dL), but, rather, was due to a lack of dose titration, an inability to significantly track patient progress, and poor patient compliance. Therefore, programs that provide the physician with the tools to identify appropriate patients for treatment, help establish the correct goals of therapy, provide a system to monitor the patient's

Table 7.1. Improving National Cholesterol Education Program Adult Treatment Panel III Guideline Adherence

1. Identify appropriate patients for risk factor reduction.
2. Motivate and educate the patient on the need for therapy.
3. Initiate the treatment that will most successfully achieve the patient's goals.
4. Track the patient's results, and adjust the treatment as needed.
5. Provide feedback to the patient and reinforce the need for risk factor modification.
6. Monitor the patient's compliance.

progress, and educate the patient to improve compliance are needed to improve NCEP ATP III guideline adherence.

The basic principles for achievement of NCEP ATP III goals are listed in Table 7.1. The in-hospital setting is an excellent opportunity to initiate a risk factor modification program. In the hospital, patients with CHD or noncoronary atherosclerosis, or who are at high risk for CHD, are relatively easily identifiable and are usually motivated to modify their risk factors. In the past, official guidelines recommended delaying the initiation of statins until 6 weeks after an acute episode and only after maximal dietary therapy had failed. There has been a fundamental shift in the new ATP III guidelines to initiate both diet and drug therapy in patients with CHD or CHD risk equivalents concomitantly, and if the patient responds adequately to dietary therapy, the drug therapy may be discontinued. This approach prevents this high-risk group from a continual cycle of attempting lifestyle changes without effectively achieving the necessary goals.

Another concern regarding the in-hospital initiation of lipid-lowering therapy was the inability to obtain accurate measures of baseline lipid levels during the acute phase of illness. However, even though lipid levels can decrease by as much as 50% within 48 hours of hospitalization for myocardial infarction, because 93% of myocardial infarction patients eventually require initiation of lipid-lowering drugs, a waiting period is of limited value in most cases. In addition, the Myocardial Ischemia Reduction with Acute Cholesterol Lowering trial has demonstrated that initiation of atorvastatin, 80 mg per day, in patients hospitalized for acute coronary syndromes results in a 16% reduction in events over a 4-month follow-up (Fig. 7.1) and is relatively safe, with a transaminase evaluation rate of only 2.8%. The in-hospital initiation of statin therapy is, therefore, both safe and effective.

Another important reason to initiate lipid-lowering therapy in the hospital is the proven concept that, when a patient is discharged on a medication from the hospital, the patient is more likely to remain on the discharged medications for longer than with medications initiated in the office. The patient in the hospital for a potentially life-threatening

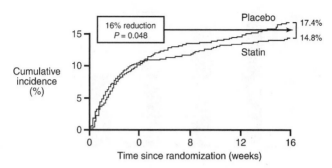

Statin = atorvastatin 80 mg

Figure 7.1. Myocardial Ischemia Reduction with Acute Cholesterol Lowering study primary outcome—time to ischemic event. A primary outcome event occurred in 228 patients in the atorvastatin group (14.8%) and 269 patients in the placebo group (17.4%), representing a risk reduction of 16%. Relative risk, 0.84; 95% confidence interval, 0.70 to 1.00. (From Fonarow GC, Gawlinski A. Rationale and design for the cardiac hospitalization atherosclerosis management program at the University of California Los Angeles. *Am J Cardiol* 2000;85:10A–17A, with permission.)

event may more fully appreciate the magnitude of benefits associated with the medications initiated in the hospital. The University of California, Los Angeles, Medical Center's Cardiac Hospitalization Atherosclerosis Management Program (CHAMP) demonstrated that a comprehensive secondary prevention program initiated in the hospital for CHD patients can improve the long-term adherence to risk factor modification. An outline of the CHAMP program is provided in Table 7.2. The CHAMP program demonstrated a significant improvement in

Table 7.2. Cardiac Hospitalization Atherosclerosis Management Program

Before discharge
   Lipid panel
   Aspirin and statin
   Exercise and diet
   Beta blocker and angiotensin-converting enzyme inhibitor if indicated
Six-wk follow-up
   Lipid panel and liver function tests
   Titrate statin to get low-density lipoprotein <100 mg/dL
   Reinforce patient adherence to lifestyle and medication

From Fonarow GC, Gawlinski A. Rationale and design for cardiac hospitalization atherosclerosis management program at the University of California Los Angeles. Am J Cardiol 2000;85:10A–17A, with permission.

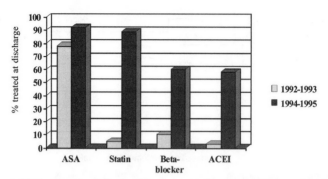

Figure 7.2. Cardiac Hospitalization Atherosclerosis Management Program: hospital discharge rates. ACEI, angiotensin-converting enzyme inhibitor; ASA, aspirin. (From Fonarow GC, Gawlinski A. Rationale and design for the cardiac hospitalization atherosclerosis management program at the University of California Los Angeles. *Am J Cardiol* 2000;85:10A–17A, with permission.)

the appropriate use of reduction at discharge (Fig. 7.2) and 1 year later. The American Heart Association (AHA) has developed a program called Get with the Guidelines that provides tracking sheets to monitor the patient's progress for all the secondary prevention goals (Fig. 7.3) and patient education materials. Quality assurance programs have been initiated throughout the nation to improve the adherence rates of the AHA secondary prevention guidelines. Various model programs involving pharmacists or nurses have been developed with increasing success rates. Since 1996, there has been a marked increase in the percent of patients discharged on a statin, but most hospitals remain far below the AHA goal of 90% of discharges of CHD patients on a statin (Fig. 7.4).

MOBILE LIPID CLINIC™ PROGRAM

The Mobile Lipid Clinic™ program was developed to integrate the necessary strategies to improve adherence to the NCEP ATP III guidelines to educate the patient, track the patient's progress, and provide feedback to the patient to reduce noncompliance. There are several computer-based patient-tracking programs available. However, most are seldom used, because the physician rapidly moves from room to room, seeing a large number of patients in a limited amount of time and, therefore, has little extra time to enter data in a personal com-

Primary and Secondary CVD Patient Tracking Form

American Heart Association®

Fighting Heart Disease and Stroke

Patient Name _____

Patient Age _____ Patient Sex _____

Pre-existing ☐ CVD conditions ☐ Diabetes ☐ Other _____

Indicate acceptable range in grey areas.

Risk Interventions		Initial Status	Patient Goal	Date	Date	Date	Date
Smoking		smoker		smoking	smoking	smoking	smoking
Complete Cessation		non-smoker		not smoking	not smoking	not smoking	not smoking
Blood Pressure • ≤ 140/90 mm Hg or • <130/85 mm Hg if heart failure, renal insufficiency or diabetes		mm Hg mm Hg					
Cholesterol Primary • LDL <160 mg/dL (If ≤1 risk factor) or • LDL <130 mg/dL (If ≥2 risk factors) **Secondary** • LDL <100 mg/dL Primary & Secondary • HDL >35 mg/dL • TG <200 mg/dL	Total	mg/dL mg/dL					
	LDL	mg/dL mg/dL					
	HDL	mg/dL mg/dL					
	TG	mg/dL mg/dL					
Physical Activity Duration P1: 30–60 min. P2: 30 min. Frequency 3–4 times/week	DUR.	min min					
	FRQ.	times/wk times/wk					
Weight Management BMI: 21–25 kg/m² Height:	Weight	lbs lbs					
	BMI	kg/m² kg/m²					
Diabetes Management Near Normal: • Glucose • HbA1c (<7)	Glucose	mg/dL mg/dL					
	HbA1c	% %					
Estrogens *Primary-* Consider ERT in all postmenopausal women *Secondary-* Estrogen Replacement		Yes / No	Compliant? Rx	Y / N Rx	Y / N Rx	Y / N Rx	Y / N Rx
Antiplatelet Agents/ Anticoagulants		Yes / No	Compliant? Rx	Y / N Rx	Y / N Rx	Y / N Rx	Y / N Rx
Ace Inhibitors Post-MI		Yes / No	Compliant? Rx	Y / N Rx	Y / N Rx	Y / N Rx	Y / N Rx
Beta-Blockers Post-MI		Yes / No	Compliant? Rx	Y / N Rx	Y / N Rx	Y / N Rx	Y / N Rx

(In Cholesterol Primary column: "Test send out")

Figure 7.3. Primary and secondary cardiovascular disease (CVD) patient tracking form. BMI, body mass index; DUR, duration; FRQ, frequency; HbA$_{1c}$, glycosylated hemoglobin; HDL, high-density lipoprotein; LDL, low-density lipoprotein; MI, myocardial infarction; Rx, medications; TG, triglyceride. (From the American Heart Association, 1999, with permission.)

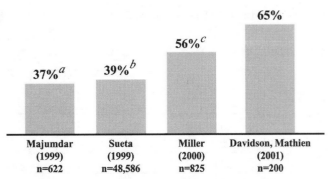

Figure 7.4. Percentage of patients receiving lipid-lowering medications.
[a]Patient population: acute myocardial infarction patients with previously established coronary artery disease (CAD) eligible for lipid-lowering medications.
[b]Patient population: patients with *International Classification of Diseases, Ninth Revision* diagnosis code consistent with CAD by review of medical records.
[c]Patient population: patients with arteriographic evidence of CAD.

puter (PC). The Mobile Lipid Clinic[TM] program is designed for handheld devices (e.g., Palm, Visor) that the physician can use readily to input data, receive useful information regarding a patient's risk and goals, and develop an individual treatment program that can be tracked easily on a longitudinal basis. Last, the program provides the physician with the ability to generate a letter to educate patients and remind them of follow-up visits.

The Mobile Lipid Clinic[TM] has two independent programs: a CHD risk calculator and a patient management and tracking system. The CHD risk calculator is designed for the physician who does not want to maintain a patient's medical information and treatment plan on a handheld device but wants an easy means of calculating a patient's global risk, identifying correct NCEP ATP III goals, and educating the patient in the importance of risk factor modification.

The following is an example of the functionality of the CHD risk calculator. Figure 7.5A shows the screen of a 55-year-old man with a family history of premature CHD, a height of 5'7", a weight of 180 lb, and a blood pressure of 120/80 mm Hg. After entering a total cholesterol of 245 mg per dL, a high-density lipoprotein (HDL) of 39 mg per dL, and a triglyceride of 201 mg per dL, the LDL, non-HDL, and total cholesterol to HDL ratios are automatically calculated. After tapping

CHD Risk Calculator

Age: 55   Sex: ▼ Male
☑ FH CHD   ☐ BP Rx   ☐ CHD
☐ Smoker   ☐ LVH   ☐ PVD
☐ Diabetes   ☐ AFib   ☐ CVA

Height: 5 ft 7 in Weight: 180 lbs
BP: 120 / 80
Chol: 245   HDL: 39   TriG: 201
LDL: 177 NonHDL: 206 Ratio: 6.28

(Risk)

A

CHD Risk Calculator

Age: 55   Sex: Male

CV Risk Adjusted Age	70
10 Year Probability	13%
10 Year Low Probability	7%
10 Year ATP III Probability	16%
NCEP LDL Goal	130mg/dL
At NCEP LDL Goal	No
LDL Reduc. to Meet Goal	22%
NCEP NonHDL Goal	160mg/dL
At NCEP NonHDL Goal	No
NonHDL Reduc. to Meet Goal	23% ↓

(Done)

B

Figure 7.5. Coronary heart disease risk calculator. **A:** Patient criteria entered (see text). **B:** Risks shown based on criteria. See text for details.

on the risk rectangle, the patient's cardiovascular (CV) risk–adjusted age, Framingham 10-year risk, ATP III Framingham risk, and NCEP ATP III LDL goal automatically appear on the screen. The screen also determines whether the NCEP goal has been achieved and the percent LDL and percent non-HDL reduction necessary to achieve the goal. The program also calculates body mass index (BMI) with the associated relative risk of type 2 diabetes, and the 10-year Framingham stroke risk with the low-risk goal for the patient's age (Fig. 7.5B).

Each of the calculations is used either to establish a patient's goal for treatment or as an educational tool to help the physician communicate the importance of risk modification. The CV risk–adjusted age is a useful means to explain to a patient the significance of his or her 10-year Framingham score. A decrease in age from 70 years to 55 years is probably more motivating than informing a patient that his or her risk can be reduced from 13% to 7% with lipid modification. The BMI-associated risk of type 2 diabetes is useful to motivate the patient to lose weight, and the stroke risk is available as a tool to convince the patient to modify other risk factors, such as smoking and hypertension. Some patients may be more motivated by a higher risk of stroke than by an increased risk of CHD.

A physician can quickly demonstrate to the patient the magnitude of benefit of lowering the total cholesterol and raising the HDL. Lowering the total cholesterol from 245 mg per dL to 145 mg per dL, raising the HDL from 39 mg per dL to 43 mg per dL, and lowering the triglycerides from 201 mg per dL to 175 mg per dL results in a new CV

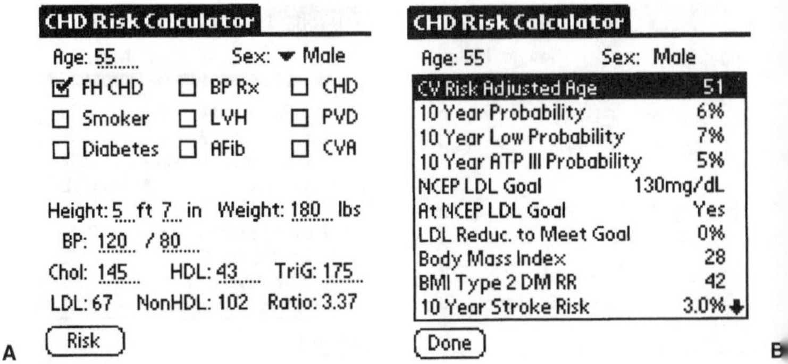

Figure 7.6. Coronary heart disease risk calculator. By lowering total cholesterol, raising high-density lipoprotein (HDL), and lowering triglycerides **(A)**, cardiovascular (CV) risk–adjusted age and risk of coronary heart disease (CHD) decrease **(B)**. See text for details.

risk–adjusted age of 51 years and a 10-year probability of CHD decreasing from 16% to 5% (Fig. 7.6). This information is not stored in the handheld device but can provide an easy means to calculate the global risk score to determine the patient's NCEP ATP III goals and motivate the patient to comply with the physician's recommended treatment program.

The Mobile Lipid Clinic™ patient mode program is a comprehensive approach to CHD risk modification. The functionality of the program is as follows:

After entering the appropriate data, the program calculates

- CV risk–adjusted age.
- 10-year probability of CHD based on the traditional Framingham score. If the patient has clinical atherosclerosis, a 2-year risk for an event can be calculated instead.
- 10-year low probability of CHD for the person's age based on the Framingham score. If the person has clinical atherosclerosis, a 2-year low risk of recurrent events can be calculated instead.
- 10-year probability of CHD based on the NCEP ATP III adapted Framingham score. (If atherosclerosis or diabetes is present, this score is not calculated.)
- The NCEP ATP LDL goal for the patient.
- Whether the patient is at the LDL goal.
- The NCEP non-HDL goal, if the triglycerides are above 200 mg per dL.

- Whether the patient is at the non-HDL goal.
- The percent reduction in LDL or non-HDL (if triglycerides are greater than or equal to 200 mg per dL) to achieve the goal.
- The coronary calcium-adjusted age, by using the patient's calcium score percentile in conjunction with the Framingham score.
- The coronary calcium-adjusted 10-year probability of CHD by combining the coronary calcium percentile for age plus the Framingham score.
- BMI.
- BMI with the relative lifetime risk of developing type 2 diabetes compared to a BMI less than 21 kg per m^2.
- Ankle-brachial index (ABI) and revise the LDL goal to less than 100 mg per dL if the ABI is less than 0.9.
- Framingham 10-year risk of stroke.
- A low 10-year risk of stroke for the patient's age as a goal.
- Whether the metabolic syndrome is preset (based on having at least three of the five criteria).

Therefore, the Mobile Lipid Clinic™ program provides all data necessary to fully comply with NCEP ATP III guidelines. The main value of the program is the ability to track the patient's progress and provide feedback to the patient to enhance long-term compliance. Once data are initially entered in the handheld device, the program stores the data on both the handheld device and, with the hot-sync software, the PC, similar to a contact list. The PC can print out an individualized summary letter to the patient as well as educational material for lifestyle changes or information about specific drug therapies. The Mobile Lipid Clinic™ program also reminds the patient of his or her next visit and tracks patients who miss follow-up office visits.

After the patient's demographic data have been entered in the handheld device, the patient's name and phone number are added to a list of patients in the program. If the patient is a new patient, the first screen will appear to determine the patient's medical history, focusing on risk factors (Fig. 7.7). The physician should tap on all the boxes that apply to the patient, using the NCEP ATP III or Framingham definitions, which follow.

- Family history—if a parent or sibling developed coronary artery disease before age 55 years in a male relative or before age 65 years in a female relative
- LVH—left ventricular hypertrophy, by electrocardiogram definition (Table 7.3)

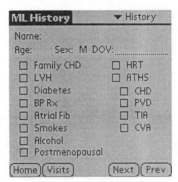

Figure 7.7. Mobile Lipid Clinic™ program History screen. See text for details.

- Diabetes—fasting glucose greater than or equal to 126 mg per dL
- BP Rx—on medication to lower elevated blood pressure
- Atrial fibrillation—chronic or frequent intermittent atrial fibrillation
- Smoker—current cigarette smoker, any cigarette during the past 30 days
- Postmenopausal—the cessation of menses for 12 months
- HRT—hormone replacement therapy, oral or transdermal
- ATHS—clinical atherosclerosis:
    1. Coronary artery disease: previous myocardial infarction, percutaneous coronary intervention, or coronary bypass surgery

Table 7.3. Voltage Criteria for Diagnosis of Left Ventricular Hypertrophy

	Sensitivity (%)	Specificity (%)
Limb lead criteria		
$R_1 + S_3 > 25$ mm	10.6	100
$RaV_L > 7.5$ mm	22.5	96.5
$RaV_L > 11$ mm	10.6	100
$RaV_F > 20$ mm	1.3	99.5
Precordial lead criteria		
$SV_1 + RV_5$ or $RV_6 > 35$ mm	42.5	95
SV_1 or $V_2 + RV_5$ or $RV_6 > 35$ mm	55.6	88.5
$SV_1 + RV_5$ or $RV_6 > 30$ mm	55.6	89.5
Greatest R + greatest S > 45 mm	45	93
RV_5 or $RV_6 > 26$ mm	25	98.5

RV = residual volume; SV = stroke volume.
Source: Romhilt et al.

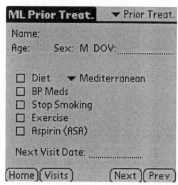

Figure 7.8. Mobile Lipid Clinic™ program Prior Treat screen. See text for details.

2. Peripheral vascular disease: claudication, peripheral vascular intervention, ABI less than 0.9, previous carotid endarterectomy, greater than 50% carotid artery stenosis, abdominal aortic aneurysm repair, or aneurysm greater than or equal to 4 cm
3. Previous transient ischemic attack or cerebral vascular accident

By tapping next to or selecting Prior Treat from the list on the bottom of the previous screen, the user sees the previous visit's treatment plan (Fig. 7.8). If this is the first visit, the physician can enter the prior treatment program or leave the fields blank. The Prior Treat screen includes

- Diet—previous dietary therapy recommendation. There are several diet choices.
- BP Rx—the present blood pressure medication can be typed or written.
- DM Rx—the present diabetes medication can be typed or written.
- Exercise—indicates previous instruction to exercise.
- Aspirin—present aspirin use.
- Stop smoking—indicates previous instruction to stop smoking.

Figure 7.9 shows a pick list of all the available lipid-lowering drugs. The generic name, dose of drug, and dosing frequency can be indicated.

Figure 7.10 shows the screen that begins the physical examination data collection for the present visit. All data that are known should be entered. The blood pressure in the right and left arms and the systolic pressure in both ankles, as determined by a Doppler, are necessary to calculate the ABI. To calculate the Framingham risk score, only a single blood pressure measurement in either arm is sufficient. Weight

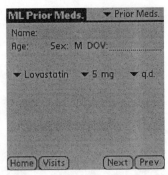

Figure 7.9. Mobile Lipid Clinic™ program Prior Meds screen. See text for details.

should be recorded in pounds (lb), and the waist should be measured at the umbilicus. The height is recorded in feet and inches.

Figure 7.11 shows the screen that records the required laboratory tests (labs) needed by the calculation to make a risk assessment. The absolute required labs are total cholesterol, triglycerides, and HDL. LDL, non-HDL, and cholesterol ratio (total cholesterol to HDL ratio) are calculated automatically and do not have to be entered. Glucose is included in the required labs, because a glucose of greater than 110 mg per dL is one of the five criteria for metabolic syndrome (other criteria are waist greater than 40 in. for a man, waist greater than 35 in. for a woman, triglycerides greater than or equal to 150 mg per dL,

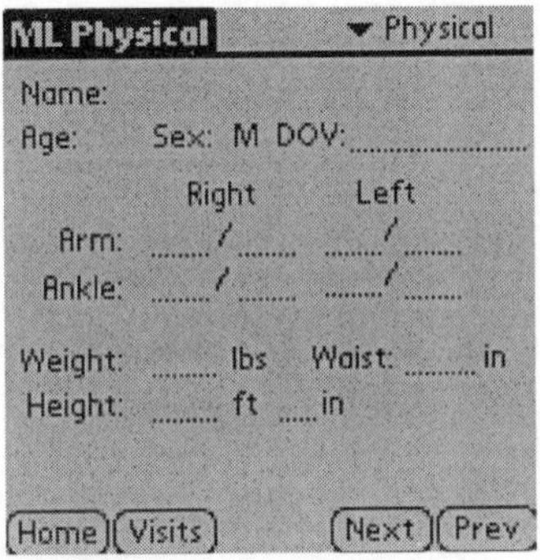

Figure 7.10. Mobile Lipid Clinic™ program Physical screen. See text for details.

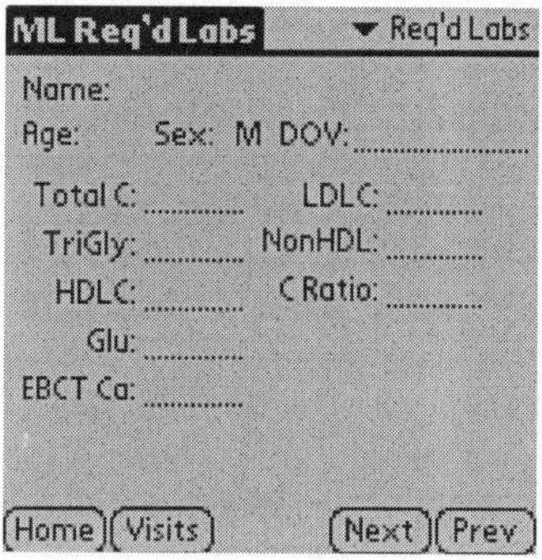

Figure 7.11. Mobile Lipid Clinic™ program Req'd (required) Labs (laboratory tests) screen. See text for details.

HDL less than 40 for a man, HDL less than 50 for a woman, and blood pressure greater than 130/85 mm Hg). The electron beam computed tomography calcium score is included, because the percentile for the patient's calcium score will adjust the Framingham risk score and the CV risk–adjusted age accordingly (see Chapter 1).

There is a series of optional labs that may be recorded and stored in the patient's database (Fig. 7.12) but are not involved in the risk assessment. These labs include

- HgA$_{1c}$—hemoglobin A$_{1c}$
- Homocys—homocysteine
- Hs-CRP—high-sensitivity C-reactive protein

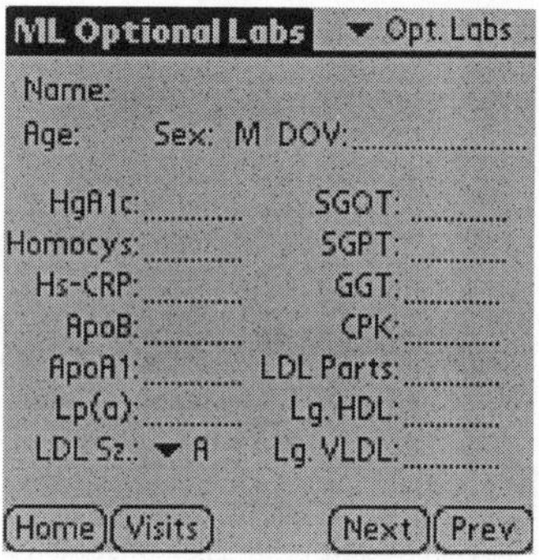

Figure 7.12. Mobile Lipid Clinic™ program Optional Labs screen. See text for details.

- Apo B—apolipoprotein B
- Apo A1—apolipoprotein Al
- Lp(a)—lipoprotein(a)
- LDL size—LDL particle size; can choose A or B as determined by Berkeley Heart Lab, VAP, or nuclear magnetic resonance (NMR) (see Lipoprotein Subfractions in Chapter 5).
- SGOT—serum glutamic-oxaloacetic transaminase—liver function safety test
- SGPT—serum glutamic-pyruvic transaminase—liver function safety test
- GGT—γ-glutamyl transferase—liver function safety test
- CPK—creatinine phosphokinase—muscle safety test
- LDL Parts—LDL particle number, as determined by LipoMed NMR (see Lipoprotein Subfractions in Chapter 5)
- Lg HDL—large HDL, as determined by LipoMed NMR
- Lg VLDL—large VLDL, as determined by LipoMed NMR

The calculation engine provides the risk assessment on the next screen (Fig. 7.13). The risk assessment includes

- CV risk–adjusted age.
- 10-year CHD risk by the Framingham score.
- 10-year low CHD risk by the Framingham score.
- 10-year CHD risk by the Adapted Framingham score used by NCEP ATP III.
- NCEP ATP III LDL goal and non-HDL goal, if triglycerides are greater than 200 mg per dL.

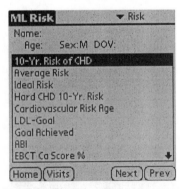

Figure 7.13. Mobile Lipid Clinic™ program Risk assessment screen. See text for details.

- BMI.
- Relative lifetime risk of developing type 2 diabetes compared to a BMI of less than or equal to 21 kg per m².
- 10-year stroke risk based on the Framingham calculation.
- 10-year low stroke risk based on the Framingham calculation.
- Metabolic syndrome—present or absent. The risk assessment may say "maybe" if the patient has two criteria and not all criteria are entered (e.g., the glucose or waist measurement is missing, but the patient has a triglyceride greater than 200 mg per dL and a blood pressure of greater than or equal to 135/85 mm Hg, but the HDL is normal).

An alternative way of navigating through a visit is to use the pull-down list from the upper right corner.

The next screen (Fig. 7.14) begins the "new" treatment plan for the patient, based on the examination and data from the visit. This screen will become the Prior Treat screen on the next visit. On this screen, a physician can choose several diet therapy options.

- Diet:
  Therapeutic Lifestyle Diet. If selected, a dietary program will be printed once the handheld program is hot-synced with the PC and provided to the patient with the report.
  Therapeutic Lifestyle Diet Plus (to include more soluble viscous fiber and plant sterols or stanols).
  The Mediterranean Diet.
  A low-carbohydrate diet—50 g per day.
  A moderate-carbohydrate diet—100 g per day.

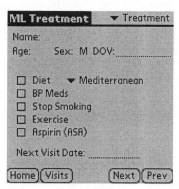

Figure 7.14. Mobile Lipid Clinic™ program Treatment screen. See text for details.

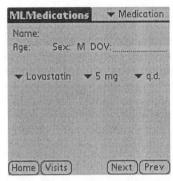

Figure 7.15. Mobile Lipid Clinic™ program Medications screen. See text for details.

Low-calorie diets:
    1,200 calories per day
    1,400 calories per day
    1,600 calories per day
A list of high soy-protein food production.
A list of high-sodium, high-potassium foods and the Dietary Approach to Prevent Hypertension diet.
- BP Rx—blood pressure medication, if initiated or changed, can be recorded.
- DM Rx—diabetes medication, if initiated or changed, can be recorded.
- Exercise—if selected, a walking or jogging program will be provided to the patient on part of the report.
- Aspirin—if aspirin therapy is indicated.
- Stop smoking—if selected, will provide a smoking cessation educational guide to the patient.
- Next visit date—once the screen is tapped, a calendar will appear and the next visit date can be recorded.

The final screen is the medication screen (Fig. 7.15). If a lipid-lowering medication is added or changed, the pick list will appear, and the modification can be made by tapping on the new medication or dose. Once all information is entered, the physician can print a report for the patient after the hot-sync or mail the report to the patient at a later date. The latter is probably most effective if the physician is busy going from patient to patient and does not have the time to print the reports. The generated report mailed to a patient is perhaps even

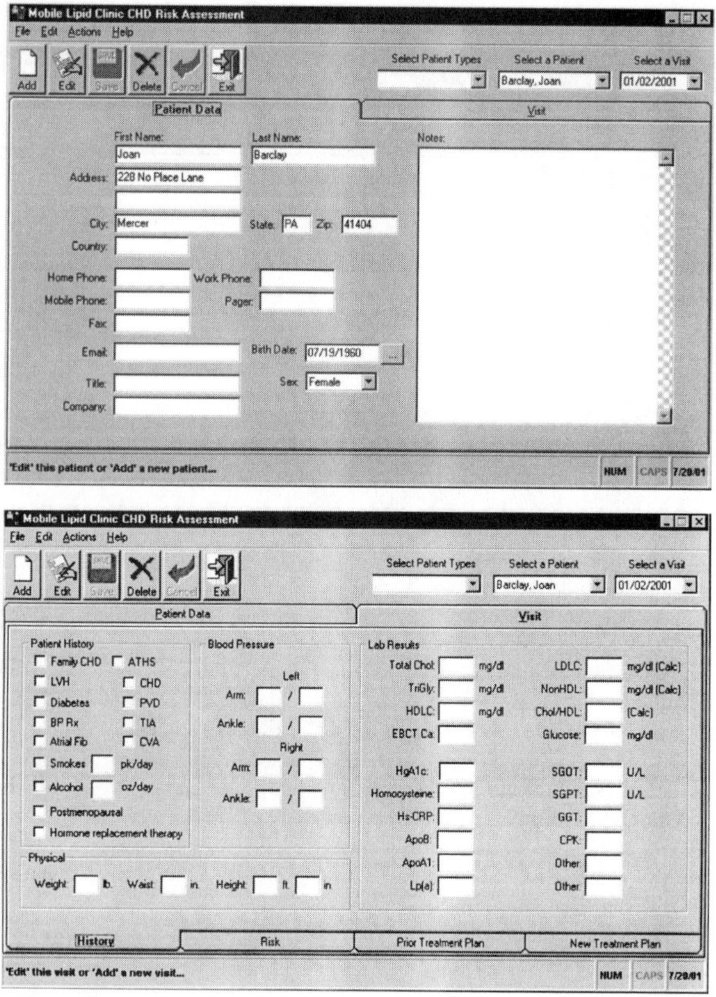

Figure 7.16. Patient coronary heart disease risk database. See text for details.

more effective because it may remind the patient of the treatment plan and of the scheduled next visit. The Mobile Lipid Clinic™ program prints a full report in a letter format to the patient that includes the recommended lifestyle changes in more detail and also provides

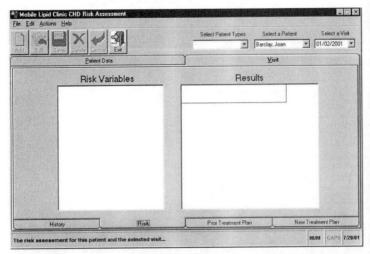

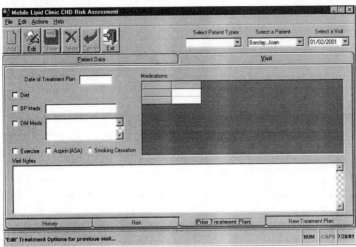

Figure 7.17. Additional screen shots from patient coronary heart disease risk database. See text for details.

instructions on the proper use of the drug treatment and potential side effects.

The Mobile Lipid Clinic™ program was designed to assist physicians in CV risk factor modification by providing an easy-to-use

Table 7.4. The ABCs of Primary and Secondary Prevention of Coronary Heart Disease

Aspirin/angiotensin-converting enzyme inhibitors
Beta blockers
Cholesterol lowering
Dietary reduction of saturated fat
Exercise
Folate to reduce homocysteine
Glucose control in diabetes
High-density lipoprotein raising
Ischemia management
Justify to the patient the importance of risk reduction
Knowing the global risk score
Lowering of blood pressure
Monounsaturated fats (olive oil, nuts)
Noninvasive measures for preclinical disease (e.g., ankle-brachial index)
Omega-3 fatty acids
Plant sterols or stanols
Quality of life improvement—cardiac rehabilitation
Reduction of body weight
Smoking cessation
Triglyceride lowering
Use nurses and dietitians to help educate the patient
Vegetables and fiber
Wine in moderation
Xanthoma evaluation to diagnose familial hypercholesterolemia
Youth screening of risk factors (especially with strong family history status)
Zero risk factors as a goal (except for age)

mobile tool to assess the patient's risk, provide individualized treatment plans, and track the patient's progress to reduce noncompliance. The desktop PC also contains a patient risk database (Figs. 7.16 and 7.17) that can identify patients not at goal or who have missed appointments. The database can also be queried for the various criteria entered, and these data can be used by the physician to longitudinally follow many different variables in the patient population. Other tools to consider to improve adherence to primary and secondary prevention guidelines are the ABCs listed in Table 7.4. The AHA also provides a patient-friendly web site called One of a Kind at www.americanheart.org that can help improve patient compliance with lifestyle changes. The end result is, one hopes, improved quality of care and a true focus by the physician on CV risk factor modification in his or her practice.

SELECTED READING

Birtcher KK, Bowden C, Ballantyne CM, Huyen M. Strategies for implementing lipid-lowering therapy: pharmacy-based approach. *Am J Cardiol* 2000;85[Suppl]:30A–35A.

Brown SB, Cofer LA. Lipid management in a private cardiology practice (the Midwest Heart experience). *Am J Cardiol* 2000;85:18A–22A.

Cabana MD, Rand CS, Powe NR, et al. Why don't physicians follow clinical practice guidelines? A framework for improvement. *JAMA* 1999;282:1458–1465.

Crouse JR III, Byington RP, Hoen HM, Furberg CD. Reductase inhibitor monotherapy and stroke prevention. *Arch Intern Med* 1997;157:1305–1310.

DeBusk RF, Miller NH, Superko HR, et al. A case-management system for coronary risk factor modification after acute myocardial infarction. *Ann Intern Med* 1994;120:721–729.

DiMatteo MR. Enhancing patient adherence to medical recommendations. *JAMA* 1994;271:79–83.

Fanarow GC, Gawlinski A. Rationale and design for the cardiac hospitalization atherosclerosis management program at the University of California Los Angeles. *Am J Cardiol* 2000;85:10A–17A.

Hillert B, Remonte S, Rodgers G, et al. Improving patient outcomes by pooling resources (the Texas Heart Care Partnership Experience). *Am J Cardiol* 2000;85:43A–51A.

Jackson G. The role of statins in acute coronary syndromes: managing the unmet need. *Int J Clin Pract* 2000;54:445–449.

McBride P, Underbakke G, Plane MB, et al. Improving practice prevention systems in primary care. The health education and research trial (HEART). *J Fam Pract* 2000;49:115–125.

Mehta RH, Das SS, Tsai TT, et al. Quality improvement initiative and its impact on the management of patients with acute myocardial infarction. *Arch Intern Med* 2000;160:3057–3062.

Merenich JA, Lousberg TR, Brennan SH, et al. Optimizing treatment of dyslipidemia in patients with coronary artery disease in the managed-care environment (the Rocky Mountain Kaiser Permanente experience). *Am J Cardiol* 2000;85[Suppl]:36A–42A.

Pearson TA, Laurora I, Chu H, et al. The lipid treatment assessment project (L-TAP). A multicenter survey to evaluate the percentages of dyslipidemic patients receiving lipid-lowering therapy and achieving low-density lipoprotein cholesterol goals. *Arch Intern Med* 2000;160:459–467.

Schectman G, Wolff JC, Byrd JG, et al. Physician extenders for cost-effective management of hypercholesterolemia. *J Gen Intern Med* 1996;11:227–286.

Dietary Therapies

THERAPEUTIC LIFESTYLE CHANGES DIET—1200

	Day 1	Day 2	Day 3	Day 4	Day 5	Day 6	Day 7
Breakfast	1 c bran cereal 1 c fat-free milk 1 sm banana Coffee, black or w/ fat-free milk	1/4 c egg substitute 2 slices whole grain toast 2 tsp margarine[a] 6 oz orange juice Coffee, black or w/ fat-free milk	1 c oatmeal 2 Tbsp raisins 1 c fat-free milk 6 oz orange juice Coffee, black or w/ fat-free milk	Cheese toast: 1 slice whole grain bread, 1 slice fat-free cheese 1 c fat-free milk 4 oz orange juice Coffee, black or w/ fat-free milk	Sandwich: 1 poached egg, 1 slice Canadian bacon, 1/2 English muffin 1/4 cantaloupe 1 c fat-free milk Coffee, black or w/ fat-free milk	1 c shredded wheat 1 c fat-free milk 1 c strawberries Coffee, black or w/ fat-free milk	1/4 c egg substitute 1 slice whole grain toast 1 tsp margarine[a] 1 c fat-free milk 1/8 honeydew melon Coffee, black or w/ fat-free milk
Lunch	2 oz hamburger from extra-lean ground beef 1 bun 1 lettuce leaf 3 slices tomato Mustard Peach	1/2 c low-fat cottage cheese 1/2 c sliced tomato 12 saltine crackers 30 grapes	2 oz sliced turkey 2 slices rye bread 1 lettuce leaf 3 slices tomato 2 tsp reduced-calorie mayonnaise 2 sm plums	1/4 c tuna 1 Tbsp reduced-calorie mayonnaise 2 slices whole grain bread Carrot & celery sticks Pear	Chicken fajita: 1 oz chicken, 1 flour tortilla, sliced onions and peppers cooked in 1 tsp oil 1/2 c rice 1/2 c pinto beans w/ chopped onion	1 Tbsp natural peanut butter 2 tsp jam 1 slice whole grain bread Carrot & celery sticks Orange	Chicken salad sandwich: 2 oz chopped chicken, 1 Tbsp reduced-calorie mayonnaise, 2 slices whole grain bread, 1 lettuce leaf, 3 slices tomato 1 1/4 c cubed watermelon

Dinner	3 oz grilled skinless chicken breast 1 baked potato 2 tsp margarine[a] 1 c green beans Salad (lettuce, tomato, onion) 1 Tbsp olive oil/vinegar	3 oz baked skinless turkey breast 1 ear corn on cob 1 tsp margarine[a] 1/2 c peas 1 tsp margarine[a] 1 c yellow squash (prepared w/ 1 tsp olive oil)	4 oz salmon 2 tsp margarine[a] 2/3 c rice 1 c broccoli 1 tsp margarine[a]	2 skinless chicken thighs 1/2 c mashed potato w/ 1 tsp margarine[a] 1 c green beans w/ 1 tsp margarine[a]	3 oz baked flounder w/ 1 tsp margarine,[a] 1 Tbsp bread crumbs 1 broiled tomato w/ 1 Tbsp parmesan cheese 1/2 c cut-up fruit	Stir fry: 3 oz flank steak, 2 tsp oil, onions, pea pods, peppers, carrots, zucchini 2/3 c rice	3 oz roasted turkey Baked sweet potato 1 tsp margarine[a] 1/2 c brussels sprouts 1 tsp margarine[a] 1 roll 1 tsp margarine[a]
Snack	1 graham cracker 4 oz fat-free milk	3/4 oz pretzels	2 1/2 c fat-free popcorn	1/2 c ice milk 1 c strawberries	8 animal crackers	Peach	1/2 c sorbet

[a]Margarine used should be Benecol or Take Control.

THERAPEUTIC LIFESTYLE CHANGES DIET—1400

	Day 1	Day 2	Day 3	Day 4	Day 5	Day 6	Day 7
Break-fast	1 c bran cereal 1 c fat-free milk 6 oz orange juice 1 sm banana Coffee, black or w/ fat-free milk	1/4 c egg substitute 2 slices whole grain toast 2 tsp margarine[a] 6 oz orange juice 1/4 cantaloupe Coffee, black or w/ fat-free milk	1 c oatmeal 2 Tbsp raisins 1 c fat-free milk 6 oz orange juice Coffee, black or w/ fat-free milk	Cheese toast: 1 slice whole grain bread, 1 slice fat-free cheese 1 c fat-free milk 4 oz orange juice Coffee, black or w/ fat-free milk	Sandwich: 1 poached egg, 1 slice Canadian bacon, 1 English muffin 1/4 cantaloupe 4 oz orange juice 1 c fat-free milk Coffee, black or w/ fat-free milk	1 c shredded wheat 1 c fat-free milk 1 c strawberries Coffee, black or w/ fat-free milk	1/4 c egg substitute 2 slices whole grain toast 2 tsp margarine[a] 1 c fat-free milk 1/8 honeydew melon 4 oz orange juice Coffee, black or w/ fat-free milk
Lunch	3 oz hamburger from extra-lean ground beef 1 bun 1 lettuce leaf 3 slices tomato Mustard Peach	1/2 c low-fat cottage cheese 1/2 c sliced tomato 12 saltine crackers 30 grapes Carrot & celery sticks	2 oz sliced turkey 2 slices rye bread 1 lettuce leaf 3 slices tomato 2 tsp reduced-calorie mayonnaise Apple	1/4 c tuna 1 Tbsp reduced-calorie mayonnaise 2 slices whole grain bread Carrot & celery sticks Pear	Chicken fajita: 1 oz chicken, 1 flour tortilla, sliced onions and peppers cooked in 1 tsp oil 1/2 c rice 1/2 c pinto beans w/ chopped onion	2 Tbsp natural peanut butter 1 tsp jam 2 slices whole grain bread Carrot & celery sticks Orange	Chicken salad sandwich: 2 oz chopped chicken, 1 Tbsp reduced-calorie mayonnaise, 2 slices whole grain bread, 1 lettuce leaf, 3 slices tomato 1 1/4 c cubed watermelon

Dinner	3 oz grilled skinless chicken breast 1 baked potato 2 tsp margarine[a] 1 c green beans Salad (lettuce, tomato, onion) 1 Tbsp olive oil/vinegar	3 oz baked skinless turkey breast 1 ear corn on cob 1 tsp margarine[a] 1/2 c peas 1 tsp margarine[a] 1 c yellow squash (prepared w/ 1 tsp olive oil) 2 plums	4 oz salmon 2 tsp margarine[a] 1 c rice 1 c broccoli 1 tsp margarine[a] 1/12 of an angel food cake 1/2 c raspberries	2 skinless chicken thighs 1 c green beans w/1 tsp margarine[a] 1/2 c mashed potato w/ 1 tsp margarine[a] 1 roll 1 tsp margarine[a]	3 oz baked flounder w/ 1 tsp margarine,[a] 1 Tbsp bread crumbs 1 broiled tomato w/1 Tbsp parmesan cheese 1/2 c cut-up fruit	Stir fry: 3 oz flank steak, 2 tsp oil, onions, pea pods, peppers, carrots, zucchini 2/3 c rice	3 oz roasted turkey Baked sweet potato 1 tsp margarine[a] 1/2 c brussels sprouts 1 tsp margarine[a] 1 roll 1 tsp margarine[a]
Snack	1 graham cracker 4 oz fat-free milk	3/4 oz pretzels	2 1/2 c fat-free popcorn	1/2 c ice milk 1 c strawberries	8 animal crackers 1 sm banana	Peach	1/2 c sorbet

[a] Margarine used should be Benecol or Take Control.

THERAPEUTIC LIFESTYLE CHANGES DIET—1600

	Day 1	Day 2	Day 3	Day 4	Day 5	Day 6	Day 7
Breakfast	1 c bran cereal 1 c fat-free milk 8 oz orange juice 1 sm banana Coffee, black or w/ fat-free milk	1/4 c egg substitute 2 slices whole grain toast 2 tsp margarine[a] 8 oz orange juice 1/4 cantaloupe Coffee, black or w/ fat-free milk	1 c oatmeal 2 Tbsp raisins 1 c fat-free milk 8 oz orange juice 1 slice whole wheat toast 1 tsp margarine[a] Coffee, black or w/ fat-free milk	Cheese toast: 2 slices whole grain bread, 2 slices fat-free cheese 1 c fat-free milk 8 oz orange juice Coffee, black or w/ fat-free milk	Sandwich: 1 poached egg, 1 slice Canadian bacon, 1 English Muffin 1/4 cantaloupe 8 oz orange juice 1 c fat-free milk Coffee, black or w/ fat-free milk	1 c shredded wheat 1 c fat-free milk 1 c strawberries 6 oz orange juice Coffee, black or w/ fat-free milk	1/4 c egg substitute 2 slices whole grain toast 2 tsp margarine[a] 8 oz orange juice 1 c fat-free milk 1/8 honeydew melon Coffee, black or w/ fat-free milk
Lunch	3 oz hamburger from extra-lean ground beef 1 bun 1 lettuce leaf 3 slices tomato Mustard Peach 1 oz pretzels	Turkey sandwich: 2 oz turkey, 2 slices whole wheat bread, 2 tsp mayonnaise, 3 slices tomato & lettuce Carrot & celery sticks 30 grapes	2 oz sliced turkey 2 slices rye bread 1 lettuce leaf 3 slices tomato 2 tsp reduced-calorie mayonnaise 2 sm plums	1/4 c tuna 1 Tbsp reduced-calorie mayonnaise 2 slices whole grain bread Carrot & celery sticks Pear	Chicken fajita: 2 oz chicken, 2 flour tortillas, sliced onions and peppers cooked in 1 tsp oil 1/2 c rice 1/2 c pinto beans w/ chopped onion	2 Tbsp natural peanut butter 1 Tbsp jam 2 slices whole grain bread Carrot & celery sticks 1 c fat-free milk Orange	Chicken salad sandwich: 2 oz chopped chicken, 1 Tbsp reduced-calorie mayonnaise, 2 slices whole grain bread, lettuce leaf, 3 slices tomato 11/4 c cubed watermelon

Dinner	3 oz grilled skinless chicken breast 1 baked potato 2 tsp margarine[a] 1 c green beans 1 tsp margarine[a] Salad (lettuce, tomato, onion) 1 Tbsp olive oil/vinegar	3 oz baked skinless turkey breast 1 ear corn on cob 1 tsp margarine[a] 1/2 c peas 1 tsp margarine[a] 1 c yellow squash (prepared w/ 1 tsp olive oil)	4 oz salmon 2 tsp margarine[a] 1 c rice 1 c broccoli 1 tsp margarine[a] 1/12 of angel food cake 1/2 c raspberries	2 skinless chicken thighs 1 c mashed potato w/1 tsp margarine[a] 1 roll 1 tsp margarine[a] 1 c green beans w/ 1 tsp margarine[a]	3 oz baked flounder w/ 1 tsp margarine,[a] 1 Tbsp bread crumbs 1 broiled tomato w/ 1 Tbsp parmesan cheese, 1 tsp margarine[a] 1/2 c cut-up fruit	Stir fry: 3 oz flank steak, 2 tsp oil, onions, pea pods, peppers, carrots, zucchini 1 c rice	3 oz roasted turkey Baked sweet potato 2 tsp margarine[a] 1 c brussels sprouts 1 tsp margarine[a] 1 roll 1 tsp margarine[a]
Snack	1 graham cracker 1/2 c fat-free milk	3/4 oz pretzels	2 1/2 c fat-free popcorn 2 tsp margarine[a]	1/2 c ice milk 1 c strawberries	8 animal crackers	Peach	1 c sorbet

[a]Margarine used should be Benecol or Take Control.

THERAPEUTIC LIFESTYLE CHANGES DIET—2000

	Day 1	Day 2	Day 3	Day 4	Day 5	Day 6	Day 7
Breakfast	1 c bran cereal 1 c fat-free milk 8 oz orange juice 1 sm banana 1 slice whole wheat toast 1 tsp margarine[a] Coffee, black or w/ fat-free milk	1/4 c egg substitute 2 slices whole grain toast 2 tsp margarine[a] 6 oz orange juice Coffee, black or w/ fat-free milk	1 c oatmeal 2 Tbsp raisins 1 c fat-free milk 8 oz orange juice 1 slice whole wheat bread 1 tsp margarine[a] Coffee, black or w/ fat-free milk	Cheese toast: 2 slices whole grain bread, 2 slices fat-free cheese 1 c fat-free milk 8 oz orange juice Coffee, black or w/ fat-free milk	Sandwich: 1 poached egg, 1 slice Canadian bacon, 1 English muffin 1/4 cantaloupe 8 oz orange juice 1 c fat-free milk Coffee, black or w/ fat-free milk	1 c shredded wheat 1 c fat-free milk 1 c strawberries 8 oz orange juice 2 slices whole wheat toast 2 tsp margarine[a] Coffee, black or w/ fat-free milk	1/4 c egg substitute 2 slices whole grain toast 2 tsp margarine[a] 8 oz orange juice 1 c fat-free milk 1/8 honeydew melon Coffee, black or w/ fat-free milk
Lunch	3 oz hamburger from extra-lean ground beef 1 bun 1 lettuce leaf 3 slices tomato 2 tsp mayonnaise Peach 1 oz pretzels	Turkey sandwich: 2 oz turkey, 2 slices whole wheat bread, 2 tsp mayonnaise, 3 slices tomato & lettuce Carrot & celery sticks 30 grapes 1 c fat-free yogurt	4 oz sliced turkey 4 slices rye bread 1 lettuce leaf 6 slices tomato 4 tsp reduced-calorie mayonnaise 2 sm plums	1/2 c tuna 2 Tbsp reduced-calorie mayonnaise 4 slices whole grain bread Carrot & celery sticks Pear	Chicken fajita: 2 oz chicken, 2 flour tortillas, sliced onions and peppers cooked in 1 tsp oil 1/2 c rice 1/2 c pinto beans w/ chopped onion 1/4 avocado 1 sm mango	2 Tbsp natural peanut butter 1 Tbsp jam 2 slices whole grain bread Carrot & celery sticks 1 c fat-free milk Orange	Chicken salad sandwich: 2 oz chopped chicken, 1 Tbsp reduced-calorie mayonnaise, 2 slices whole grain bread, 1 lettuce leaf, 3 slices tomato 2 oz baked potato chips 11/4 c cubed watermelon

Dinner	3 oz grilled skinless chicken breast 1 baked potato 2 tsp margarine[a] 1 c green beans Salad (lettuce, tomato, onion) 1 Tbsp olive oil/vinegar 1/2 c carrots 1 pear	3 oz baked skinless turkey breast 1 ear corn on cob 1 tsp margarine[a] 1/2 c peas 1 tsp margarine[a] 1 c yellow squash (prepared w/ 1 tsp olive oil)	4 oz salmon 2 tsp margarine[a] 1 c rice 1 c broccoli 1 tsp margarine[a] 1 c yellow squash 1 tsp olive oil 1/12 of angel food cake 1/2 c raspberries	3 skinless chicken thighs 1 c mashed potato w/ 1 tsp margarine[a] 1 roll 1 tsp margarine[a] 1 c green beans w/ 1 tsp margarine[a]	3 oz baked flounder w/ 1 tsp margarine,[a] 1 Tbsp bread crumbs 1 broiled tomato w/ 1 Tbsp parmesan cheese, 1 tsp margarine[a] 1 c peas 1 slice whole grain bread 1/2 c cut-up fruit	Stir fry: 3 oz flank steak, 2 tsp oil, onions, pea pods, peppers, carrots, zucchini 1 1/2 c rice	3 oz roasted turkey Baked sweet potato 2 tsp margarine[a] 1 c brussels sprouts 1 tsp margarine[a] 1 roll 1 tsp margarine[a] Apple
Snack	2 graham crackers 1 c fat-free milk	2 ginger snap cookies 1 c sorbet	2 1/2 c fat-free popcorn 2 tsp margarine[a]	1/2 c ice milk 1 c strawberries	8 animal crackers 6 oz low-fat yogurt	Peach	1 c sorbet 2 fig bar cookies

[a]Margarine used should be Benecol or Take Control.

MEDITERRANEAN DIET

	Day 1	Day 2	Day 3	Day 4	Day 5	Day 6	Day 7
Breakfast	1 c high-fiber cereal 1 c fat-free milk 1 banana 3/4 c strawberries	1 c low-fat yogurt 2 slices whole wheat bread 2 tsp tub margarine[a] Apple	1 c oatmeal 1 c fat-free milk 2 Tbsp raisins 1 slice whole wheat toast 1 tsp tub margarine[a]	1 c low-fat yogurt 1 English muffin 2 tsp tub margarine[a] 1/4 cantaloupe	1 c high-fiber cereal 1 c fat-free milk 1/2 c blueberries 1 slice whole wheat toast w/ jam	1 c low-fat yogurt 1 bran muffin 1 tsp tub margarine[a] 1/8 honeydew melon	1 egg 2 slices whole wheat toast 2 tsp tub margarine[a] Orange
Lunch	1/6 cheese & spinach quiche Tossed salad 1 Tbsp olive oil/vinegar Grapes	Grilled vegetables: 1 sm zucchini, 1 sm yellow squash, 1 sm potato, 1/2 sm eggplant, 1/2 red pepper 1 Tbsp olive oil 2 oz mozzarella	Baked potato w/ 2 oz cheese & 1/2 c broccoli Salad w/ 1 Tbsp olive oil/vinegar Peach	Large Greek salad: 2 oz Feta cheese, 10 Greek olives, 2 Tbsp olive oil/vinegar 2 slices pita bread	Salad: 2 whole tomatoes sliced, 4 oz mozzarella, fresh basil leaves, 2 Tbsp olive oil/balsamic vinegar 2 slices Italian bread 2 tsp olive oil	Grilled skinless chicken breast on whole wheat bun w/ lettuce, tomato, 1 tsp mayonnaise Baked potato wedges: 1 med potato, 2 tsp olive oil, 1/2 c broccoli sprinkled w/ 2 tsp parmesan cheese	3/4 c low-fat cottage cheese 1 1/2 c sliced melon 8 low-fat crackers 1/2 c pudding made with fat-free milk

Snack	1 1/2 oz box raisins	1/4 c peanuts	Trail mix (no coconut)	6 dried apricot halves	2 plums	Grapes	1/4 c dried sour cherries
Dinner	1 c minestrone soup, 2 slices bread, 2 tsp olive oil, Salad, 3 oz grilled salmon, 1 c green beans w/ 1 Tbsp slivered almonds, Orange	1/4 of large vegetarian pizza, Salad w/ 1 Tbsp olive oil/vinegar, 1 1/4 c watermelon	2 c lentil soup, Salad: Raw spinach, 1/2 tomato, 1/4 c water chestnuts, onion, 1 Tbsp pine nuts, 1 Tbsp olive oil/vinegar, 2 slices bread, 2 tsp olive oil, Pear	3 oz flounder, 1/2 c carrots, onions, peppers, garlic, 1 tsp olive oil mixed w/ 1 c rice, 1 c split pea soup (no ham), 1/2 c spinach, 1/8 honeydew melon	Cook together: 2 oz skinless chicken, 2 sm potatoes, 1 carrot, onion, peppers, 1 c tomato, 1 tsp olive oil; serve over 1 c couscous prepared w/ olive oil	1 c black beans prepared w/ garlic, 1 tsp olive oil, 1 1/2 c rice, 2 Tbsp chopped onion; Salad (on lettuce leaf): 1 tomato sliced, 1/4 avocado sliced, 1 tsp olive oil	2 c pasta w/ 1–2 c marinara sauce w/ cubed eggplant (no meat); Salad: Lettuce, tomato, onion, 1 Tbsp parmesan cheese, 1 Tbsp olive oil/vinegar, 2 slices bread, 2 tsp olive oil
Snack	1/4 c soy nuts	Peach	6 ginger snaps, 1 c fat-free milk	1/4 c peanuts	1/2 c fat-free vanilla frozen yogurt, 1/2 c sliced strawberries, 1 Tbsp chopped walnuts	1/4 c sunflower seeds	16 black olives

aMargarine used should be Benecol or Take Control.

50-G CARBOHYDRATE GUIDELINES

To keep your carbohydrate intake within 50 g, the following foods should be avoided:

Drinks containing sugar (soda pop, sweetened teas, powdered drinks, sports drinks)
Desserts
Breads, cereals, rice, pasta, noodles, muffins, doughnuts
Snack foods (chips, pretzels, crackers)
Starchy vegetables (potatoes, corn, peas, dried beans)
Milk and yogurt
Fruits and fruit juices

The following foods are not high in carbohydrate but are high in saturated fat and should be limited: high-fat cheeses, luncheon meats, hot dogs, butter, cream, stick margarine, high-fat meats (e.g., ribs, steak, sausage, bacon).

Go with these foods:

Vegetables	Meats	Dairy	Condiments	Beverages
Asparagus	Chicken or turkey with no skin	Low-fat cottage cheese	Avocado	Water
Bean sprouts	Cornish hen (no skin)	Part-skim mozza-rella	Olives	Unsweetened tea
Broccoli	Fish (not fried)	Two percent milk	Nuts	Coffee (black)
Brussels sprouts	Shellfish	cheeses	Liquid oils	Diet sodas
Cabbage	Tuna	Parmesan	Tub margarine	Sugar-free pow-dered drinks
Cauliflower	Egg whites		Squeeze margarine	Sugar-free gelatins
Celery	Egg substitutes		Seeds (sesame, pumpkin, sun-flower)	Fat-free broth or bouillon
Cucumber	Eggs (not more than 2 per week)		Peanut butter (natu-ral)	
Eggplant	Beef steak [round, sir-loin, cubed, flank, tenderloin (all fat trimmed off]		Italian salad dress-ing	
Green or string beans			Oil and vinegar	
Green onions or spring onions			Mayonnaise	
Greens (collard, kale, mustard, turnip)	Beef roast [rib, chuck, rump (no fat)]			
Leeks	Extra lean or round ground beef			
Mushrooms	Lean pork (tenderloin)			
Okra	Ham			
Onions	Canadian bacon			
Pea pods	Veal (lean chop, roast)			
Peppers	Lamb [roast, chop, leg (no fat)]			
Radishes				
Salad greens (endive, escarole, let-tuce, romaine, spinach)				
Sauerkraut				
Spinach				
Summer squash				
Tomato				
Turnips				
Water chestnuts				
Watercress				
Wax beans				
Zucchini				

50-G CARBOHYDRATE DIET

	Day 1	Day 2	Day 3	Day 4	Day 5	Day 6	Day 7
Breakfast	1/2 c egg substitute 2 tsp margarine[a] 2 strips turkey bacon	Omelet: 1/2 c egg substitute & fat-free cheese	1/2 c Eggbeaters	1/2 c egg substitute prepared w/ 2 tsp margarine[a] 2 slices turkey bacon	Western omelet: 1/2 c Eggbeaters, green pepper, onion, tomato, 2 tsp margarine[a]	1/2 c Eggbeaters prepared w/ 2 tsp margarine[a] 3 slices Canadian bacon	Western omelet: 1/2 c Eggbeaters, green pepper, onion, tomato
Lunch	2 grilled chicken breasts 1 c steamed broccoli 2 tsp margarine[a] Salad[b] 2 Tbsp Italian salad dressing	Chef salad: 2 oz sliced turkey, 2 oz sliced ham, 2 slices fat-free cheese, 2 c lettuce, 1 c tomato, onions, celery, carrots, 4 Tbsp French salad dressing	6 oz grilled flank steak (marinated in 2 Tbsp oil/vinegar) 1 c cauliflower Salad[b] 1 Tbsp oil/vinegar 2 tsp margarine[a]	1 c cottage cheese 1 whole tomato sliced Salad[b] 1 Tbsp oil/vinegar	6 oz sliced turkey breast 1 c cooked spinach 2 tsp margarine[a] Salad[b] 1 Tbsp olive oil/vinegar	Tuna fish salad on lettuce leaf w/ 1 tomato quartered: 1 c tuna, 2 Tbsp mayonnaise, chopped celery & onion	5 oz extra-lean ground beef patty 1 whole tomato sliced Lettuce leaf 1 Tbsp mayonnaise 1/2 c cottage cheese
Snack	1/4 c (2 oz) almonds	1/4 c walnuts	1/4 c sunflower seeds	1/4 c peanuts	1/4 c sunflower seeds	1/4 c almonds	20 green olives

Dinner	6 oz broiled salmon 1 Tbsp margarine[a] (used in preparation) 1 c zucchini & yellow squash sautéed in 1 Tbsp olive oil Salad[b] 1 Tbsp olive oil/vinegar	Baked skinless chicken (2 thighs & 1 leg) 1 c cooked spinach 2 tsp margarine[a] Salad[b] 2 Tbsp Italian salad dressing	Spinach salad: 2 c raw spinach, 4 strips turkey bacon, 1/2 c water chestnuts, 1/2 onion sliced, 1 egg, 4 Tbsp Italian salad dressing	Broiled orange roughy w/ 1 Tbsp margarine[a] 1 c brussels sprouts 2 tsp margarine[a] Salad[b] 2 Tbsp Italian salad dressing	Stir fry: 6 oz round steak, 3 onions (spring), 1/4 c pea pods, 1/2 red pepper, 1/2 c mushrooms Salad[b] 1 Tbsp oil/vinegar	2–3 oz grilled chicken breast 1 c green beans 2 tsp margarine[a] Cole slaw (1 c shredded cabbage w/ 2 Tbsp mayonnaise)	5 oz ham steak 1 c cauliflower 1 tsp margarine[a] Salad[b] 2 Tbsp French salad dressing
Snack	2 celery stalks w/ 4 Tbsp natural peanut butter	1/4 c peanuts	20 black olives	2 celery stalks w/ 4 Tbsp natural peanut butter	1/4 c walnuts	2 celery stalks w/ 4 Tbsp natural peanut butter	1/4 c sunflower seeds

[a]Margarine used should be Benecol or Take Control.
[b]Salad = lettuce, 1/2 tomato, onions.

100-G CARBOHYDRATE DIET

	Day 1	Day 2	Day 3	Day 4	Day 5	Day 6	Day 7
Breakfast	1/2 c egg substitute, 2 tsp margarine[a], 2 strips turkey bacon, 1 slice whole grain bread	Omelet: 1/2 c egg substitute, 2 slices fat-free cheese, 1 slice whole grain bread, 2 tsp margarine[a]	Cheese toast: 1 slice whole wheat bread, 2 slices fat-free cheese	1/2 c egg substitute, 2 slices turkey bacon, 1 slice whole grain bread, 2 tsp margarine	Western omelet: 1/2 c Eggbeaters, green pepper, onion, tomato, 1 slice whole grain bread, 2 tsp margarine[a]	1/2 c Eggbeaters, 3 slices Canadian bacon, 1 slice whole grain bread, 2 tsp margarine[a]	Cheese toast: 1 slice whole wheat bread, 2 slices fat-free cheese, 1/2 banana
Lunch	2 grilled chicken breasts, 1/2 c mashed potatoes, 1 c steamed broccoli, 2 tsp margarine[a], Salad[b], 2 Tbsp Italian salad dressing	Chef salad: 2 oz sliced turkey, 2 oz sliced ham, 2 slices fat-free cheese, 2 c lettuce, 1 c tomato, onions, celery, carrots, 4 Tbsp French salad dressing	6 oz grilled flank steak (marinated in 2 Tbsp oil/vinegar), Vegetable medley, 2 tsp margarine[a], Salad[b], 2 Tbsp French dressing	1 c cottage cheese, 1 whole tomato sliced, Salad[b], 2 Tbsp French dressing	6 oz sliced turkey breast, 1 c cooked spinach, 2 tsp margarine[a], Salad[b], 1 Tbsp olive oil/vinegar, Apple	Tuna fish salad on lettuce leaf w/ 1 tomato quartered: 1 c tuna, 2 Tbsp mayonnaise, chopped celery & onion, 1 slice whole grain bread	5 oz extra-lean ground beef patty, 1 whole tomato sliced, Lettuce leaf, 1 tsp mayonnaise, 1/2 c cottage cheese, 1 slice whole grain bread

Snack	1/4 c (2 oz) almonds	1/4 c walnuts	1/4 c sunflower seeds	1/4 c peanuts	1/4 c sunflower seeds	1/4 c almonds	20 green olives
Dinner	6 oz broiled salmon, 1 tsp margarine[a] (used in preparation), 1 c zucchini & yellow squash sautéed in 1 tsp olive oil, Salad[b], 1 Tbsp olive oil/vinegar, Peach	Baked skinless chicken (2 thighs & 1 leg), 1 c cooked carrots, 2 tsp margarine[a], Salad[b], 2 Tbsp Italian salad dressing	Spinach salad: 2 c raw spinach, 4 strips turkey bacon, 1/2 c water chestnuts, 1/2 onion sliced, 1 egg, 4 Tbsp Italian salad dressing, Orange	Broiled orange roughy w/ 1 Tbsp margarine[a], 1 c brussel sprouts, 2 tsp margarine[a], Salad[b], 2 Tbsp Italian dressing, 2 plums	Stir fry: 6 oz round steak, 1/2 c broccoli, 1/2 c cauliflower, 3 onions (spring), 1/4 c pea pods, 1/2 red pepper, 1/2 c mushrooms, Salad[b], 2 Tbsp French dressing	2–3 oz grilled chicken breast, 1 c green beans, 2 tsp margarine[a], Cole slaw (1 c shredded cabbage w/ 2 Tbsp mayonnaise), 1 c whole strawberries	5 oz ham steak, 2 sm red potatoes, 1 c cauliflower, 2 tsp margarine[a], Salad[b], 2 Tbsp French salad dressing
Snack	2 celery stalks w/ 4 Tbsp natural peanut butter	1/4 c peanuts	20 black olives	2 celery stalks w/ 4 Tbsp natural peanut butter	1/4 c walnuts	2 celery stalks w/ 4 Tbsp natural peanut butter	1/4 c sunflower seeds

[a] Margarine used should be Benecol or Take Control.
[b] Salad = lettuce, 1/2 tomato, onions.

THERAPEUTIC LIFESTYLE CHANGES DIET—2 PLANT STANOLS AND HIGH FIBER

	Day 1	Day 2	Day 3	Day 4	Day 5	Day 6	Day 7
Breakfast	1 c bran cereal 1 c fat-free milk 1/4 cantaloupe 1 sm banana 1 slice whole wheat toast 1 tsp margarine[a] Coffee, black or w/ fat-free milk	1/4 c egg substitute 2 slices whole grain toast 2 tsp margarine[a] 1 sm banana Peach Coffee, black or w/ fat-free milk	1 c oatmeal 2 Tbsp raisins 1 c fat-free milk 1/4 c cantaloupe 1 slice whole wheat bread 1 tsp margarine[a] Coffee, black or w/ fat-free milk	Cheese toast: 2 slices whole grain bread, 2 slices fat-free cheese 1 c fat-free milk Apple Coffee, black or w/ fat-free milk	Sandwich: 1 poached egg, 1 slice Canadian bacon, 1 English muffin 1/2 cantaloupe 1 c fat-free milk Coffee, black or w/ fat-free milk	1 c shredded wheat 1 c fat-free milk 1 c strawberries 2 slices whole wheat toast 3 tsp margarine[a] 6 prunes Coffee, black or w/ fat-free milk	1/4 c egg substitute 2 slices whole grain toast 2 tsp margarine[a] 1 c fat-free milk 1/4 honeydew melon Coffee, black or w/ fat-free milk
Lunch	3 oz hamburger from extra-lean ground beef 1 bun, whole grain 1 lettuce leaf 3 slices tomato 2 tsp mayonnaise 1/2 c baked beans Peach	Turkey sandwich: 2 oz turkey, 2 slices whole wheat bread, 2 tsp mayonnaise, 3 slices tomato & lettuce 1/2 c three-bean salad Carrot & celery sticks 30 grapes	3 oz sliced turkey 3 slices rye bread 1 lettuce leaf 6 slices tomato 3 tsp reduced-calorie mayonnaise 1 c bean soup 2 sm plums	1/2 c tuna 2 Tbsp reduced-calorie mayonnaise 3 slices whole grain bread 1 c lentil soup Carrot & celery sticks Pear	Chicken fajita: 2 oz chicken, 2 flour tortillas, sliced onions and peppers cooked in 1 tsp oil 1/2 c rice 1 c pinto beans w/ chopped onion 1/4 avocado 1 sm mango	2 Tbsp natural peanut butter 1 Tbsp jam 2 slices whole grain bread Carrot & celery sticks 1 c fat-free milk Orange	Chicken salad sandwich: 2 oz chopped chicken, 1 Tbsp reduced-calorie mayonnaise, 2 slices whole grain bread, 1 lettuce leaf, 3 slices tomato 1 c bean soup 11/4 c cubed watermelon

Dinner	3 oz grilled skinless chicken breast 1 baked potato 2 tsp margarine[a] 1 c green beans Salad (lettuce, tomato, onion) 1 Tbsp olive oil/vinegar 1/2 c carrots 1 pear	3 oz baked skinless turkey breast 1 ear corn on cob 1 tsp margarine[a] 1/2 c peas 1 tsp margarine[a] 1 c yellow squash (prepared w/ 1 tsp olive oil)	4 oz salmon 2 tsp margarine[a] 1 c rice 1 c broccoli 1 tsp margarine[a] 1 c yellow squash 1 tsp olive oil 1/12 of angel food cake 1/2 c raspberries	3 skinless chicken thighs 1 c mashed potato w/ 1 tsp margarine[a] 1 roll 1 tsp margarine[a] 1 c green beans w/ 1 tsp margarine[a]	3 oz baked flounder w/ 2 tsp margarine,[a] 1 Tbsp bread crumbs 1 broiled tomato w/ 1 Tbsp parmesan cheese, 1 tsp margarine[a] 1 c peas 1 c cut-up fruit	Stir fry: 3 oz flank steak, 2 tsp oil, onions, pea pods, peppers, carrots, zucchini (at least 2 c) 1 1/2 c rice	3 oz roasted turkey 1 baked sweet potato 2 tsp margarine[a] 1 c brussels sprouts 1 tsp margarine[a] 1 roll, whole grain 1 tsp margarine[a] Apple
Snack	2 graham crackers 1 c fat-free milk	1/2 c dried apricots 1 c fat-free yogurt	2 1/2 c fat-free popcorn 2 tsp margarine[a]	1/2 c ice milk 1 c strawberries	1/2 c oat bran cereal 6 oz fat-free milk	Peach	1 c sorbet 2 fig bar cookies

[a]Margarine used should be Benecol or Take Control.

Quit Smoking Action Plan[*]
✝ AMERICAN LUNG ASSOCIATION.

INTRODUCTION

The American Lung Association developed this booklet under the guidance of a team of experts on cigarette smoking. It offers specific recommendations for selecting a personalized *Quit Smoking Action Plan* to free yourself of cigarettes and stay that way.

HOW TO USE THIS BOOKLET

To help you better understand your options, the material in this booklet is presented in the following 3 steps of a *Quit Smoking Action Plan*, along with charts to guide you through each step.

Step 1—Preparing to quit
Step 2—Using medications
Step 3—Staying smoke-free

A DEADLY COMBINATION: ADDICTION AND BEHAVIOR

Nicotine is a powerful drug that raises mood, reduces anxiety, and, in those accustomed to it, increases alertness. Over time, it causes changes in smokers' brains that make them need nicotine. Then, when they try to quit, smokers have unpleasant symptoms such as irritability, craving for cigarettes, or difficulty concentrating.

An additional obstacle to quitting is the many daily behavior patterns that smokers may not even realize they have, such as morning or

---

[*]From the American Lung Association, with permission. ©1998 American Lung Association.

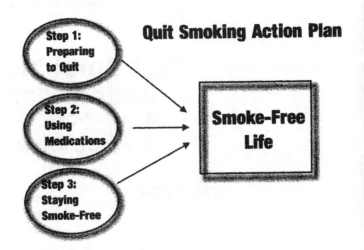

before-bed cigarette routines, or smoking with friends, coworkers, or spouses. These links can be numerous and strong, but your *Quit Smoking Action Plan* should help you deal with them.

People who are fairly dependent on cigarettes need to incorporate multiple sources of help in their quitting plan to maximize their odds of success. Those who are less dependent on cigarettes may be successful by using only a few sources of help. However, the more help you have, the better your chances of quitting and staying smoke-free.

BE A SMART QUITTER!

There are many programs to help you quit smoking. The cost of these programs may vary from almost nothing to hundreds of dollars. A higher cost does not guarantee success. Many health plans and work sites provide free quit-smoking programs, and some health plans cover the cost of medications to help you quit. Check with your insurance carrier or employer for more information.

Before investing your time or money in a program ask questions such as

- Is there a cost to you?
- Is the program convenient for you?
- Is the staff well trained and professional?
- Does the program meet your needs?

- What is the success rate of this program?

A program representative should be able to answer your questions. If they can't, keep looking. There are no tricks or magic bullets to make you stop smoking. If a program seems too easy, guarantees you will quit, or claims a success rate that sounds unrealistic, look elsewhere.

EXAMINING YOUR OPTIONS

The charts on the next few pages review your options for each of the 3 steps of your *Quit Smoking Action Plan*. Although there are many sources of help available, it's best to choose what feels right to you. The more comfortable you are with the methods you use, the better the chances that you will stick with them.

STEP #1: PREPARING TO QUIT

What You Need to Do

1. Identify your personal reasons for quitting.

2. Set a quit date, usually within 10 days to several weeks. If you smoke mostly at work, try quitting on a weekend. If you smoke mostly when relaxing or socializing, quit on a weekday.

3. Identify your barriers to quitting (such as your spouse smokes or you've relapsed before due to depression or weight gain). You'll find sources of help in this booklet to overcome these barriers.

4. Make *specific* plans *ahead of time* for dealing with temptations. Identify two or three coping strategies that work for you (such as taking a walk or calling a friend).

5. Get cooperation from family and friends. They can't quit for you, but they can help by not smoking around you, providing a sympathetic ear and encouragement when you need it, and leaving you alone when you need some space. (See Step #1 chart, Preparing to Quit.)

STEP #2: USING MEDICATIONS

What You Need to Know

When you smoke a cigarette, a high concentration of nicotine enters your body rapidly and travels to your brain. Nicotine medications provide you with a safer alternative source of nicotine that enters the body less rapidly and in a lower concentration than cigarettes. There is much unfounded concern about the safety of nicotine medications even though they have been extensively tested and used by millions of people. Unlike cigarettes, which contain thousands of harmful chemicals, nicotine medications contain small doses of nicotine alone to combat cravings and urges to smoke.

To optimize your chances of success, generally medications should be a component of your *Quit Smoking Action Plan.* However, not everyone who decides to quit smoking will want or need to use them. Depending on the medication you use, you may need a prescription. As with any medication, consult the package directions or your pharmacist before using. If you are pregnant, consult your physician; if you are taking other medications, consult the doctor who prescribed them or your pharmacist.

Your goal in using nicotine medication is to stop smoking completely. If you plan to take nicotine medications, begin using them on your quit date. If you continue to have strong urges to smoke or are struggling to stop smoking completely, ask your health care provider about additional help.

If you take the non-nicotine medication, it should be started approximately 7 to 10 days before your target quit date. (See Step #2 chart, Using Medications.)

Other Tips for Using Medications

- Ask your physician or pharmacist for advice if you are uncertain about which medication to use.

- Learn to use the medication you choose (e.g., apply patches properly, use nicotine gum, nasal spray, or inhaler as recommended on package labeling).

- Many experts believe nicotine medications are often taken for too short a time to be of full benefit to users. For this reason, your healthcare provider may advise you to use your medication for a longer period or in combination with another medication. However, if you take these medications on your own, do not deviate from package directions.

STEP #3: STAYING SMOKE-FREE

What You Need to Remember

After quitting and getting through the first couple of weeks, staying off cigarettes is critical—and not always easy. Research indicates that continued support and encouragement from health providers, family, friends, and other sources are extremely helpful.

Your friends and family won't automatically know how to encourage you. Talk to them ahead of time about what they can do. Also, think about who you want to give you encouragement—someone who will stay positive even if you have some problems along the way. (See Step #3 chart, Staying Smoke-Free.)

The average person makes two to four attempts at quitting before they are able to stay smoke-free. If you return to smoking, it doesn't mean you can't quit. It just means you need to try again by figuring out what caused you to slip and improving your plan for next time.

You may want to use medications this time if you have tried to quit without them in the past. Or you may want to try a different group, individual counselor, or other source of help if you've been unsuccessful at quitting on your own.

Some smokers wrongly believe they can reduce their health risks and continue to smoke by substituting other forms of tobacco. Low tar/nicotine cigarettes are not safer than cigarettes, nor do they reduce your risk of smoking-related disease. Smokeless tobacco, pipes, and cigars also are not safe.

Step #1: Preparing to Quit

Description and Examples	Pros and Cons	Comments
Group programs American Lung Association's Freedom From Smoking® group program offers seven sessions to help you set and follow your *Quit Smoking Action Plan*. Also offered by many hospitals, medical facilities, and by voluntary agencies.	**Pros** • Supportive, encouraging environment • Opportunity for building skills needed to quit smoking **Cons** • Meeting schedule may not be flexible enough for some • A group may not be available when you need it	**Comments/limitations:** Best for those who work well with others. The groups focus on helping you change your smoking behaviors. May also be helpful for those whose family or friends are unlikely to provide support. Usually meets for four to seven sessions, with each session lasting 1 to 2 hours.

continued

Step #1: Preparing to Quit *Continued*

Description and Examples	Pros and Cons	Comments
Individual counseling from healthcare provider Many healthcare providers offer individual quit-smoking programs that help you develop a *Quit Smoking Action Plan*. They should also provide encouragement for staying smoke-free and plans for coping with relapse.	**Pros** • Flexible • Personalized to your needs • Opportunity for building skills needed to quit smoking **Cons** • No opportunity for peer support, sharing • Usually requires an appointment	**Comments/limitations:** This may be best if you have a good relationship with your healthcare provider. Best for people who prefer to work independently rather than in group settings. The more counseling sessions you attend, the better your chances of staying smoke-free.
Books, manuals, audiotapes, videotapes, and Internet resources ALA's *7 Steps to a Smoke-Free Life* is one of many excellent sources available. These should be educational, informative, and discuss the key parts of a *Quit Smoking Action Plan*. May be a starting point for additional help.	**Pros** • Convenient • Private • May be especially appropriate for those who like to work on their own or enjoy "do-it-yourself" projects **Cons** • Success depends on continued use • Many are superficial and do not provide needed key elements	**Comments/limitations:** Although you may prefer to quit on your own, quitting without preparing an action plan is unlikely to be successful. The American Lung Association provides a variety of materials and programs, including special programs for pregnant women, African-American smokers, and other populations.

continued

Step #1: Preparing to Quit *Continued*

Description and Examples	Pros and Cons	Comments
Telephone counseling Many health providers and work sites offer telephone counseling to provide assistance in developing and following through with your *Quit Smoking Action Plan.* (Additionally, telephone counseling to provide encouragement for staying smoke-free is described in Step #3 chart, Staying Smoke-Free.) Many states have smokers' help lines. For more information, call: American Lung Association 1-(800) LUNG-USA	**Pros** • Convenient • Flexible • Personal and private • Useful in rural areas or anywhere access to counseling services is limited **Cons** • Phone counselor may change from contact to contact • Lack of fixed schedule may be discouraging to some	**Comments/limitations:** Telephone counseling services are also sometimes used to help you stay smoke-free. Ask your healthcare provider or check your phone book for availability of these services in your area.

Step #2: Using Medications

Description and Examples	Pros and Cons	Comments
Nicotine patch NicoDerm® CQ Nicotrol® Nicotine Transdermal Patch (prescription required) Habitrol® (prescription required) ProStep® (prescription required) Patches deliver nicotine through the skin in different strengths, over different lengths of time.	**Pros** • Easy to use • Only needs to be applied once a day • Some available without a prescription • Few side effects **Cons** • Less flexible dosing • Slow onset of delivery • Mild skin rashes and irritation	**Comments/limitations:** Patches vary in strengths and the length of time over which nicotine is delivered. Depending on the brand you use, may be left on for anywhere from 16 to 24 hours. Some smokers who use these products can stop them abruptly, while others prefer to reduce their dosage slowly.

continued

Step #2: Using Medications *Continued*

Description and Examples	Pros and Cons	Comments
Nicotine polacrilex (nicotine gum) Nicorette® The term "gum" is misleading. Although it actually is a gum-like substance impregnated with small amounts of nicotine, nicotine gum is not chewed like regular gum. Instead, you chew it briefly and then "park" it between your cheek and gum. The nicotine is absorbed through the lining of the mouth.	**Pros** • Convenient • Flexible dosing • Faster delivery of nicotine than the patches **Cons** • May be inappropriate for people with dental problems and those with temporomandibular joint (TMJ) syndrome • Cannot eat or drink while the medication is in your mouth • Frequent use during the day required to obtain adequate nicotine levels	**Comments/limitations:** Many people use this medication incorrectly. Most of the time the gum is in your mouth, it should be "parked" between your cheek and gum. Read package directions carefully for a full explanation. To achieve greatest benefit, you generally should chew nine or more pieces per day.
Nicotine nasal spray Nicotrol® NS (prescription required) Delivers nicotine through the lining of the nose when you squirt it directly into each nostril.	**Pros** • Flexible dosing • Can be used in response to stress or urges to smoke • Fastest delivery of nicotine of currently available products • Reduces cravings within minutes **Cons** • Nose and eye irritation is common, but usually disappears within 1 week • Frequent use during the day required to obtain adequate nicotine levels	**Comments/limitations:** Unlike nasal sprays used to relieve allergy symptoms, the nicotine spray is not meant to be sniffed. Rather, it is sprayed once into each nostril once or twice an hour. Take a deep breath, hold it, spray once into each nostril and exhale through the mouth. Ask your pharmacist for help in using the product correctly.

continued

Step #2: Using Medications *Continued*

Description and Examples	Pros and Cons	Comments
Nicotine inhaler Nicotrol® Inhaler (prescription required) A plastic cylinder containing a cartridge that delivers nicotine when you puff on it. Although similar in appearance to a cigarette, the inhaler delivers nicotine into the mouth, not the lung, and enters the body much more slowly than the nicotine in cigarettes.	**Pros** • Flexible dosing • Mimics the hand-to-mouth behavior of smoking • Few side effects • Faster delivery of nicotine than the patches **Cons** • Frequent use during the day required to obtain adequate nicotine levels • May cause mouth or throat irritation	**Comments/limitations:** Puffing must be done frequently, far more often than your cigarette. Each cartridge lasts for 80 long puffs; each cartridge is designed for 20 minutes of use. A minimum of six cartridges per day is needed for 3 to 6 weeks, then the patient starts tapering off. You do not need to inhale deeply to achieve an effect. Small doses of nicotine provide a sensation in the back of the throat similar to cigarette smoke.
Non-nicotine medication Zyban® (bupropion hydrochloride) sustained-release tablets (prescription required) Currently the only non-nicotine medication shown to be effective for quitting smoking. Treatment must be started at least 1 week before your target quit date.	**Pros** • Easy to use • Pill form • Few side effects • Can be used in combination with nicotine patches **Cons** • Should not be used by patients with eating disorders, seizure disorders, or those taking certain other medications • Lack of flexibility of use	**Comments/limitations:** This is the first medication to help quit smoking that is available in tablet form. Its primary role is to act on brain chemistry to bring about some of the same effects that nicotine has when people smoke. A small risk of seizure is associated with use of this medication. The main ingredient in Zyban has been available for many years as a treatment for depression under the trade name Wellbutrin. However, it works well in people with no depression as an aid to quit smoking.

Step #3: Staying Smoke-Free

Source of Help	Pros and Cons
Preventing relapse	
The group program, individual counseling from a healthcare provider, telephone counseling, or self-help materials you choose should include information on how to prevent a relapse and what to do if a relapse occurs.	Refer to Step #1: Preparing to Quit
Encouragement from family and friends	**Pros** • Convenient/available • Understand you well and can anticipate your needs • Reinforce your desire to quit when you feel tempted to smoke again **Cons** • May become overly critical if your quit attempt fails • If they try to quit for you instead of for themselves, they may relapse and undermine your efforts
Work site and community	**Pros**
Many work sites and communities offer quit-smoking programs. These often include group programs such as those offered by the American Lung Association or support programs such as Nicotine Anonymous. Smoke-free work site and community promotional campaigns may also include "buddy systems" and other activities to help people stay smoke-free.	• Helpful to have encouragement in the places—your job or community—where you spend most of your time • Helpful—and healthful—to work in smoke-free workplace **Cons** • Programs may not be available or may be hard to find in your area • Work site may not be smoke-free or may not encourage nonsmoking
Telephone encouragement or "health lines"	**Pros** • Convenient • Private • Provide support when family and friends do not or cannot
In addition to telephone counseling for developing a *Quit Smoking Action Plan*, many employers, health maintenance organizations, communities, and makers of nicotine and non-nicotine medications offer ongoing telephone counseling to encourage staying smoke-free.	**Cons** • May not be available in your health plan, company, or community

CONCLUSION

The information you have just read is meant to provide the knowledge you need to prepare and use your *Quit Smoking Action Plan*. Some of the main messages to keep in mind are

- You can quit! Millions—approximately half of all smokers in the United States—already have.

- The more dependent you are on cigarettes, the harder it is to quit.

- Don't be afraid to ask for help.

- The more sources of help you use, the better your chance of success.

By reading this booklet and understanding the roles of behavior, medications, and support, you have taken a major step toward becoming smoke-free. You may want to show this information to your healthcare provider and make notes of any questions you have now.

In addition, a listing of national organizations has been included to provide you with more sources of help and guidance. Good luck and good health!

RESOURCES

American Lung Association
Call 1-800-LUNG-USA to contact your local American Lung Association office.
Internet: http://www.lungusa.org
America Online: Keyword: ALA

The American Academy of Family Physicians
Department of Public Health & Scientific Affairs & Health Education
Kansas City, MO
(800) 274-2237, ext. 5500

Action on Smoking and Health
2013 H Street
Washington, D.C. 20077-2410
(202) 659-4310

American Academy of Otolaryngology Head and Neck Surgery
One Prince Street
Alexandria, VA 22314
(703) 836-4444

American Cancer Society
1599 Clifton Road, NE
Atlanta, GA 30329
(404) 320-3333

American Heart Association
7272 Greenville Avenue
Dallas, TX 75231
(800) AHA-USA1 (242-8721)

Centers for Disease Control and Prevention
National Center for Chronic Disease Prevention and Health Promotion
Office on Smoking and Health
Mailstop K-50
4770 Buford Highway, NE
Atlanta, GA 30341-3724
(800) CDC-1311

National Cancer Institute
Bethesda, MD 20894
(800) 4-CANCER (422-6237)

National Heart, Lung, and Blood Institute
Building 31, Room 4A21
Bethesda, MD 20892
(301) 496-4236

National Institute on Drug Abuse
Drug Abuse Information and Treatment Referral Line
11426 Rockville Pike, Suite 410
Rockville, MD 20852
(800) 662-4357
(800) 662-9832 (Spanish)
(800) 228-0427 (hearing impaired)

Nicotine Anonymous
P.O. Box 591777
San Francisco, CA 94159-1777
(415) 750-0328

The Mobile Lipid Clinic™ Palm Program

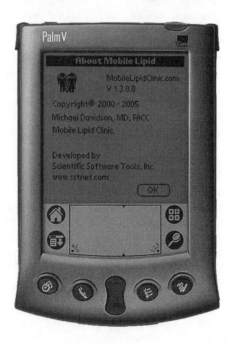

**By
Pam Scheese,
Scientific Software Tools, Inc.**

Sponsored by
AstraZeneca

WHAT'S NEW IN VERSION 1.3.0.0

Version 1.3.0.0 includes risk calculations based on the NCEP Report "Implications of Recent Clinical Trials for the National Cholesterol Education Program Adult Treatment Panel III Guidelines" by S. M. Grundy et al. The program will present therapeutic optional goals for patients within certain risk groups. The treatments also record the assigned treatment goal for the data presented at the specific visit allowing tracking of patient goals.

INTRODUCTION

The Mobile Lipid Clinic™ Palm program affords the physician the convenience of having patient data in his or her pocket. It provides a means for the physician to enter basic patient data, such as name, address, phone numbers, and a general note about the patient.

Test results and physical data are entered for each patient visit. Family history, blood pressures, and coronary heart disease–related parameters can all be entered. Once sufficient risk factor parameters are entered, the physician can obtain a risk evaluation based on the data from the specified visit. By communicating the results to the patient, the physician can reinforce the need to improve his or her lifestyle and maintain the medication program prescribed by the physician. The physician can also use this data to evaluate the treatment program for the specified patient.

PALM INSTRUCTIONS

The objectives of this tutorial are to guide you through the procedures to add and edit a patient's

- Personal information
- Visit information, including vitals, history, medications, and treatments for each visit
- Risk assessment
- New treatments and medications recommended from that risk assessment

BEFORE WE BEGIN

AutoKeyboard Feature

The AutoKeyboard feature, when turned on, allows the user to use a keyboard to tap information into the Palm quickly and easily. Experienced Palm users may even prefer this as a more expedient way of entering information. The following screens will demonstrate how to use this feature. You will need to refer back to these pages when you arrive at these screens during the tutorial.

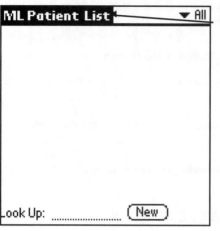

When in this screen, tap on **ML Patient List**.

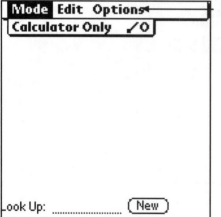

In this screen, tap on **Options**.

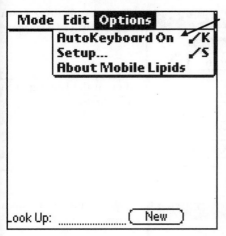

To turn the AutoKeyboard feature on, simply tap on **AutoKeyboard**.

The AutoKeyboard feature is now turned on. To turn it off, tap **AutoKeyboard Off**. Every time you tap on **AutoKeyboard**, the program will toggle back and forth between **On** and **Off**. To return to the **ML Patient List** screen without toggling the option, simply tap on **Options**.

By setting this option to **On**, you can now use the AutoKeyboard feature in any screen. If you are in an alpha field, the alpha keyboard will appear. If you are in a numeric field, the numeric keyboard will appear.

Tap on **Setup** to determine

- **Language**
- **Guideline**
- **Exam Units**
- **Lab Units**

The following screen will appear.

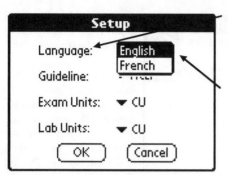

Tap on the drop down arrow next to **Language**.

Tap on the language you wish to use.

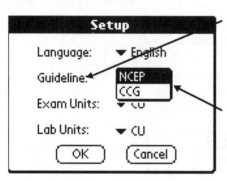

Tap on the drop down arrow next to **Guideline**

Tap on the guideline you wish to use.

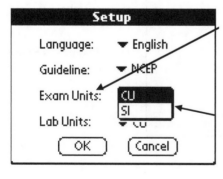

Tap on the drop down arrow next to **Exam Units**.

Tap on the exam units you wish to use.

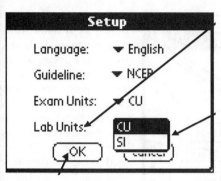

Tap on the drop down arrow next to **Lab Units**.

Tap on the lab units you wish to use.

Tap on **OK** when you are done selecting.

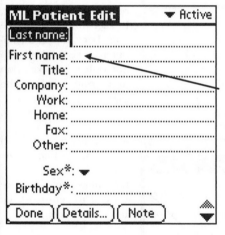

When any screen first comes up, the cursor will be in the very first field. The AutoKeyboard feature will not automatically come up in this instance. You must tap on the next field for it to open. Tap on the field next to **First name**.

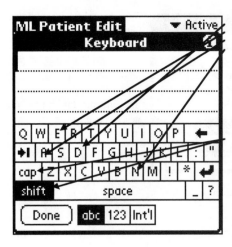

Notice that the keyboard setup is the identical to that of a computer keyboard. To enter a name, simply spell it out by tapping on the appropriate letters. Once the first letter is tapped, the keyboard will automatically shift to show lower case letters. If you need to capitalize another letter, simply tap the **cap** or **shift** keys to return to the upper case letters.

Note that the cap key will remain dark if you tap it. It acts the same as the Caps Lock key on a computer keyboard. If you do not wish this locked, tap on it again to release the caps lock feature.

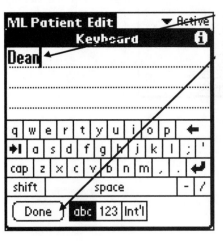

As you tap, the word will appear in the lines at the top.

Tap **Done** when you are finished to return to the data entry screen.

ML Patient Edit ▼ Active

Last name: ....

First name: Dean

Title: ....

Company: ....

Work: ....

Home: ....

Fax: ....

Other: ....

Sex*: ▼

Birthday*: ....

(Done) (Details...) (Note)

Now you can go back up and fill out the first entry on the page.

In a numeric field such as **Zip Code**, the numeric keyboard will come up when you tap on the field.

ML Patient Edit ▼ Active

Keyboard ℹ

\$	€	£	¥		1	2	3		-	+	←
[	]	{	}		4	5	6		/	*	:	↹
<	>	\	=		7	8	9		↵
@	~	&	#		(	0	)		.	,	space	%

(Done) [abc | 123 | Int'l]

This works the same way the alpha keyboard works.

Please note that the right side of the numeric keyboard is used only for entering these characters into a field. They do not actually calculate when using the AutoKeyboard feature.

You also have the ability to toggle between the two keyboards. This is very useful when entering a street address.

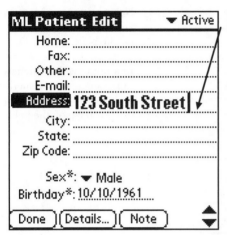

When you tap on this field, the alpha keyboard will appear first. Simply toggle over to the numeric keyboard to tap in the number and then toggle back to the alpha keyboard for the street name.

Using the AutoKeyboard feature should save time, especially for users who have not previously used a Palm Pilot.

Information Tips

Through the Mobile Lipid Clinic™ Palm program, there are tips that will help you to fill out information and to explain what will happen when certain buttons are tapped.

These can be accessed by tapping the 🛈 icon. For example, when you are in the **ML Patient Details** screen, use the following procedure.

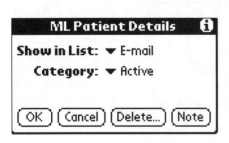

Tap here on the icon.

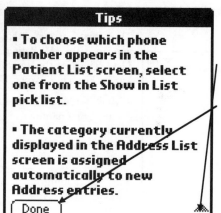

This explains the objectives of the previous screen.

Use the down arrow to view more information.

Tap on **Done** to return to the previous screen.

There are many **Tips** like this one throughout the program. Look for them when you are not sure what you should do or what the result of what you do will be.

ACCESSING MOBILE LIPID

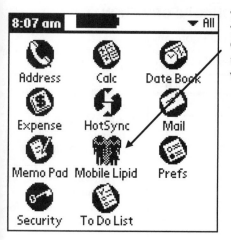

Turn your Palm Pilot on. To start the Mobile Lipid Clinic™ Palm program, tap the **Mobile Lipid** icon with the stylus.

ML PATIENT LIST SCREEN

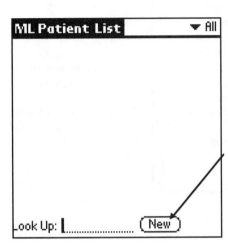

The first screen that appears is the **ML Patient List**. This is the main screen. From here, you can

- View patients by last name, first name
- Add a new patient
- Add or read a note on a specific patient

Start by adding a new patient. Tap on **New**.

PERSONAL INFORMATION

Adding a Patient's Personal Information

This screen is the **ML Patient Edit** screen. From this screen you can

- Add/edit personal information
- Edit **Details** relating to patient's file
- Add/edit **Notes**

The asterisks next to **Sex** and **Birthday** indicate that this data is required for risk calculations.

You are not required to fill out all information. However, it is recommended that you fill out as much information as possible. Certain data are required, such as

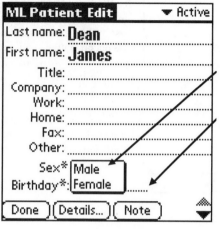

- **Last name**
- **First name**
- **Sex** (tap on down arrow for choices, and then tap on appropriate choice)
- **Birthday** (tap on the line to the right of **Birthday** and calendar will appear as shown in the following screen)

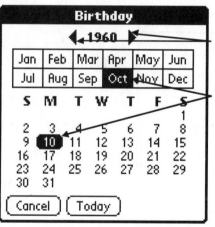

Calendar starts at the year 1960. To increase/decrease year, tap on left/right arrows.

Tap on appropriate **month** and **day**. You will return to the **ML Patient Edit** screen when you tap on a specific day.

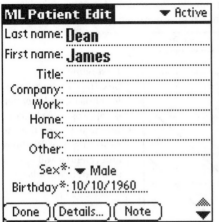

All other data are optional. However, it is recommended that **Work** and **Home** phone numbers are entered since these are the most common ways of contacting a patient. **Other** is for additional phone number, such as a cell phone.

Fill out any additional information deemed to be significant.

In this example, the **Home** phone number is entered.

Tap on the down arrow to move on to the next screen.

Although all of this information is optional, it is recommended that the

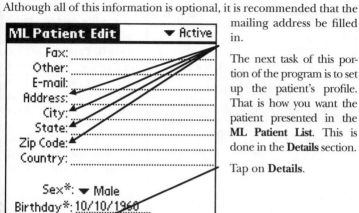

mailing address be filled in.

The next task of this portion of the program is to set up the patient's profile. That is how you want the patient presented in the **ML Patient List**. This is done in the **Details** section.

Tap on **Details**.

Here you are presented with the **ML Patient Details** pop-up screen.

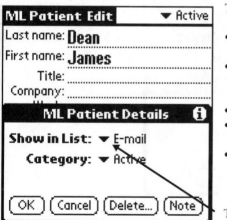

This allows you to

- Customize the **ML Patient List** display
- Select the patient's category (**Active** or **Inactive**)
- **Delete** the patient
- Add a general note regarding the patient
- **Cancel** without saving any changes

Tap on the down arrow for the **Show in List** field.

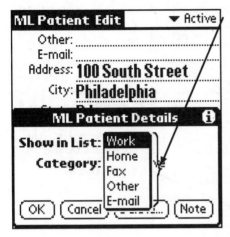

This is a list from which you will decide which information will show in the **ML Patient List**. You can only choose one. It should be the most used contact number or e-mail address. For this exercise, choose a phone number or e-mail address you entered in the **ML Patient Edit** screen.

In this exercise, **Home** is chosen, as it was the only phone number that was entered for this patient.

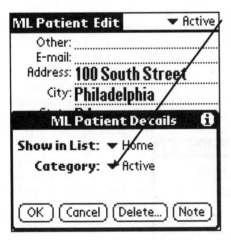

Tap on the arrow next to **Active**.

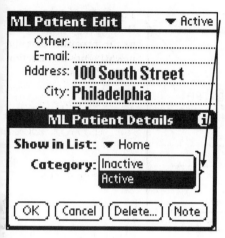

Initially, the patient should always be **Active**. This is the default choice. However, at some point, the patient may become inactive for one reason or another, and you will no longer wish his name to appear in the **Active** list. Tap on **Inactive**, and that patient's information will then only be accessed through the **Inactive** list. For this exercise, be sure the patient is **Active**.

The patient's profile has now been set up to reflect that

- The patient's **Home** phone number will appear in the **ML Patient List**
- The patient is **Active**

ML Patient Edit	▼ Active
Last name: **Dean**	
First name: **James**	
Title:	
Company:	

ML Patient Details   🛈

Show in List: ▼ Home

Category: ▼ Active

(OK) (Cancel) (Delete...) (Note)

The basic patient information has been set up. It is time to take a look at how the **ML Patient List** appears with this new patient's information.

Tap on **OK**.

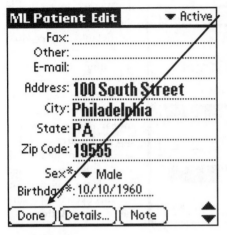

Tap on **Done**. By tapping **Done**, you are indicating to the program that the new patient's information is ready to be stored.

If the record does not contain the **Last Name**, **Sex**, or **Birthday** when you tap on **Done** in the previous screen, this screen will appear.

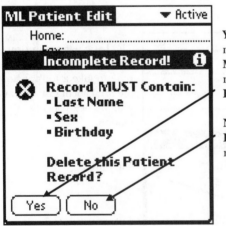

Yes will delete all information just entered in **ML Patient Edit** and return you to the **ML Patient List**.

No will return you to **ML Patient Edit** to enter the required information.

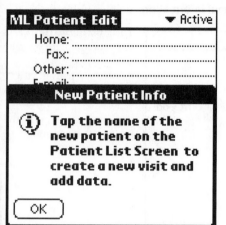

This message box appears to let you know that this patient will now be added to the list. It also gives instructions about how to create a new visit and add or change data.

Tap **OK** to continue to the **ML Patient List**.

Now you are back at the very first screen with a patient listed. Note a phone number is visible with an **H** to indicate that it is the **Home** number.

Suppose the patient has changed his mind about how he wishes to be contacted and new information needs to be added. To do this, tap on the patient's name.

Editing a Patient's Personal Information

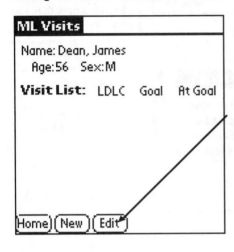

This is the **ML Visits** screen. From here you can

- Create a patient visit
- Edit patient information

You are going to edit the patient information by tapping on **Edit**.

This patient has decided he would like to be contacted via his e-mail address. This creates the need to

- Add the e-mail address
- Change his **Show in List** choice
- It's also a good idea to make a note that this is the patient's preference.

First add the e-mail address by locating the proper field. Tap the down arrow in the bottom right corner.

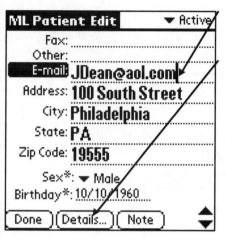

Enter the new e-mail address in the appropriate field.

Tap on **Details**.

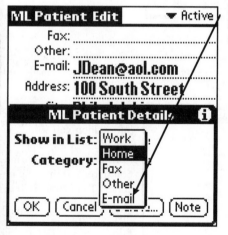

Now change the **Show in List** choice to **E-Mail** by tapping on it.

Adding a Patient Note

It may be a good idea to include a note to indicate that the patient has requested that he be contacted only through his e-mail account.

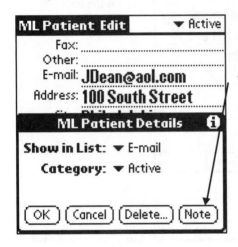

Tap on **Note**.

Often, there is the need to keep general notes regarding the patient. This program has provided a way to enter and access these notes quickly and easily from the **ML Patient List**.

Here you can enter any information you wish. You can add to it any time you wish. Enter some information here, and then tap on either **Done** or **Delete**. Both will return you to the first screen of **ML Patient Edit**. However, **Delete** will remove the **Note** and **Done** will save it.

Then tap **Done** in **ML Patient Edit** to return to the **ML Patient List**.

Notice that the **Home** phone number had been replaced by the patient's e-mail address. Also, there is an indicator on the right of the e-mail address. This will allow you to go directly to the note section to read a note without the need to enter the **ML Patient Edit** screens. If there is no existing note, this area will be blank. However, if you tap on that blank area, the program will take you into the note area.

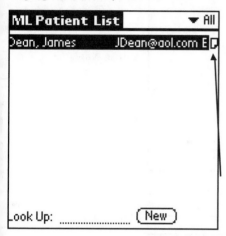

Tap on this indicator now.

You can add to or delete the note if you wish. For now, just tap on **Done**. You will return directly to the **ML Patient List**.

Deleting a Patient

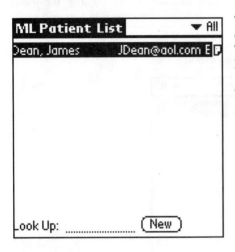

The need may arise to delete a patient completely. This is accomplished using **ML Patient Edit** screens.

Tap on the patient's name that you wish to delete.

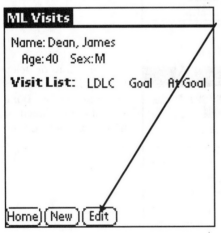

Tap on **Edit**.

When you get to the **ML Patient Edit** screen, tap on **Details**.

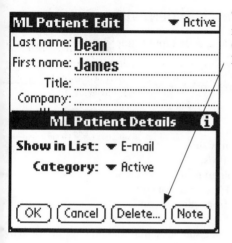

To remove the patient from the Mobile Lipid Clinic™ program, tap on **Delete**.

Here you are given the choice to

- Tap **Cancel** and not delete
- Tap **OK** to delete this patient from the Palm Pilot

This note allows the option to save the archived copy in the Desktop PC. By checking this box, you are allowing the copy on the PC to remain saved even through the HotSync between the Palm Pilot and the PC. From that point, this information will only be accessible through the desktop. For now, tap on **Cancel** to not delete.

ADDING A PATIENT VISIT

The **Patient Visit** part of the Mobile Lipid Clinic™ Palm program has multiple screens.

- History of patient and patient's family
- Prior treatments
- Prior medications
- Physical for current visit
- Required labs for current visit
- Optional labs for current visit
- Risk assessment determined from current visit
- Medication determined from current visit
- Treatment determined from current visit

In order to obtain a full risk assessment, all information must be correctly filled out, except the **Optional Labs**. That information is statistical only.

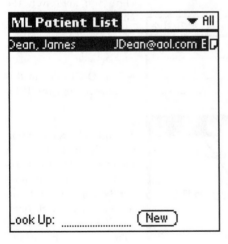

To start, make sure you are in the **ML Patient List**.

Tap on the name of the patient to whom you wish to add a visit.

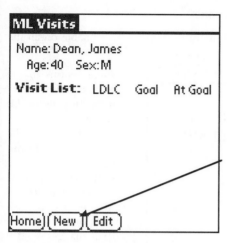

From here, you can

- Return to the **ML Patient List** by tapping on **Home**
- Enter information from an office visit by tapping on **New**
- Edit personal information by tapping on **Edit**

Tap on **New** to add a visit.

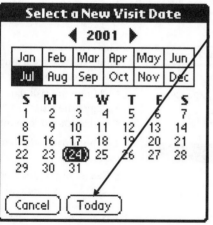

The calendar screen appears with the current date highlighted. If the visit is this day, then tap on **Today**.

To change this date, simply use the left/right arrows to change the year, tap on the appropriate month, and then tap on the day.

The next screen will appear in either instance.

Navigating in the Visit Screens

The five buttons at the bottom of this screen are available on all the visit screens.

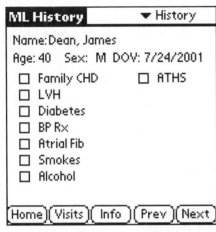

- **Home** returns to the **ML Patient List**.
- **Visits** lists visits for this patient.
- **Prev** returns to the previous screen in visit sequence.
- **Next** moves to the next screen in sequence.
- **Info** opens a **Visit Info** box to allow detail changes regarding this visit.

Tap on **Info** now to view this screen.

This is a quick way to do some things regarding this visit date. You can

- Change the visit date
- Delete the visit
- Add a note to the visit

The buttons on the bottom will

- **Cancel** out of this message box without saving changes.
- **Delete** this visit.
- Add a **Note** specific to this visit.
- **OK** leaves this message box and saves any changes made.

Directions for each are given in the **Tips** box. Tap on the 🛈 to view. When you return to this screen, tap **Cancel** to return without making changes.

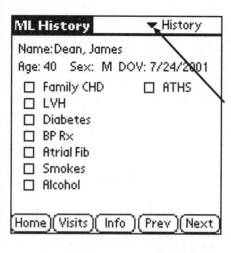

You will return to the **ML History** screen.

The **Patient Visit** screens also allow movement through screens in any order you wish. To do this, tap on the down arrow next to **History**.

By tapping on any one of these choices, you will go straight to that particular screen. For instance, by tapping on **Prior Meds**, the program will automatically go to **Prior Meds**, skipping **Prior Treat**. This will become very useful once you become familiar with the program and know exactly what fields you wish to go to for a patient.

For now, tap on **History** to move through the program in sequence.

ML History Screen

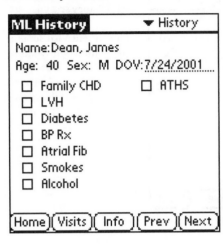

This screen is used to enter data about the patient's history and current condition. This screen looks slightly different for female patients to include details specific to women. These are

- Postmenopausal
- HRT

Tap in the appropriate boxes to indicate those items that apply to this patient. A **check mark** in a box indicates **yes**; a **blank** box indicates **no**.

When some fields are filled out, additional fields will appear

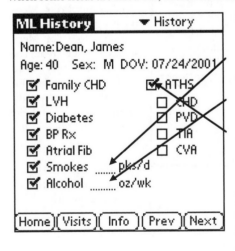

- **Smokes**: Packs per day [range is 0 to 6 packs per day (use decimal for partial pack)]
- **Alcohol**: Ounces per week (range is between 0 and 96 ounces per week)
- **ATHS**: When this is checked, other options appear. Check those that apply to the patient.

Note: If the **ATHS** box is checked, the **Risk Assessment** is based on a patient having atherosclerosis (ATHS).

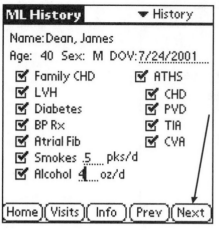

Finish filling out this screen.

Note: For the purposes of this exercise, all boxes have been checked off.

Tap **Next** in the bottom right corner.

ML Prior Treatment Screen

This screen is used to view the patient's prior treatment plan from the last visit. If this is the patient's first visit, it becomes the **Baseline**. If there is information regarding prior visits in the system, the most recent prior visit date will default into the **Date of Prior Treatment** field. Treatment goals for that visit will also be displayed, if available. For the baseline visit, the treatment goals are blank.

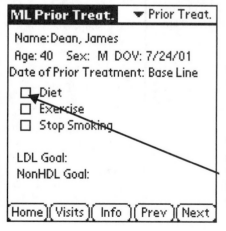

The first option, **Diet**, allows further information to be entered if this box is checked. Check that box now.

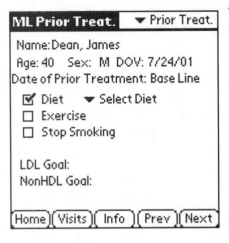

Tap on the down arrow to the left of **Select Diet**.

This gives you all the available diet choices. Simply tap on the appropriate diet.

To view more choices, tap on the down arrow.

If you do not wish a diet to be entered at this time, then simply tap in the box next to **Diet** to eliminate the **check mark**.

For now, tap on one of the diets.

Check anything else that would apply.

Tap **Next** to continue.

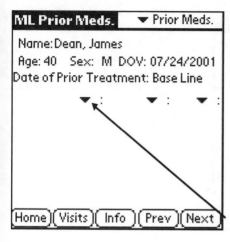

ML Prior Medications

This screen will display any medications previously prescribed. Choose medications, doses, and frequencies from the list. The columns are specified as follows:

- Column 1: Medication
- Column 2: Dosage
- Column 3: Frequency

Tap on the first down arrow on the left side to add a medication.

This is a list of the medications known by the program. Notice that the top line is a blank, which is the first choice in each column.

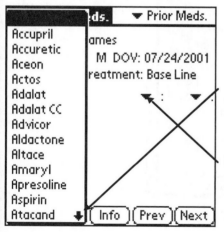

Tap on the down arrow at the bottom right corner of the list box to view more choices.

Select a medication if it applies.

Then tap on the down arrow in the second column.

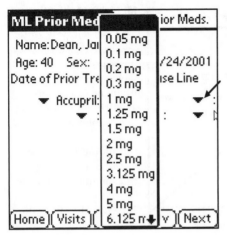

Choose the appropriate dosage for the list supplied.

Then tap on the down arrow in the last column.

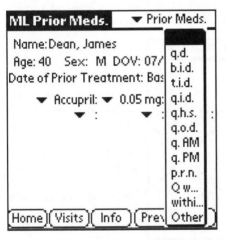

Select the appropriate frequency from the list supplied.

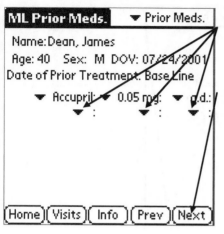

If there is a second medication, then tap on the second down arrow in each column and proceed as before.

Tap on **Next** to continue.

ML Physical Screen

This screen is used to enter data collected during the physical exam.

Enter at least one arm **blood pressure**. To complete the ankle-brachial index calculation, all four blood pressures should be provided.

Then enter the patient's

- **Weight**: Range is 0 to 500 lb
- **Height**: Range is 1'0" to 7'11"0
- **Waist**: Range is 10 to 60 in

Your screen should resemble the following screen.

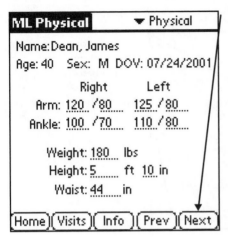

Tap **Next** to continue.

ML Required Labs Screen

This screen is used to enter the lab results that are required to obtain a full risk assessment. If all the inputs are not provided, the risk assessment will be incomplete.

See Table 1 for a list of the input ranges in both **Conventional** and **SI Units**.

If you enter an invalid number—that is, a number that is not within the range given—an error message will appear when you try to move on the next field.

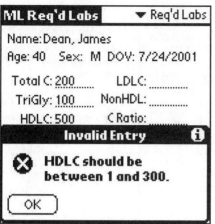

This message appears if you have entered a value that is out of range. You can

- Enter a value that is in range
- Enter no value (Blank)

Tap **OK** to continue

ML Req'd Labs   ▼ Req'd Labs

Name: Dean, James
Age: 40   Sex: M DOV: 07/24/2001

Total C: <u>200</u>   LDLC: <u>119</u>
TriGly: <u>203</u>   NonHDL: <u>160</u>
HDLC: <u>40</u>   C Ratio: <u>5.00</u>
Glu: <u>80</u>
EBCT Ca: <u>50</u>

(Home)(Visits)(Info)(Prev)(Next)

Finish filling out the information on the left side of this screen. **LDLC**, **Non-HDL**, and the **C Ratio** are calculated from **Total C**, **TriGly**, and **HDLC** inputs. Note that those fields will not populate until all the others are filled out.

Tap **Next** to continue.

ML Optional Labs Screen

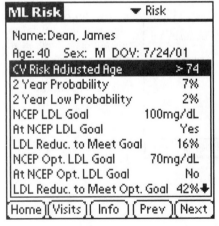

These lab results are not required for any calculations. They are for statistical use only.

See Table 1 for a list of the input ranges in both **Conventional** and **SI Units**.

ML Risk Assessment Screen

Note: If a patient has no preexisting ATHS, assessments are based on 10 years. If the patient has ATHS, assessments are based on 2 years. This patient has ATHS.

ML Risk	▼ Risk
Name: Dean, James	
Age: 40 Sex: M DOV: 7/24/01	
CV Risk Adjusted Age	> 74
2 Year Probability	7%
2 Year Low Probability	2%
NCEP LDL Goal	100mg/dL
At NCEP LDL Goal	Yes
LDL Reduc. to Meet Goal	16%
NCEP Opt. LDL Goal	70mg/dL
At NCEP Opt. LDL Goal	No
LDL Reduc. to Meet Opt. Goal	42%↓
Home Visits Info Prev Next	

If required information was not entered, **na** will appear in the appropriate calculated field. Note that there are optional treatment goals available for this assessment. Not all assessments will produce optional treatment goals. See the section ML Treatment Screen for additional information about optional treatment goals.

Tap on the down arrow to view the remainder of the assessment.

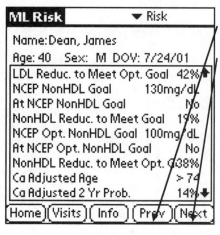

To view the previous page, tap on **Prev**.

Tap **Next** to continue.

ML Medications Screen

This screen is used to enter any medications that are to be prescribed to the patient based on the results of this visit.

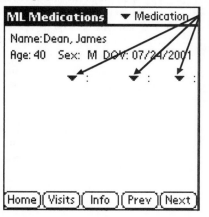

As previously done, use the down arrows to choose the medication, dosage, and frequency assigned at this visit.

Tap **Next** to continue.

ML Treatment Screen

This screen is used to enter a new treatment plan based on the results of this visit.

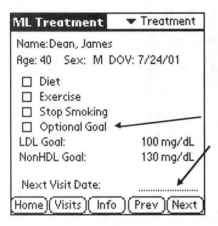

This screen works exactly the same as the **Prior Treatment** screen.

Enter any treatments suggested during this visit. Optional goals may be available based on the risk assessment. You may select the optional treatment goals by tapping on the **Optional Goal** check box.

Enter the next scheduled appointment if appropriate.

This completes the nine screens for a given visit. Tap on **Visits** to return this patient's **Visit List** or **Home** to return to the **Patient List** screen.

CALCULATOR ONLY MODE

There may be times when you may wish to just use the calculator part of this program to obtain a quick assessment without saving a patient and his or her data in the program. The Mobile Lipid Clinic ™ Palm program accommodates this.

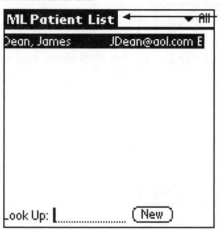

To access just the calculator, tap on **ML Patient List**.

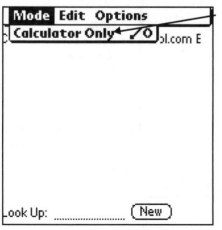

Now tap on **Calculator Only**.

This screen is basically the same as the **ML Patient History** screen. Notice that where the patient's name was in the previous screen now reads **CALCULATOR ONLY MODE.** There are only four screens available in this mode.

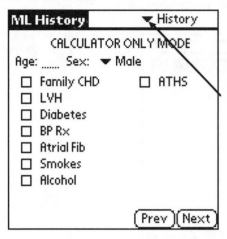

Tap on the arrow to the left of **History** to view the list.

You can enter information regarding

- **History**
- **Physical**
- **Req'd Labs**
- **Risk**

Move through these screens by

- Selecting the screen you wish in this list
- By tapping on **Next**

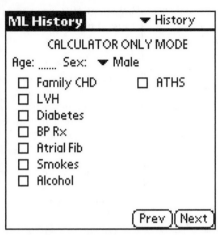

As there is no patient information screen in the **CALCULATOR ONLY MODE**, it is necessary to fill in the age and choose the sex in this screen.

- It does not have the patient's name
- You will need to enter **Age**
- Use the down arrow here to toggle between **Male** and **Female**

Enter data about the individual's history and current condition. As in the **ML Patient History** screen, if the patient is female, **Postmenopausal** and **HRT** are also included in this list.

Tap in the appropriate boxes to indicate those items that apply to this individual. A **check mark** in a box indicates **yes**; a **blank** box indicates **no**.

As in the **ML Patient History** screen, when **Smokes**, **Alcohol**, and **ATHS** are checked, more information is requested. Fill these out appropriately and then tap **Next**.

ML Physical ▼ Physical

CALCULATOR-ONLY MODE

Age: ...... Sex: ▼ Male

	Right	Left
Arm:	...... /	...... / ......
Ankle:	...... /	...... / ......

Weight: .... lbs

Height: .... ft ...... in

Waist: .... in

(Prev)(Next)

Again, this screen looks no different than the **Patient Visit** screen.

Enter at least one arm **blood pressure**. In order to complete the ankle-brachial index calculation, all four blood pressures should be provided.

Then enter the patient's

- **Weight**: Range is 0 to 500 lb
- **Waist**: Range is 10 to 60 in
- **Height**: Range is 1'0" to 7'11"0

When this screen is filled out, tap on **Next**.

ML Req'd Labs ▼ Req'd Labs

CALCULATOR ONLY MODE

Age: 46 Sex: ▼ Male

Total C:	LDLC: ....
TriGly:	NonHDL: ....
HDLC:	C Ratio: ....
Glu:	
EBCT Ca:	

(Prev)(Next)

Input ranges are as follows:

- **Total C**: 50 to 1000 mg/dL
- **LDLC**: Calculated
- **TriGly**: 1 to 10,000 mg/dL
- **NonHDL**: Calculated
- **HDLC**: 1 to 300 mg/dL
- **C Ratio**: Calculated
- **Glu**: 1 to 600 mg/dL
- **EBCT Ca**: 0 to 10,000

If the numbers entered are not reasonable, though within range, two question marks (??) will appear in one or all of the calculated fields.

Fill this information out and tap on **Next** to see the **Risk** screen.

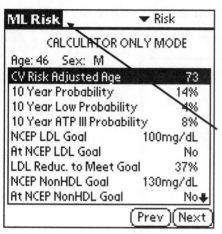

Tap on the down arrow in the bottom right corner to view more risk information.

You can move throughout these four screens as much as you like to adjust information.

To return to **Patient** mode, tap on **ML Risk**.

To toggle back to **Patient Mode**, simply tap on **Patient Mode**. Be aware that all information entered in **Calculator Mode** will be lost when you do this. It is not the intention of **Calculator Only** mode to save any data. Tapping on **Patient Mode** returns you to the **ML Patient List**.

RETURNING TO PALM PILOT HOME SCREEN

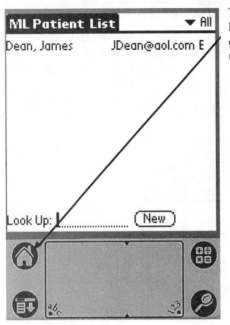

To return to your **Palm Pilot Home** screen, tap on the house in the bottom part of the screen.

TABLES

Table 1. Lab Value Ranges and Conversion Factors

Test result	Lab tests CU	Lab tests SI	Conversion	CU Min	CU Max	SI Min	SI Max
Total C	mg/dL	mmol/L	0.0259	50.00	1000.00	1.30	25.90
TriGly	mg/dL	mmol/L	0.0113	1.00	10000.00	0.01	113.00
HDLC	mg/dL	mmol/L	0.0259	1.00	300.00	0.03	7.77
Glu	mg/dL	mmol/L	0.0555	1.00	600.00	0.06	33.30
EBCT Ca	N/A	N/A	1	0.00	10000.00	0.00	10000.00
LDLC	mg/dL	mmol/L	0.0259	25.00	700.00	0.65	18.13
NonHDLC	mg/dL	mmol/L	Calc	N/A	N/A	N/A	N/A
C Ratio	N/A	N/A	Calc	N/A	N/A	N/A	N/A
ApoA1	mg/dL	g/L	0.01	1.00	700.00	0.01	7.00
ApoB	mg/dL	g/L	0.01	1.00	700.00	0.01	7.00
CPK	units/L	U/L	1	0.00	10000.00	0.00	10000.00
Hs-CRP	mg/L	g/L	10	0.00	50.00	0.00	500.00
GGT	units/L	U/L	1	0.00	50.00	0.00	50.00
HgA1c	%	Proportion	0.01	0.00	100.00	0.00	1.00
Homocys	mg/L	umol/L	7.397	1.00	50.00	7.40	369.85
LDL Size	nm	nm	1	100.00	5000.00	100.00	5000.00
Lg. HDL	mg/dL	mmol/L	0.0259	1.00	2000.00	0.03	51.80
Lg. VLDL	mg/dL	mmol/L	0.0259	0.00	1000.00	0.00	25.90
Lp(a)	mg/dL	umol/L	0.0357	0.00	1000.00	0.00	35.70
SGOT (AST)	units/L	U/L	1	1.00	1000.00	1.00	1000.00
SGPT (ALT)	units/L	U/L	1	1.00	1000.00	1.00	1000.00

ALT, alanine aminotransferase; Apo, apolipoprotein; AST, aspartate aminotransferase; EBCT Ca, electron beam computed tomography calcium score; C Ratio, total cholesterol/high-density lipoprotein cholesterol ratio; CPK, creatine phosphokinase; GGT, gamma-glutamyl transpeptidase; Glu, glucose; HDLC, high-density lipoprotein cholesterol; HgA1c, hemoglobin A_{1c}; Homocys, homocysteine; Hs-CRP, high-sensitivity C-reactive protein; LDLC, low-density lipoprotein cholesterol; Lg., large; Lp(a), lipoprotein(a); N/A, not applicable; SGOT, serum glutamic oxaloacetic transaminase; SGPT, serum glutamic pyruvic transaminase; Total C, total cholesterol; TriGly, triglycerides; VLDL, very-low-density lipoprotein.

Table 2. Diabetes Medications

Actos	Humulin N
Amaryl	Humulin R
Apo-Tolbutamide	Humulin U
Avandamet	Iletin II Lente
Avandia	Iletin II NPH
DiaBeta	Iletin II Regular
Diabinese	Lantus
Diamicron	Metaglip
Glucophage	Micronase
Glucophage XR	Novolin R
Glucotrol XL	NovoLog
Glucovance	Orinase
Glynase PresTab	Prandase
Glyset	Prandin
Humalog	Precose
Humalog Mix 75/25	Starlix
Humulin 70/30	Tolinase
Humulin L	Humulin N

Table 3. Cardiovascular Medications

Advicor	Mevacor
Aggrastat	Niacin
Altocor	Niaspan
Aspirin	Novasen
Cordarone	Plavix
Coumadin	Pravachol
Crestor	Questran
Ecotrin	Questran Light
Ezetrol	Slo-Niacin
Lanoxin	Sotacor
Lescol	Tricor
Lescol XL	Welchol
Lipidil	Zetia
Lipitor	Zocor
Lopid	

Table 4. Blood Pressure Medications

Accupril	Diovan	Monitan
Accuretic	Diovan HCT	Monocor
Aceon	Diuril	Monopril
Adalat	Dyazide	Monopril-HCT
Adalat CC	DynaCirc	Mykrox
Adalat XL	DynaCirc CR	Nimotop
Aldactazide	Enduron	Normodyne
Aldactone	Esidrix	Norvasc
Altace	HydroDIURIL	Oretic
Apo-Methyldopa	Hygroton	Plendil
Apresoline	Hytrin	Prinivil
Atacand	Hyzaar	Prinzide
Atacand HCT	Imdur	Procardia
Atacand Plus	Inderal	Procardia XL
Avalide	Inderal LA	Renedil
Avapro	Inderide	Sectral
Benicar	Inderide LA	Sular
Betaloc	Inhibace	Tarka
Blocadren	Inspra	Teczem
Calan	Isoptin	Tenex
Calan-SR	Isoptin SR	Tenoretic
Capoten	Isordil	Tenormin
Capozide	Kerlone	Teveten
Cardene	Lasix	Teveten HCT
Cardene SR	Levatol	Tiazac
Cardizem	Lexxel	Timolide 10-25
Cardizem CD	Loniten	Toprol XL
Cardizem SR	Lopressor	Trandate
Cardura	Lopressor HCT	Trasicor
Cartia XT	Lotensin	Uniretic
Cartrol	Lotensin HCT	Univasc
Catapres	Lotrel	Vascor
Catapres-TTS	Lozide	Vaseretic
Chlorthalidone	Lozol	Vasotec
Combipres	Mavik	Verelan
Coreg	Maxzide	Verelan PM
Corgard	Micardis	Visken
Corzide	Micardis HCT	Wytensin
Covera HS	Microzide	Zaroxolyn
Coversyl	Midamor	Zebeta
Cozaar	Minipress	Zestoretic
Demadex	Minizide	Zestril
Dilacor XR	Moduretic	Ziac

Table 5. Other Medications

Viagra

Table 6. Drug Dosages

0.05 mg	250 mg	2 mg/240 mg
0.1 mg	300 mg	2 mg/500 mg
0.2 mg	320 mg	2.5 mg/500 mg
0.3 mg	360 mg	4 mg/240 mg
0.5 mg	400 mg	4 mg/500 mg
1 mg	420 mg	5 mg/6.25 mg
1.2 mg	500 mg	5 mg/12.5 mg
1.25 mg	600 mg	5 mg/50 mg
1.5 mg	625 mg	5 mg/500 mg
2 mg	750 mg	7.5 mg/12.5 mg
2.5 mg	850 mg	10 mg/2.5 mg
3.125 mg	1,000 mg	10 mg/5 mg
3.6 mg	1,250 mg	10 mg/12.5 mg
4 mg	1,500 mg	10 mg/25 mg
5 mg	1,750 mg	10 mg/100 mg
6.125 mg	1,875 mg	15 mg/25 mg
6.25 mg	2,000 mg	20 mg/5 mg
7.5 mg	2,500 mg	20 mg/10 mg
8 mg	2,750 mg	20 mg/12.5 mg
10 mg	3,000 mg	20 mg/25 mg
12 mg	3,125 mg	25 mg/15 mg
12.5 mg	3,250 mg	25 mg/25 mg
15 mg	3,500 mg	37.5 mg/25 mg
16 mg	3,750 mg	40 mg/12.5 mg
20 mg	1 g	50 mg/12.5 mg
25 mg	2 g	50 mg/15 mg
30 mg	3 g	50 mg/25 mg
32 mg	4 g	50 mg/50 mg
40 mg	5 g	80 mg/12.5 mg
45 mg	8 g	100 mg/25 mg
50 mg	12 g	150 mg/12.5 mg
54 mg	15 g	160 mg/12.5 mg
60 mg	16 g	160 mg/25 mg
75 mg	20 g	180 mg/5 mg
80 mg	<10 units/d	300 mg/12.5 mg
81 mg	11–25 units/d	500 mg/10 mg
90 mg	26–50 units/d	500 mg/20 mg
100 mg	51–75 units/d	600 mg/12.5 mg
120 mg	76–100 units/d	600 mg/25 mg
150 mg	>100 units/d	750 mg/20 mg
160 mg	1 mg/240 mg	1,000 mg/20 mg
180 mg	1 mg/500 mg	2,000 mg/40 mg
200 mg	1.25 mg/250 mg	
240 mg	2 mg/180 mg	

Table 7. Drug Frequencies

q.d.	q. AM
b.i.d.	q. PM
t.i.d.	p.r.n.
q.i.d.	q week
q.h.s.	w/ meals
q.o.d.	Other

The Mobile Lipid Clinic™ Desktop Program

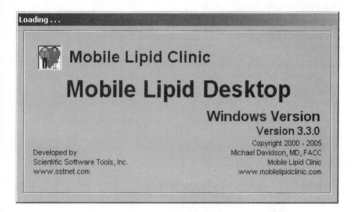

By
Pam Scheese,
Scientific Software Tools, Inc.

Sponsored by
AstraZeneca

WHAT'S NEW IN VERSION 3.3.0

Version 3.3.0 includes risk calculations based on the NCEP Report "Implications of Recent Clinical Trials for the National Cholesterol Education Program Adult Treatment Panel III Guidelines" by S. M. Grundy et al. The program will present therapeutic optional goals for patients within certain risk groups. The treatments also record the assigned treatment goal for the data presented at the specific visit, allowing tracking of patient goals.

INTRODUCTION

The desktop program provides a means for the office staff or doctor to enter basic patient data, such as name, address, phone numbers, and a general note about the patient. Test results and physical data are entered for each patient visit. Family history, blood pressures, and CHD-related parameters are then stored in a database for the risk evaluation.

Once sufficient risk factor parameters are entered, the physician can obtain a risk evaluation based on the data from the specified visit. The physician can see the risk variables, the points associated with each of the variables, and the evaluation results. The physician can use this data to evaluate the treatment program for the specified patient. Report of individual visits, as well as a history report, can be printed and given to the patient for further reinforcement.

A trend graph is available to patients who wish to follow the progress of their treatment. A graph of total cholesterol trends is also available to analyze patient progress, treatment evaluation, and patient education. Both can also be printed out for the patients' information.

DESKTOP INSTRUCTIONS

The objectives of this tutorial are to guide you through the procedures to add and edit a patient's

- Patient data, including all pertinent personal information
- Visit data, including vitals, history, medications, and treatments for each visit
- Risk assessment
- New treatments and medications recommended from the risk assessment

BEFORE WE BEGIN

It is assumed that the user has the general knowledge required to operate a PC.

Program Options

There are four program options—language, guideline, exam measurement units, and lab measurement units—each of which should be reviewed and set before you use the program for the first time.

To set these options, go to the **File** menu and select **Options**.

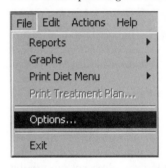

The **Options** dialog box will appear as shown:

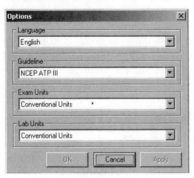

There are two languages options: **French** and **English**. Select the language of your choice.

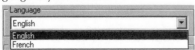

There are two guideline options, **NCEP ATP III** and **Cholesterol Canadian Guidelines**. It is *strongly recommended* that you select the guideline for your practice and never change it. Changing guidelines after patient data have been entered can lead to erroneous target goals for any existing patient. Select the guideline of your choice:

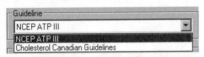

The system supports two measuring systems—**Conventional Units** and **SI Units**—for both exam data and lab data.
Select the exam units of your choice:

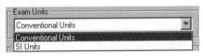

Select the lab units of your choice:

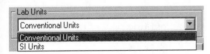

When your selections are completed, you will need to apply the changes using the button on the bottom of the dialog box.

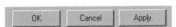

The **OK** button will apply the changes and close the dialog box. The **Cancel** button will discard the changes and return the option to its state before you started making changes. The **Apply** button will make the changes but leave the dialog box on the screen.

You can change the language and guideline options anytime you wish. However, it is strongly recommended that once the exam and lab units are specified, you do not change these options. Changing the exam and lab units after you start using the program can lead to small conversion errors in data already entered into the system.

General Program Instructions

There are some basic toolbar buttons that will be used throughout this program. Below is a snapshot of these buttons and the three dropdown lists that will always be viewable at the top of the screen. Not all buttons will be useable at all times. As you will note in this snapshot, the **Save** and **Cancel** buttons are grayed out, indicating that they will not operate at this time.

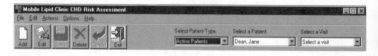

Toolbar Buttons

  This button is used to add new patients and visits.

  This button is used to edit an existing patient or visits.

  This button is used to save patient or visit information.

  This button is used to delete a patient or visit.

  This button will cancel out of whatever action you are currently doing.

  This button will exit you from the program.

Dropdown Lists

To access a dropdown list, place the cursor on the down arrow to the right of the list and click your mouse.

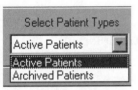

This is the **Patient Type** dropdown list. On the desktop there are two kinds of patients, **Active** and **Archived**.

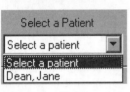

This is the **Patient** dropdown list. Patients will be in alphabetical order.

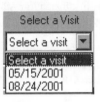

This is the **Visit** dropdown list. Visits will be listed in chronological order.

Tabs

Look at this program as a sort of file drawer. Directly underneath the toolbar buttons and dropdown lists, are file tabs for **Patient Data** and **Visit**.

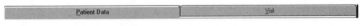

The **Patient Data** folder contains all fields relating to a patient's personal information. The **Visit** folder contains all fields relating to a specific visit, depending on which visit date appears in the **Visit** dropdown list. Note here that if the choice in the **Patient** dropdown list is **Select a Patient**, the **Visit** folder is unavailable. When a patient name is selected and the **Visit** folder is the active folder (the active folder will be in **bold**), more folder tabs appear at the bottom of the screen.

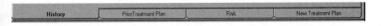

These will be reviewed in detail as this tutorial moves forward.

MEDICAL PRACTICE INFORMATION

The first information to be entered into this program is the office practice information. To do this, click on **Edit** in the menu over the toolbar.

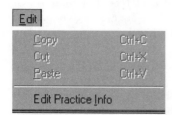

Click on **Edit Practice Info**.

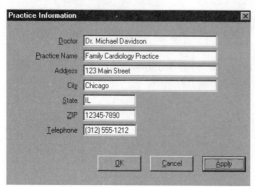

The **Practice Information** box will pop up. Fill in all fields. This information will appear on all reports.

When you are done, click on **Apply**, and then **OK**.

PATIENT DATA

When you start the program, it opens into the **Patient Data** screen. From here, you can

- **Add/edit** personal information
- **Add/edit** notes
- **Delete** a patient

Adding Patient Data

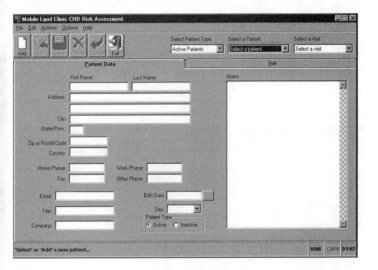

To add a new patient, click on the **Add** button. The curser will automatically appear in the **First Name** field. Type in the first name and tab to the **Last Name**. You can tab through the entire screen or place the curser where you wish to type. The only required information is

- **First Name**
- **Last Name**
- **Birth Date**
- **Sex**

All other data are optional. It is recommended that **Work** and **Home** phone numbers are entered, as these are the most common ways of contacting a patient.

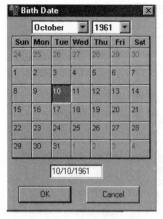

Fill out any additional information deemed to be significant and then click on the 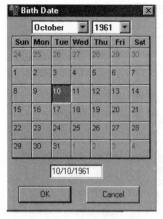 button next to the **Birth Date** field.

This box will automatically appear. The patient is assumed to be at least 40 years old, so the calendar opens at the date exactly 40 years earlier than the current date. Using the dropdown lists, select the month and year, and then click on the appropriate day.

The selected date will appear in the box below the calendar. Once the correct date is selected, click **OK**.

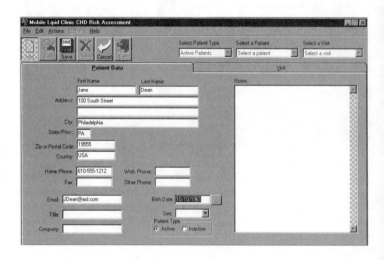

Note that the date you chose now populates the **Birth Date** field. If this is not correct, it can be changed by clicking on the ▦ button to the right of the date. This will reopen the calendar box.

Now click on the dropdown arrow in the box beside **Sex**.

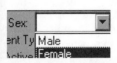   Click on the appropriate choice.

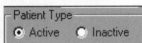

Note that the **Patient Type** defaults to **Active Patient** for all new patients.

Tab over or place the curser in the **Notes** box and type any information you wish to keep pertaining to this particular patient.

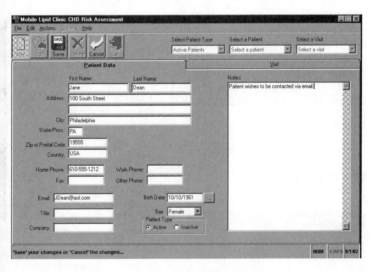

Look at the instructions in the bottom left of the screen. These indicate the options available to you. Now look at the toolbar buttons in the top left of the screen. As you can see, **Save** and **Cancel** are the only buttons not grayed out. Click on **Save** to save this data. Click on **Cancel** to erase this information and start over. Note that when you click **Cancel**, a dialogue box will appear asking for confirmation of the cancellation. Click **Yes** to confirm or **No** to continue in **Add** mode. For now, click **Yes**.

Notice now that
- **Save** and **Cancel** are the only toolbar buttons grayed out.
- The new patient's name appears in the **Select a Patient** dropdown list.
- **Select a Visit** now appears in the **Select a Visit** dropdown list. This indicates that you can now enter a visit for this new patient.

Editing Patient Data

Click on the **Edit** toolbar button.

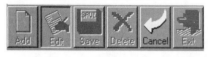

Notice that the only changes in the screen are the toolbar buttons. **Cancel** is the only one available. Now you can change personal information or add a note if you wish. As soon as you make a change in the screen, be it adding or changing something, the toolbar buttons will once again change.

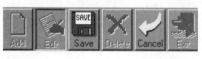

Now both the **Save** and **Cancel** buttons are available. **Save** will take you out of edit mode and keep the changes.

Cancel will take you out of edit mode without saving the changes.

Click on either **Cancel** or **Save** to return you to the previous mode.

Deleting Patient Data

Click on the **Delete** toolbar button.

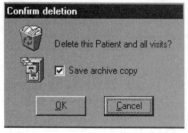

The **Confirm deletion** box will appear. You have the option to

- **Delete** this patient and all visits, and save the information in the archives (note the check in the **Save archive copy** box) by clicking **OK**.
- **Delete** this patient and all visits, and not save the information in the archives (remove the check in the **Save archive copy** box) by clicking **OK**.
- **Cancel** out of this box without deleting this patient and all visits.

This is the only warning you will receive regarding deleting a patient.

For now, click on **Cancel**.

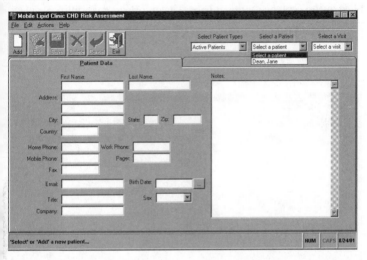

The screen will clear the patient information and return **Select a
Patient** to the **Select a Patient** dropdown list. As you can see, the
patient still remains in the list.

VISIT DATA

Adding a Visit

The **Visit** part of the Mobile Lipid Clinic™ Desktop program has several aspects.

- History of patient and patient's family
- Prior treatments
- Prior medications
- Physical for current visit
- Required labs for current visit
- Optional labs for current visit
- Risk assessment determined from current visit
- Medication determined from current visit
- Treatment determined from current visit

In order to obtain a full risk assessment, all information must be correctly filled out, except the **Optional Labs**. That information is statistical only.

Click on the **Visit** tab.

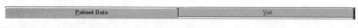

Your screen should now appear as below:

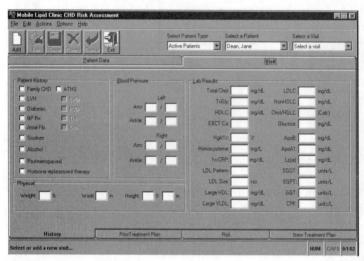

Note that the only toolbar buttons available are **Add** (a visit) and **Exit** (the program). Click on **Add** to add a new visit.

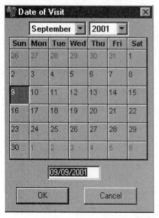

This works the same way as adding the patient's birthday. The only difference is that the default date is the current date. Change this if necessary. If this is the correct date, simply click **OK**.

Notice that the **Select a Visit** dropdown list is now populated with the chosen date.

Also notice the tabs at the bottom of the screen:

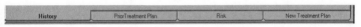

| History | PriorTreatment Plan | Risk | New Treatment Plan |

You will be using these tabs to move through the **Visit** part of the program.

History

In this tab, you will enter the patient's history, vitals, and lab results.

Patient History

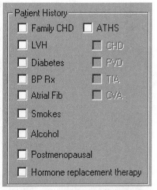

This screen is used to enter data about the patient's history and current condition. This screen looks slightly different for male patients. The two options that would **not** be included would be

- **Postmenopausal**
- **Hormone replacement therapy**

Click in the appropriate boxes to indicate those items that apply to this patient. A **check mark** in a box indicates **yes**, a **blank** box indicates **no**.

When some fields are filled out, additional fields will appear.

- **Smokes**: Packs per day [range is 0 to 6 packs per day (use decimal for partial pack)].
- **Alcohol**: Ounces per day (range is between 0 and 96 ounces per day).
- **ATHS**: When this is checked, other options appear. Check those that apply to the patient.

Note: If the **ATHS** box is checked, the **Risk Assessment** is based on a patient having atherosclerosis (ATHS).

Finish this section with the appropriate checks.

Blood Pressure

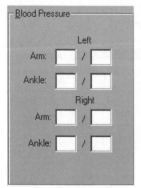

This screen is used to enter data collected during the physical exam.

Enter at least one arm **blood pressure**. To complete the ABI calculation, all four blood pressures should be provided.

Fill this screen out appropriately.

Physical

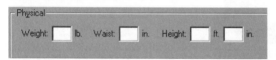

Conventional Units

- **Weight**: Range is 0 to 500 lb
- **Waist**: Range is 10 to 60 in.
- **Height**: Range is 1'0" to 7'11"0.

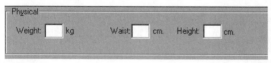

SI Units

- **Weight**: range is 0 to 266 kg
- **Waist**: range is 25 to 152 cm
- **Height**: range is 1 to 243 cm

Required Labs

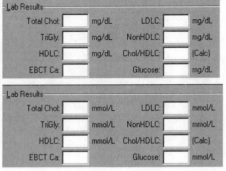

This screen is used to enter the lab results. Input ranges of required labs can be found in Table 1 at the end of this manual.

If you enter an invalid number—that is, a number that is not within the range given—an error message will appear when you try to move on the next field.

This message appears if you have entered a value that is out of range. You can

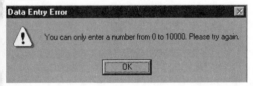

- Enter a value that is in range
- Enter no value (Blank)

Click **OK** to continue.

Optional Labs

These lab results are not required for any calculations. They are for statistical use only. Ranges for **Optional Labs** input can be found in Table 1 at the end of this manual.

Your screen should have the minimum input shown in the screen below:

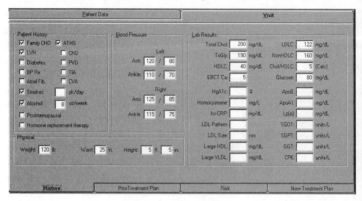

Prior Treatment

This tab is used to view the patient's prior treatment plan from the last visit. On the very first visit, there is no prior treatment date. If the patient was previously treated by another doctor, that information should be entered here. It will become the **baseline** treatment information. Once a visit is entered and saved, that visit will become the prior visit. Then each subsequent visit will become the prior visit to the next.

Prior Treatment

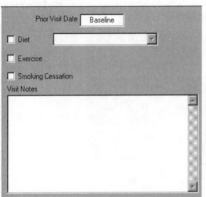

Check the box marked **Diet** and then click on the down arrow to view the choices in the dropdown list.

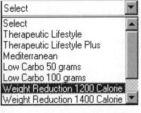

Select a diet by clicking on it.

If **Exercise** and/or **Smoking Cessation** had been prescribed, then place a **check mark** in those boxes.

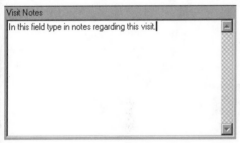

Any **Visit Notes** from a **Prior Visit** will automatically default in that box. If information is being added, then simply type it in this box.

Prior Meds

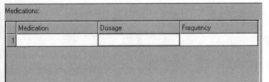

To choose a medication, click on the blank field under **Medication** to bring up the drop down list.

Select the appropriate medication. Use the up and down arrows to look through the list. A complete list of the medications can be found in Tables 2–5 at the end of the manual.

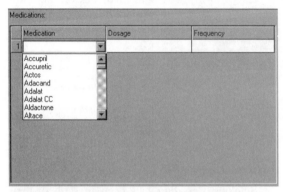

Click on the first blank field under **Dosage**.

Select the correct **Dosage**.

Click on the first blank field under **Frequency**. A complete list of the dosages can be found in Table 6 at the end of the manual.

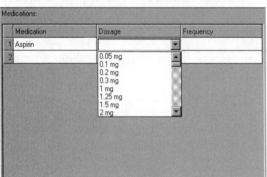

Select the correct **Frequency** by clicking on it. A complete list of frequencies can be found in Table 7 at the end of the manual.

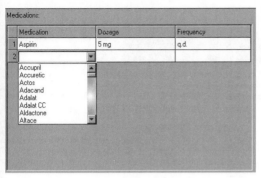

To add other medications, click on the consecutive fields in each column.

Prior Treatment Plan Goals

Version 3.3.0 allows the user to record treatment goals on a per-visit basis. When on the **Prior Treatment** screen, the goals are for display only and cannot be changed. The treatment goals will be displayed as follows:

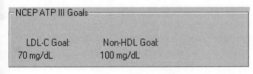

If an optional goal is used, that will be indicated by a **check box** showing the optional goal.

Risk

This part of the **Visit** folder has two sections. It allows the comparison between the variables and the results.

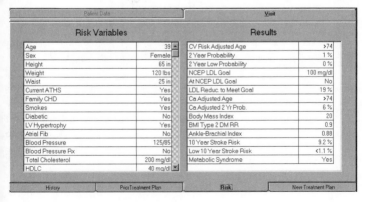

Risk Variables

Risk Variables	
Age	39
Sex	Female
Height	65 in
Weight	120 lbs
Waist	25 in
Current ATHS	Yes
Family CHD	Yes
Smokes	Yes
Diabetic	No
LV Hypertrophy	Yes
Atrial Fib	No
Blood Pressure	125/85
Blood Pressure Rx	No
Total Cholesterol	200 mg/dl
HDLC	40 mg/dl

The **Risk Variables** is a summary of the patient's history.

To view the rest of the list, click the down arrow in the lower right corner.

Results

The **Results** screen shows the calculations resulting from those variables. In this example, there is a **2-Year Probability**, and a **2-Year Low**

Results	
CV Risk Adjusted Age	>74
2 Year Probability	1 %
2 Year Low Probability	0 %
NCEP LDL Goal	100 mg/dl
At NCEP LDL Goal	No
LDL Reduc. to Meet Goal	19 %
Ca Adjusted Age	>74
Ca Adjusted 2 Yr Prob.	6 %
Body Mass Index	20
BMI Type 2 DM RR	0.9
Ankle-Brachial Index	0.88
10 Year Stroke Risk	9.2 %
Low 10 Year Stroke Risk	<1.1 %
Metabolic Syndrome	Yes

Probability of a cardiovascular incident, due to the fact of there being CHD in this patient's history.

If there were no indication of the patient having CHD, then the results would be based on a 10-year probability.

Return to the **History** tab and click on the **Edit** toolbar button.

The screen on the left indicates that this patient had an incident of ATHS, the type being coronary heart disease. Remove those checks as shown in the screen on the right. **Save** the patient's **History** record and return to the **Risk** tab.

Results	
CV Risk Adjusted Age	>74
10 Year Probability	9 %
10 Year Low Probability	1 %
10 Year ATP III Probability	4 %
NCEP LDL Goal	100 mg/dl
At NCEP LDL Goal	No
LDL Reduc. to Meet Goal	19 %
Ca Adjusted Age	>74
Ca Adjusted 10 Yr Prob.	18 %
Body Mass Index	20
BMI Type 2 DM RR	0.9
Ankle-Brachial Index	0.88
10 Year Stroke Risk	6.3 %
Low 10 Year Stroke Risk	<1.1 %
Metabolic Syndrome	Yes

Now the calculation shows only a **10-Year Probability**, a **10-Year Low Probability**, and a **10-Year ATP III Probability** because any indication of ATHS has been removed from the patient's history.

To view the remaining results, click on the down arrow in the lower right corner.

New Treatment Plan

This tab of the **Visit** is where a new treatment plan based on the results in the **Risk** tab is entered. You will notice this looks very similar to the **Prior Treatment Plan** tab. The only difference is the **Next Visit Date** field. Notice that the **Prior Treatment Diet** and **BP Meds** information has defaulted into the appropriate fields.

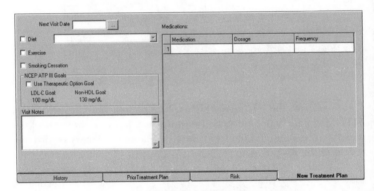

There are two ways to enter the **Next Visit Date**:
- Place the curser in the field beside **Next Visit Date** and type it in.
- Click on the ▦ button to the right of that field to bring up the calendar.

Change or add any necessary data.

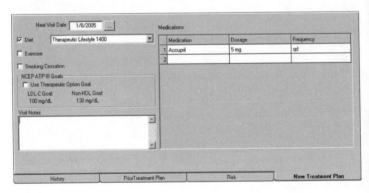

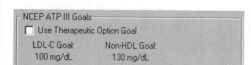

If the risk assessment has determined that an optional therapeutic goal is available, a **check box** will be shown to indicate that the option can be selected. Click on the **check box** to select the optional goal.

When the next visit is added, this information will default into the **Prior Treatment Plan** tab. Be sure to click on the **Save** toolbar button before you move on to other parts of this program.

Editing a Visit

To edit a patient visit, be sure the visit date you wish to edit is in the **Select a Visit** window.

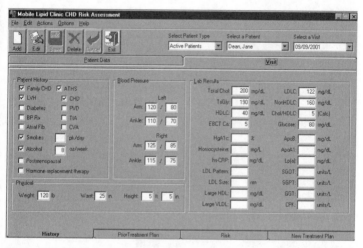

Click on the **Edit** toolbar button.

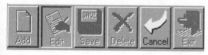

Notice that the only changes in the screen are the toolbar buttons. **Cancel** is the only one available. Now you can change visit information regarding **History**, **Prior Treatment Plan**, and **New Treatment Plan**. As soon as you make a change in the screen, be it adding a **check mark** or changing/adding data, the toolbar buttons will once again change.

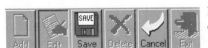

Now both the **Save** and **Cancel** buttons are available.

Save will take you out of edit mode and keep the changes.
Cancel will take you out of edit mode without saving the changes.
Changed information may affect **Risk Results**. Click on either **Cancel** or **Save** to return to the previous mode.

Deleting a Visit

To delete a patient visit, be sure the visit date you wish to delete is in the **Select a Visit** window.

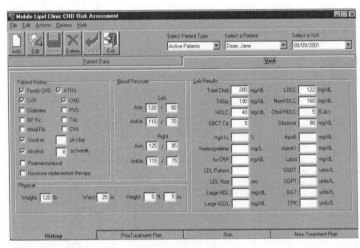

Click the **Delete** toolbar button.

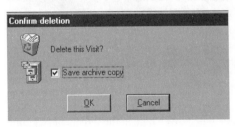

This pop-up screen will be your one chance to change your mind. Your choices are

• Click **Cancel** and do not delete this visit.
• Click **OK** and delete this visit. It will not be archived.

For the purpose of this lesson, click **Cancel**.

REPORTS AND GRAPHS

There are three reports and nine graphs from which to choose.
- **Patient Summary Report**
- **Visit Report**
- **New Treatment Plan Report**
- **Cardiovascular Age Graph**
- **Total Cholesterol Graph**
- **LDL-C Graph**
- **HDL-C Graph**
- **Non-HDL-C Graph**
- **TC/HDL-C Ratio Graph**
- **Triglycerides Graph**
- **Systolic BP Graph**
- **Glucose Graph**

They can all be viewed on screen and printed.

Reports

How to Print a Report

Reports will always appear in the **Print Preview** screen first. To print a report, click on the **Printer** icon, 🖳, in the **Print Preview** screen. It appears in the upper left corner.

Patient Summary Report

Click on **File** in the menu options above the toolbar buttons.

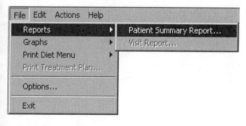

Click on **Patient Summary Report**.

The report will first appear in the **Print Preview** screen and is automatically dated with the current date.

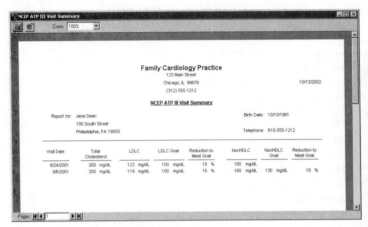

Print by clicking on the **Printer** icon.

Visit Report

Return to the **Patient Data** screen and **Select a Visit** for which you wish
to print a list of the **Risk Variables** and **Results**.

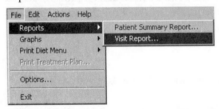

Click on **File** again. When
the dropdown list of reports
appears, select **Visit Report**.

The report will first appear in the **Print Preview** screen and is automatically assigned the current date.

Print by clicking on the **Printer** icon.

Family Cardiology Practice
123 Main Street
Chicago, IL 99876
(312) 555-1212

10/13/2002

Report for: Dean, Jane

Birth Date: 10/10/1961

Visit Date: 9/6/2001

Telephone: 610-555-1212

Risk Variables		Results	
Age	39	CV Risk Adjusted Age	55
Sex	Female	2 Year Probability	1 %
Height	70 in	2 Year Low Probability	0 %
Weight	187 lbs	NCEP LDL Goal	100 mg/dL
Waist	42 in	At NCEP LDL Goal	No
Current ATHS	Yes	LDL Reduc. to Meet Goal	16 %
Family CHD	Yes	NCEP NonHDL Goal	130 mg/dL
Smokes	No	At NCEP NonHDL Goal	No
Diabetic	No	NonHDL Reduc. to Meet Goal	19 %
LV Hypertrophy	No	Ca Adjusted Age	na
Atrial Fib	No	Ca Adjusted 2 Yr Prob.	na
Blood Pressure	120/70	Body Mass Index	27
Blood Pressure Rx	No	BMI Type 2 DM RR	4.2
Total Cholesterol	200 mg/dL	Ankle-Brachial Index	na
HDLC	40 mg/dL	10 Year Stroke Risk	2.0 %
LDLC	119 mg/dL	Low 10 Year Stroke Risk	<1.1 %
Chol Ratio	5.00 mg/dL	Metabolic Syndrome	Yes
Triglycerides	205 mg/dL		
NonHDLC	160 mg/dL		
Glucose	46 mg/dL		
Calcium Score	na		
Postmenopausal	No		
Hormone Replacment	No		

New Treatment Plan Report

Be sure a patient and visit date are selected and go to the **New Treatment Plan** tab in **Visit** folder. Make sure there is a **New Treatment Plan** entered in this tab. Click on **File**. When the dropdown list of reports appears, select **Print Treatment Plan**.

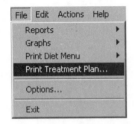

A print preview of this treatment plan will appear.

Family Cardiology Practice
123 Main Street
Chicago, IL 99876
(312) 555-1212

October 2, 2002

Jane Dean
100 South Street

Philadelphia, PA 19555

On your office visit of Thursday, September 06, 2001, you had the following lab and physical results:

Height:	70 in	Total Cholesterol:	200 mg/dL
Weight:	187 lb	HDLC:	40 mg/dL
Waist:	42 in	LDLC:	119 mg/dL
Blood Pressure:	120/70	Triglycerides:	205 mg/dL
Body Mass Index:	27	Glucose:	
CV Risk Adjusted Age:	55	Non HDLC:	160 mg/dL
		Cholesterol Ratio:	5
NCEP LDL Goal:	100 mg/dL	LDL Reduc. to Meet Goal:	16 %
NCEP NonHDL Goal:	130 mg/dL	NonHDL Reduc. to Meet Goal:	19 %

Based on these results, I am recommending the following treatment:

Diet: Low Carbo 50 grams
Medication: Lipitor 5 mg
Benicar 1 mg

I look forward to seeing you on your next visit on or about 10/18/2001.

Dr. Michael Davidson

Print this report by clicking on the print icon. Any diet associated with this treatment plan will automatically print out after the **Treatment Plan**. In this case, the **Low Carbo 50 grams** diet would print.

Graphs

Common Features

All graphs share common features. If the currently selected guideline provides a target goal for a given blood level or calculated value, then the graph will show that goal as a single line.

Selecting a Graph

One of nine specific graphs can be selected from the Graphs menu.

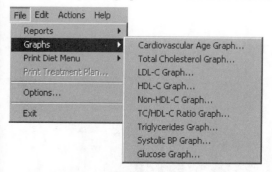

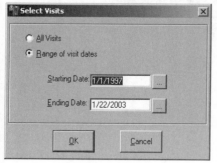

After selecting a graph, you are presented with the **Date Selection Dialog Box**. All graphs are set up for single-page printing. This allows only 15 visit points to be displayed on a single page. If the patient has more than 15 visits, you can select a range of dates from the **Date Selection Dialog Box**. If you select all dates, then the most recent 15 visits are used for the graph.

Graph Buttons

The three buttons on the bottom of the screen for each graph allow you to:

Full Screen

Expand the graph to the full screen by clicking on the **Full Screen** button. Hit **Enter** or double-click anywhere on the screen to return to the smaller screen. To close this screen, you must click on the close box (**X**) in the upper right corner.

Close

Print the graph by clicking on the **Print** button.

Print

Exit this screen without printing by clicking on the **Close** button.

Cardiovascular Age Graph

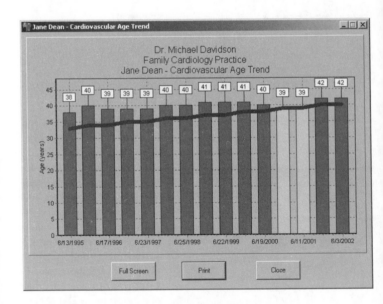

This is a graph of the cardiovascular age (CV age) values as calculated for each visit within the visit range selected. The bars represent the calculated value. The blue line is the actual age on the specific visit. Because the calculation is based on data up to and including age 74 years, it is possible for the calculation to provide a CV age of some unknown value greater than 74. In this case, the specific bar will be set to a value of 90 years. Select **Print** to print this graph or **Close** to return to the previous screen.

Total Cholesterol Graph

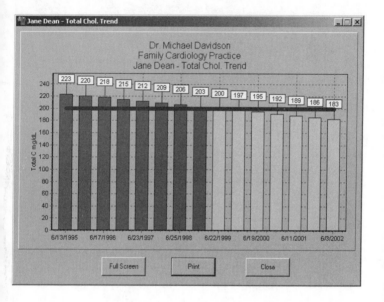

This is a graph of the total cholesterol values as measured for each visit within the visit range selected. Select **Print** to print this graph or **Close** to return to the previous screen.

LDL-C Graph

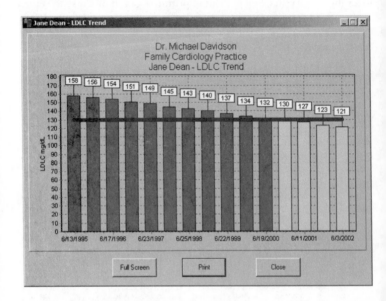

This is a graph of the low-density lipoprotein cholesterol (LDL-C) values as calculated for each visit within the visit range selected. Select **Print** to print this graph or **Close** to return to the previous screen.

HDL-C Graph

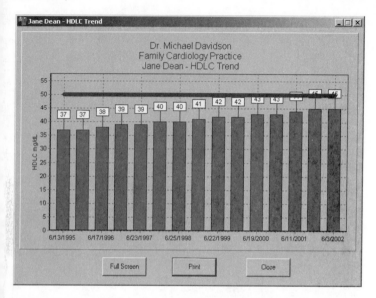

This is a graph of the high-density lipoprotein cholesterol (HDL-C) values as measured for each visit within the visit range selected. Select **Print** to print this graph or **Close** to return to the previous screen.

Non-HDL-C Graph

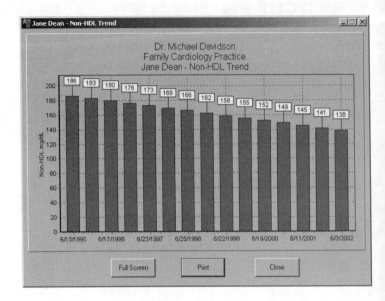

This is a graph of the non-HDL-C values as calculated for each visit within the visit range selected. Select **Print** to print this graph or **Close** to return to the previous screen.

TC/HDL-C Ratio Graph

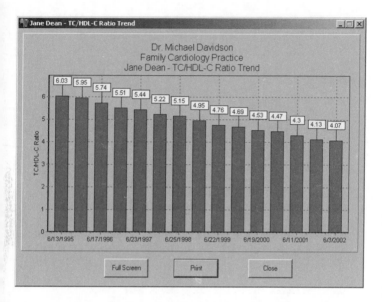

This is a graph of the total cholesterol (TC)/HDL-C ratio as calculated for each visit within the visit range selected. Select **Print** to print this graph or **Close** to return to the previous screen.

Triglycerides Graph

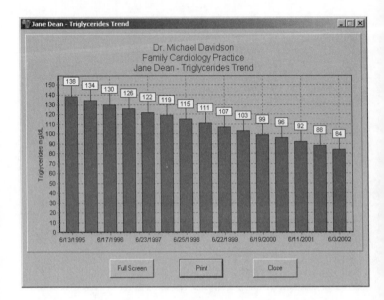

This is a graph of the triglyceride values measured for each visit within the visit range selected. Select **Print** to print this graph or **Close** to return to the previous screen.

Systolic Blood Pressure Graph

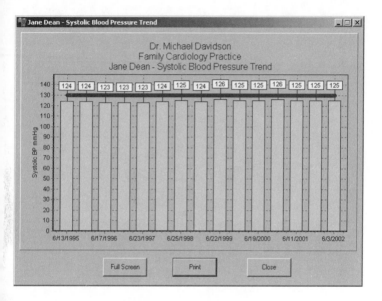

This is a graph of the systolic blood pressure values measured for each visit within the visit range selected. Select **Print** to print this graph or **Close** to return to the previous screen.

Glucose Graph

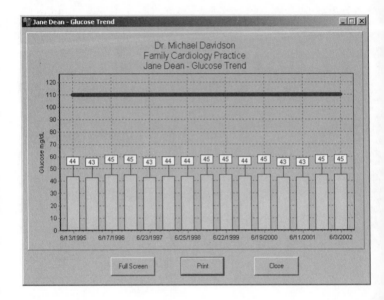

This is a graph of the glucose values measured for each visit within the visit range selected. Select **Print** to print this graph or **Close** to return to the previous screen.

Print Diet Menu

It may be necessary to print just a diet menu. To do this, return to the
Patient Data screen and click on **File**. When the dropdown list of reports
appears, select **Print Diet Menu**. Menus are available in English and
French.

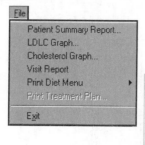

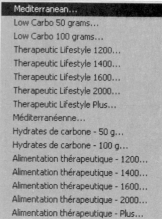

Select the diet you wish to print.

No print preview screen will appear. The selected diet menu will automatically print. This concludes the basic tutorial.

Mediterranean Diet

	Day 1	Day 2	Day 3	Day 4	Day 5	Day 6	Day 7
Breakfast	1c high fiber cereal 1c fat free milk 1 banana ¼ c strawberries	1c low fat yogurt 2 slices whole wheat bread 2 tsp tub margarine* Apple	1c oatmeal 1c fat free milk 2 Tbsp raisins 1 slice whole wheat toast 1 tsp tub margarine*	1c low fat yogurt 1 English Muffin 2 tsp tub margarine* ¼ cantaloupe	1c high fiber cereal 1c fat free milk ½ c blueberries 1 slice whole wheat toast w/jam	1c low fat yogurt 1 bran muffin 1 tsp tub margarine* 1/8 honeydew melon	1 egg 2 slices whole wheat toast 2 tsp tub margarine* Orange
Lunch	1/6 cheese & spinach quiche tossed salad 1 Tbsp olive oil/vinegar Grapes	Grilled vegetables: 1 sm zucchini 1 sm yellow squash 1 sm potato ½ sm eggplant ½ red pepper 1 Tbsp olive oil 2 oz mozzarella	Baked potato w/2 oz cheese & ½ c broccoli Salad w/1 Tbsp olive oil/vinegar Peach	Large Greek salad: 2 oz Feta cheese 10 Greek olives 2 Tbsp olive oil/vinegar 2 slices pita bread	Salad: 2 whole tomatoes sliced 4 oz mozzarella Fresh basil leaves 2 Tbsp olive oil/balsamic vinegar 2 slices Italian bread 2 tsp olive oil	Grilled skinless chicken breast on whole wheat bun w/lettuce, tomato, 1 tsp mayonnaise Baked potato wedges: 1 med potato 2 tsp olive oil ½ c broccoli sprinkled w/2 tsp parmesan cheese	¼ c low fat cottage cheese 1½ c sliced melon 8 low fat crackers ½ c pudding made with fat free milk
Snack	1½ oz boxraisins	¼ c peanuts	Trail mix (no coconut)	6 dried apricot halves	2 plums	Grapes	¼ c dried sour cherries
Dinner	1c minestrone soup 2 slices bread 2 tsp olive oil Salad 3 oz grilled Salmon 1c green beans w/ 1 Tbsp slivered almonds Orange	¼ of large vegetarian pizza Salad w/1 Tbsp olive oil/vinegar 1¼ c watermelon	2c lentil soup Salad: Raw spinach ½ tomato ¼ c water chestnuts onion 1 Tbsp pine nuts 1 Tbsp olive oil/vinegar 2 slices bread 2 tsp olive oil Pear	3 oz Flounder ½ c carots, onions, peppers, garlic, 1 tsp olive oil mixed w/1c rice 1c split pea soup (no ham) ½ c spinach 1/8 honeydew melon	Cook together: 2 oz skinless chicken 2 sm potatoes 1 carrot onion/peppers 1c tomato 1 tsp olive oil Serve over 1c couscous prepared w/olive oil	1c black beans prepared w/garlic, 1 tsp olive oil 1½ c rice 2 Tbsp chopped onion Salad (on lettuce leaf): 1 tomato sliced ¼ avocado sliced 1 tsp olive oil	2c pasta w/1-2c marinara sauce w/cubed eggplant (no meat) Salad: Lettuce, tomato, onion 1 Tbsp parmesan cheese 1 Tbsp olive oil/vinegar 2 slices bread 2 tsp olive oil
Snack	¼ c soy nuts	Peach	6 ginger snaps 1c fat free milk	¼ c peanuts	½ c fat free vanilla frozen yogurt ½ c sliced strawberries 1 Tbsp chopped walnuts	¼ c sunflower seeds	16 black olives

* Margarine used should be Benecol or Take Control

TABLES

Table 1. Lab Test Input Ranges

Test Result	Lab Tests CU	Lab Tests SI	Conversion	CU Min	CU Max	SI Min	SI Max
Total Chol	mg/dL	mmol/L	0.0259	50.00	1000.00	1.30	25.90
TriGly	mg/dL	mmol/L	0.0113	1.00	10000.00	0.01	113.00
HDLC	mg/dL	mmol/L	0.0259	1.00	300.00	0.03	7.77
Glucose	mg/dL	mmol/L	0.0555	1.00	600.00	0.06	33.30
EBCT Ca	N/A	N/A	1	0.00	10000.00	0.00	10000.00
LDLC	mg/dL	mmol/L	0.0259	25.00	700.00	0.65	18.13
NonHDLC	mg/dL	mmol/L	Calc	N/A	N/A	N/A	N/A
Chol/HDLC	N/A	N/A	Calc	N/A	N/A	N/A	N/A
ApoA1	mg/dL	g/L	0.01	1.00	700.00	0.01	7.00
ApoB	mg/dL	g/L	0.01	1.00	700.00	0.01	7.00
CPK	units/L	U/L	1	0.00	10000.00	0.00	10000.00
hs-CRP	mg/L	g/L	10	0.00	50.00	0.00	500.00
GGT	units/L	U/L	1	0.00	50.00	0.00	50.00
HgA1c	%	Proportion	0.01	0.00	100.00	0.00	1.00
Homocysteine	mg/L	umol/L	7.397	1.00	50.00	7.40	369.85
LDL Size	nm	nm	1	100.00	5000.00	100.00	5000.00
Large HDL	mg/dL	mmol/L	0.0259	1.00	2000.00	0.03	51.80
Large VLDL	mg/dL	mmol/L	0.0259	0.00	1000.00	0.00	25.90
Lp(a)	mg/dL	umol/L	0.0357	0.00	1000.00	0.00	35.70
SGOT (AST)	units/L	U/L	1	1.00	1000.00	1.00	1000.00
SGPT (ALT)	units/L	U/L	1	1.00	1000.00	1.00	1000.00

ALT, alanine aminotransferase; Apo, apolipoprotein; AST, aspartate aminotransferase; Chol/HDLC, total cholesterol/high-density lipoprotein cholesterol ratio; CPK, creatine phosphokinase; EBCT Ca, electron beam computed tomography calcium score; GGT, gamma-glutamyl transpeptidase; HDL, high-density lipoprotein; HDLC, high-density lipoprotein cholesterol; HgA1c, hemoglobin A_{1c}; hs-CRP, high-sensitivity C-reactive protein; LDL, low-density lipoprotein; LDLC, low-density lipoprotein cholesterol; Lp(a), lipoprotein(a); N/A, not applicable; SGOT, serum glutamic oxaloacetic transaminase; SGPT, serum glutamic pyruvic transaminase; Total Chol, total cholesterol; TriGly, triglycerides; VLDL, very-low-density lipoprotein.

Table 2. Diabetes Medications

Actos	Humulin L
Amaryl	Humulin N
Apo-Tolbutamide	Humulin R
Avandamet	Humulin U
Avandia	Iletin II Lente
DiaBeta	Iletin II NPH
Diabinese	Iletin II Regular
Diamicron	Lantus
Glucophage	Metaglip
Glucophage XR	Micronase
Glucotrol	Novolin R
Glucotrol XL	NovoLog
Glucovance	Orinase
Glynase PresTab	Prandase
Glyset	Prandin
Humalog	Precose
Humalog Mix 75/25	Starlix
Humulin 70/30	Tolinase

Table 3. Cardiovascular Medications

Advicor	Lopid
Aggrastat	Mevacor
Altocor	Niacin
Aspirin	Niaspan
Colestid	Novasen
Cordarone	Plavix
Coumadin	Pravachol
Crestor	Questran
Ecotrin	Questran Light
Ezetrol	Slo-Niacin
Lanoxin	Sotacor
Lescol	Tricor
Lescol XL	Welchol
Lipidil	Zetia
Lipitor	Zocor

Table 4. Blood Pressure Medications

Accupril	Diovan	Monitan
Accuretic	Diovan HCT	Monocor
Aceon	Diuril	Monopril
Adalat	Dyazide	Monopril-HCT
Adalat CC	DynaCirc	Mykrox
Adalat XL	DynaCirc CR	Nimotop
Aldactazide	Enduron	Normodyne
Aldactone	Esidrix	Norvasc
Altace	HydroDIURIL	Oretic
Apo-Methyldopa	Hygroton	Plendil
Apresoline	Hytrin	Prinivil
Atacand	Hyzaar	Prinzide
Atacand HCT	Imdur	Procardia
Atacand Plus	Inderal	Procardia XL
Avalide	Inderal LA	Renedil
Avapro	Inderide	Sectral
Benicar	Inderide LA	Sular
Betaloc	Inhibace	Tarka
Blocadren	Inspra	Teczem
Calan	Isoptin	Tenex
Calan-SR	Isoptin SR	Tenoretic
Capoten	Isordil	Tenormin
Capozide	Kerlone	Teveten
Cardene	Lasix	Teveten HCT
Cardene SR	Levatol	Tiazac
Cardizem	Lexxel	Timolide 10-25
Cardizem CD	Loniten	Toprol XL
Cardizem SR	Lopressor	Trandate
Cardura	Lopressor HCT	Trasicor
Cartia XT	Lotensin	Uniretic
Cartrol	Lotensin HCT	Univasc
Catapres	Lotrel	Vascor
Catapres-TTS	Lozide	Vaseretic
Chlorthalidone	Lozol	Vasotec
Combipres	Mavik	Verelan
Coreg	Maxzide	Verelan PM
Corgard	Micardis	Visken
Corzide	Micardis HCT	Wytensin
Covera HS	Microzide	Zaroxolyn
Coversyl	Midamor	Zebeta
Cozaar	Minipress	Zestoretic
Demadex	Minizide	Zestril
Dilacor XR	Moduretic	Ziac

Table 5. Other Medications

Viagra

Table 6. Drug Dosage

0.05 mg	250 mg	2 mg/240 mg
0.1 mg	300 mg	2 mg/500 mg
0.2 mg	320 mg	2.5 mg/500 mg
0.3 mg	360 mg	4 mg/240 mg
0.5 mg	400 mg	4 mg/500 mg
1 mg	420 mg	5 mg/6.25 mg
1.2 mg	500 mg	5 mg/12.5 mg
1.25 mg	600 mg	5 mg/50 mg
1.5 mg	625 mg	5 mg/500 mg
2 mg	750 mg	7.5 mg/12.5 mg
2.5 mg	850 mg	10 mg/2.5 mg
3.125 mg	1,000 mg	10 mg/5 mg
3.6 mg	1,250 mg	10 mg/12.5 mg
4 mg	1,500 mg	10 mg/25 mg
5 mg	1,750 mg	10 mg/100 mg
6.125 mg	1,875 mg	15 mg/25 mg
6.25 mg	2,000 mg	20 mg/5 mg
7.5 mg	2,500 mg	20 mg/10 mg
8 mg	2,750 mg	20 mg/12.5 mg
10 mg	3,000 mg	20 mg/25 mg
12 mg	3,125 mg	25 mg/15 mg
12.5 mg	3,250 mg	25 mg/25 mg
15 mg	3,500 mg	37.5 mg/25 mg
16 mg	3,750 mg	40 mg/12.5 mg
20 mg	1 g	50 mg/12.5 mg
25 mg	2 g	50 mg/15 mg
30 mg	3 g	50 mg/25 mg
32 mg	4 g	50 mg/50 mg
40 mg	5 g	80 mg/12.5 mg
45 mg	8 g	100 mg/25 mg
50 mg	12 g	150 mg/12.5 mg
54 mg	15 g	160 mg/12.5 mg
60 mg	16 g	160 mg/25 mg
75 mg	20 g	180 mg/5 mg
80 mg	<10 units/d	300 mg/12.5 mg
81 mg	11–25 units/d	500 mg/10 mg
90 mg	26–50 units/d	500 mg/20 mg
100 mg	51–75 units/d	600 mg/12.5 mg
120 mg	76–100 units/d	600 mg/25 mg
150 mg	>100 units/d	750 mg/20 mg
160 mg	1 mg/240 mg	1000 mg/20 mg
180 mg	1 mg/500 mg	2000 mg/40 mg
200 mg	1.25 mg/250 mg	
240 mg	2 mg/180 mg	

Table 7. Frequency

q.d.	q. AM
b.i.d.	q. PM
t.i.d.	p.r.n.
q.i.d.	q week
q.h.s.	w/meals
q.o.d.	Other

Canadian Guidelines for the Management and Treatment of Dyslipidemia and Prevention of Cardiovascular Disease: Summary of Recommendations

GLOBAL RISK ASSESSMENT

Risk Assessment Screening

Routinely screen the following patients: men older than age 40 years and women who are postmenopausal and/or older than age 50 years. In addition, screen those with:

- Diabetes mellitus
- Presence of risk factors such as hypertension, smoking, and abdominal obesity
- A strong family history of premature cardiovascular disease (CVD)
- Manifestations of hyperlipidemia (such as the presence of xanthelasma, xanthoma, arcus)
- Evidence of symptomatic or asymptomatic atherosclerosis
- Patients of any age may be screened at the discretion of the physician, particularly where lifestyle changes are indicated

RISK CATEGORIES

Risk	10-year risk est. of CVD	Low-density lipoprotein cholesterol (LDL-C)	Total cholesterol (TC): high-density lipoprotein cholesterol (HDL-C)
High	≥20%, diabetes or atherosclerotic diseases	<2.5 and	<4.0
Moderate	10% –<20%	<3.5 and	<5.0
Low	<10%	<4.5 and	<6.0

FACTORS INFLUENCING RISK ASSESSMENT

Metabolic Syndrome

The clustering of cardiovascular risk factors is recognized as being a major health issue. The metabolic syndrome is defined in qualitative terms and encompasses abdominal obesity, insulin resistance, elevated plasma triglyceride, low HDL-C levels, and high blood pressure.

Criteria—3 or more of the following risk determinants:

Risk factor	Defining level
Abdominal obesity	Waist circumference
Men	>102 cm
Women	>88 cm
Triglycerides	≥1.7 mmol/L
HDL-C	
Men	<1.0 mmol/L
Women	<1.3 mmol/L
Blood pressure	≥130/85 mm Hg
Fasting glucose	≥6.2 mmol/L

Apolipoprotein B

Plasma apolipoprotein B (apo B) measurement may be of use in determining coronary artery disease (CAD) risk and adequacy of treatment in subjects with the metabolic syndrome. An optimal level of apo B in a high-risk patient is less than 0.9 g/L.

Lipoprotein(a)

A lipoprotein(a) [Lp(a)] concentration greater than 30 mg/dL in an individual with a TC/HDL-C ratio greater than 5.5 or other major risk factors may indicate a need for earlier and more intensive LDL-C lowering.

Homocysteine

There is insufficient evidence to warrant broad screening of homocysteine level until the results of ongoing clinical trials show that vitamin supplementation to lower homocysteine levels decreases cardiovascular risk.

High-Sensitivity C-Reactive Protein

High-sensitivity C-reactive protein may be clinically useful in identifying individuals who are at a higher risk for CVD than that predicted by a global risk assessment, in particular those persons with a calculated 10-year risk between 10% and 20%.

Genetic Risk

When a family history of CAD (<56 years for men, 65 for women) can be ascertained unambiguously, risk for first-degree relatives is increased by a factor of 1.7 to 2.0.

Recommendations for Hormone Replacement Therapy and Cardiovascular Disease

Oral hormone replacement therapy does not reduce and may increase CVD risk.

PRECLINICAL DIAGNOSIS OF ATHEROSCLEROSIS

Detection of Atherosclerosis

Detection of atherosclerosis and diagnosis of CVD may be confirmed using the following.
Recommended:

- Physical examination
- Ankle-brachial index

Possibly useful in intermediate risk subjects:

- Carotid ultrasound—may detect subclinical atherosclerosis
- Electrocardiogram
- Graded exercise testing in men older than 40 years with risk factors

Not currently recommended, based on available evidence:

- Flow-mediated vasodilatation, plethysmography, arterial compliance
- Electron beam computed tomography

- Magnetic resonance imaging
- Intravascular ultrasound

TREATMENT

Diet

An important focus should be on decreasing caloric consumption in particular by reducing intake of refined carbohydrates and sugar to achieve and maintain a body mass index less than 27 kg/m^2.

Medication

Target lipid levels. In high-risk individuals, treatment should be started immediately, concomitant with diet and therapeutic lifestyle changes. The priority for treatment is reduction of the LDL-C to less than 2.5 mmol/L and TC/HDL-C ratio to less than 4.0. In light of the data from the Heart Protection Study, the Working Group recommends that treatment in high-risk subjects be initiated with the equivalent of 40 mg simvastatin per day, with a minimum target level for LDL-C of 2.5 mmol/L.

Generic name	Trade name	Recommended dose range
Statins		
Atorvastatin	Lipitor	10–80 mg
Fluvastatin	Lescol	20–80 mg
Lovastatin	Mevacor	20–80 mg
Pravastatin	Pravachol	10–40 mg
Rosuvastatin	Crestor	10–40 mg
Simvastatin	Zocor	10–80 mg
Bile acid binding resins		
Cholestyramine	Questran	2–24 g
Colestipol	Colestid	5–30 g
Cholesterol absorption inhibitors		
Ezetimibe	Ezetrol	10 mg
Fibrates		
Bezafibrate	Bezalip	400 mg
Fenofibrate	Lipidil	67–200 mg
Gemfibrozil	Lopid	600–1200 mg
Niacin		
Nicotinic acid		1–3 g

Jacques Genest, Jiri Frohlich, George Fodor, Ruth McPherson

Index

Note: Page numbers followed by *t* indicate tables; those followed by *f* indicate figures.